Slimming
The Complete Guide

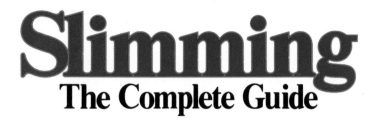

Slimming
The Complete Guide

By the Experts of Slimming Magazine

Introduction by Audrey Eyton

COLLINS

Slimming Magazine contributors

Editors: Sybil Greatbatch and Vera Segal
Writer: Gaynor Hagan
Diets and recipes: Joyce Hughes B.Sc.
Calorie research: Glynis McGuinness
Consultants to Slimming Magazine:
Professor John Yudkin
Derek Miller
Dr Henry Jordan
Editor of Slimming Magazine: Patience Bulkeley
Editorial consultant: Audrey Eyton

First published in 1982
Reprinted 1982
Reprinted 1983
by William Collins Sons & Co Ltd
London · Glasgow · Sydney
Auckland · Johannesburg

© Slimming Magazine, S.M. Publications Limited 1982

Designed by Sackville Design Group Ltd
32-34, Great Titchfield Street, London W1P 7AD
Art director: Al Rockall
Editor: Heather Thomas

ISBN pb 0 00 411813 8
ISBN hb 0 00 411675 5

Printed and bound by South China Printing Co., Hong Kong

Contents

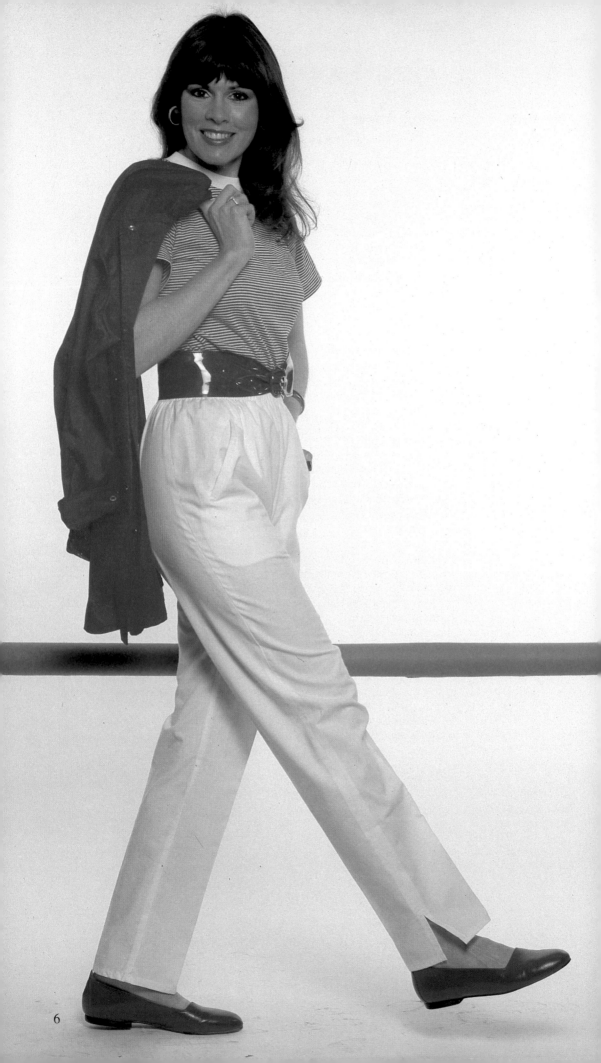

6

Introduction

by Audrey Eyton,
founder-editor of Slimming Magazine
and now Editorial Consultant

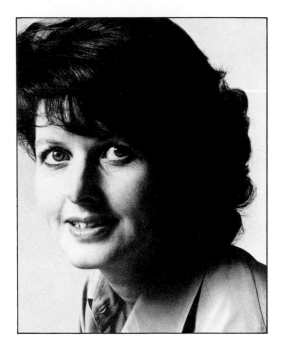

What she eats, how often and how much, are the most closely guarded secrets of almost every woman's life. Any expert who has tried to explore eating behaviour is aware of this, and since its first publication in 1969 *Slimming Magazine,* perhaps more than any other investigator, has had cause to discover just why this reticence can present so many women with such a major problem.

There is only one way in which any of us can determine what is normal in any area of life and that is by observing what other people do. Without the reassurance that 'most other people do, too', we would soon start to suspect our own behaviour to be disquietingly abnormal. Right from the start, slimmers have talked to us about both their successes and failures, and we have listened. Two years after *Slimming Magazine* was established we began to set up a network of slimming clubs throughout Great Britain. These clubs, whose members' weight problems range from a few pounds to many stones, also helped us in our research.

So what is 'normal' when it comes to the subject of eating? Ten years ago when scientists first started to explore this area, no one really knew. The only available guide was what could be ascertained from studying general nutritional advice and dietitians' diet sheets. From all this, one could only deduce that the eating pattern of the normal woman, as opposed to oneself, was like this: the normal woman eats three meals a day and nothing else. Her meals are mainly of high-protein food and vegetables, and she rarely eats canned, frozen and packaged foods, let alone things like chocolate or marmalade sandwiches. Her eating habits are totally dependent on nutritional requirements, not mood; and she rarely, if ever, departs from her regular sensible pattern.

Where is this normal woman? Our own research into eating habits has failed to reveal her to us in person. Instead, to our relief, we have discovered that a long list of eating habits that we attributed to our own abnormalities turns out to be reassuringly normal. Evening snacking is normal. That odd urge to wander into the kitchen, despite a perfectly satisfying dinner, is so common that only the exceptional and somewhat abnormal woman never experiences it. Frequent urges to nibble food are normal — natural, too, since primitive woman probably ate more like a horse in the literal sense, constantly snacking and grazing on anything available. Chocolate cravings are normal; we hardly ever meet a person who never has them. Premenstrual eating binges are normal — so common that we now tend to warn all slimmers about 'those few days each month when you may find it almost impossible to keep to your diet'.

The list of suspect abnormalities that we have been able to re-categorize as standard behaviour is almost endless. So when we devised and tested our diets, we took all this normal behaviour into account. None of the diets in this book are cranky or gimmicky; they are all effective and attractive slimming regimes which can do their job because their flexibility allows them to cater for individual tastes. You should find that at least one will suit your lifestyle and eating habits.

Stepping up your daily level of activity can speed up your weight loss from dieting. This book will also help you to tone up muscles, lose flab and encourage you to make exercise *and* healthy eating an integral part of your new slim outlook and lifestyle.

Our policy has always been to base our diets and slimming advice on sound scientific fact. However, we have always tried to add to this the human touch — the understanding of people with a weight-gaining tendency who have succeeded in getting and staying slim. The main reason why we remain undismayed by over-indulgent days, sudden cravings and mood-based eating urges is that we know them all to be normal habits which we have to moderate rather than eradicate completely. We are all normal, thank goodness, and we can all lose excess weight if we really set out minds to it. So we wish you success in your slimming campaign — you *can* do it too!

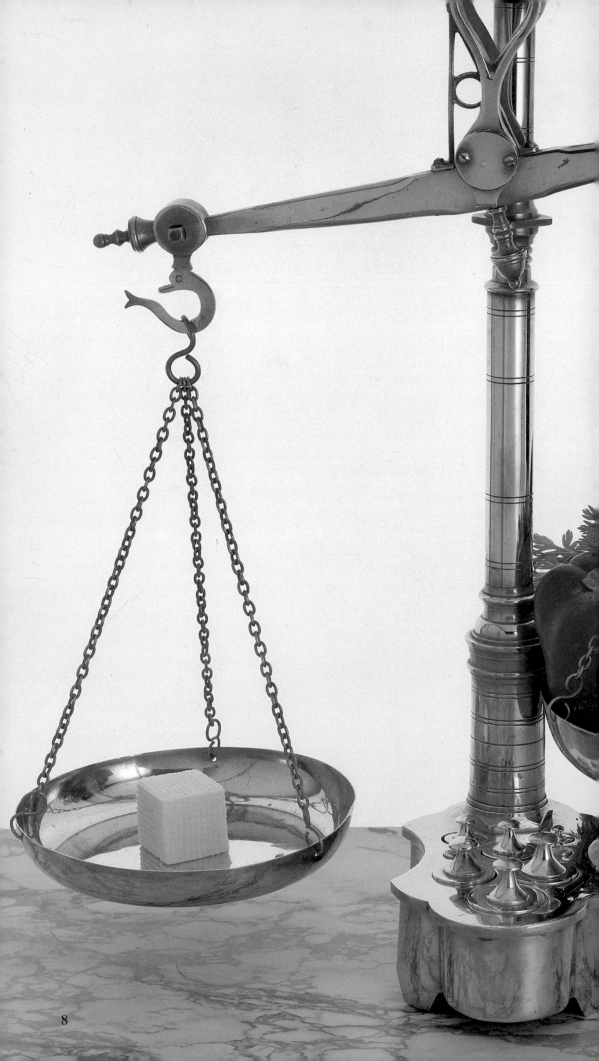

CHAPTER 1

Why do you gain weight?

If you eat more calories than your body uses in a day, you will get fat. However, if you eat fewer calories than your body uses in a day, you will lose weight. The more active you are, the more calories you burn up and the quicker you will slim. This, in a nutshell, is what weight control is all about. Many people face a weight problem at some time in their lives. Some progress from being a chubby baby to a plump teenager and end up as a buxom adult. Others are slim until a certain event, such as getting married or having children, changes their life and their shape, but how is it, exactly, that some of us gain too much weight and then find difficulty in losing it?

We are all born with an in-built fat-storing mechanism which in primitive times was part of our survival kit. When food was plentiful, early men and women would build up their body reserves by eating as much as they could. Thus when food was scarce, the body had a store of fat to draw upon to survive hard times. Those who could store fat easily were the lucky ones who lived to pass this mechanism genetically down through the subsequent generations.

That storage system is still with us, although the vicissitudes of primitive life are not. In affluent societies, food shortages, which use up body stores of fat, no longer occur. Those modern men and women who have inherited an effective fat-storage mechanism are now, perhaps, the less lucky sector of the population. They build up stores of surplus fat easily, but Nature's need to draw upon that supply has gone. Even those people who do not store fat so readily can

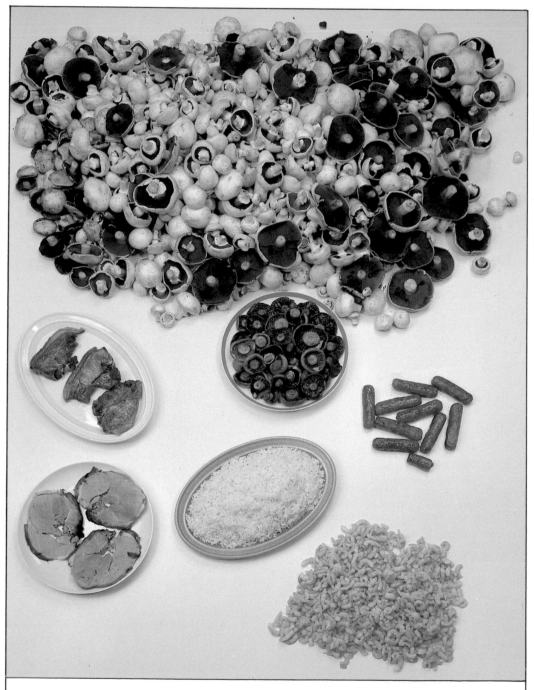

You are looking at 1,000 calories' worth each of well-grilled large pork sausages, boiled rice, well-grilled pork chops, lean roast pork and shrimps. This mountain of raw mushrooms is the same number of calories — 1,000 — as the fried plateful of mushrooms.

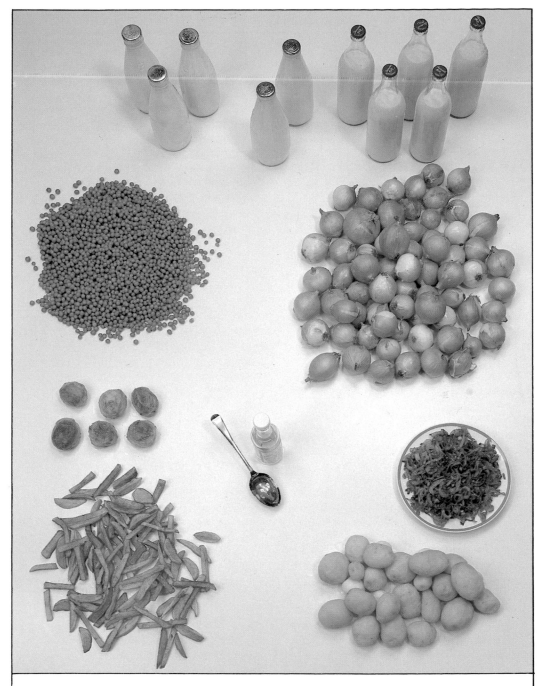
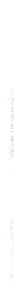

Here is around 1,000 calories' worth of skimmed milk, whole milk (silver top) and full cream milk (gold top). Which would you rather choose?

We also show potatoes, boiled, chipped and roast, some boiled peas, oil and onions, raw and fried, all in 1,000 calorie quantities.

put on excess weight because in these affluent times we simply eat too much and do not take enough exercise to burn up the calories.

The energy that we take in as food and use up in activity is measured in calories or joules. In scientific terms, a calorie is a unit of energy: the amount that, if converted into heat, would raise the temperature of one gram of water through one degree Centigrade. However, this is a very small unit in terms of what the body uses, so when we are measuring food intake and energy expenditure we use a unit that is 1,000 times larger..This bigger unit is referred to by

scientists as a kilocalorie (shortened to a 'kcal'). However, in everyday language, people do not bother with the 'kilo' prefix, and throughout this book we use calories to mean kilocalories. A calorie is equal to 4.184 joules.

To discover the number of calories in any type of food, it has to be burned and the amount of heat released measured exactly. This figure is then adjusted slightly because the body does not burn the protein in food completely. When you say that a slice of bread or an apple has a certain number of calories you really mean that it has the

11

potential to produce these calories if eaten and then completely metabolized (or burned) by the body. Thus calories are an imaginary but perfectly practical measure of the potential energy in food. Getting slim and maintaining your ideal body weight is a question of getting the calorie balance right, so let us now look at both sides of the balancing scale.

Controlling your intake of calories

All slimming diets are designed to reduce calorie intake. Each method has its devotees, but controlling calories is the secret behind each one (see *Cutting down the calories you eat*). If you do not exceed your calorie allowance you can eat anything you fancy and still shed weight.

It is thought that the average woman uses (or burns up) around 2,000 calories a day, and the average man between 2,500 and 3,000 a day, although this varies among individuals. Nearly all men, and most women, can shed weight if they reduce their calorie intake to 1,500 a day. The body will then have to feed on its stores of energy — those bulges of surplus fat — to find the additional 500 calories or more that it needs to function. Particularly for those who are heavily overweight, 1,500 calories a day is the ideal level to achieve a satisfactory weight loss at the start of a slimming campaign. Generally, the more overweight you are, the more rapidly you will shed weight when you start dieting.

However, some women find it difficult to shed a satisfactory amount of weight at this level of calorie intake, and those likely to experience the greatest difficulty are the ones carrying only a little surplus weight. To lose this, we recommend a total daily calorie intake of 1,000.

During prolonged periods of dieting, the body tends to adjust gradually to the lowered calorie intake and economizes in the number of calories it needs for bodily functions and activity. This is another throwback to that primitive mechanism of adjustment to scarcity in order to survive, but in these days of plenty, it indicates that after several months of dieting there may be a slowing-down of weight loss. There are two solutions to this: cutting back even further on calorie intake or increasing your level of activity. Generally speaking, 1,000 calories a day is regarded as the lowest level at which a person should diet without medical supervision. This does not mean, however, that you are courting disaster by eating a couple of hundred calories less on days when you find it easy to be strict with yourself. Although for convenience we put daily limits on

calories, it is the total over a week or more that really counts: thus if you eat 600 calories today and 1,400 tomorrow your weight loss will be exactly the same as if you were eating 1,000 calories each day.

Providing you know yourself to be in sound health, and you are carrying genuine surplus fat, there should be no need to go knocking on your doctor's door to ask permission to limit your food intake to 1,000 calories a day. How you spend your calories is, of course, vitally important. They must provide all the vitamins, minerals, protein and other nutrients essential for good health. The secret of good nutrition is, basically, variety, and if you eat several different foods at one meal and several different meals in one day, you are not likely to suffer from a nutritional deficiency. Each food provides a different combination of nutrients, and we usually end up getting all the essentials that our bodies need without even trying. However, because we usually eat less food when dieting it is worth giving nutritional facts a little more thought. Make sure that you include in your diet some low-fat protein foods, such as white fish, lean meat, offal, cottage cheese and skimmed milk; these all supply many nutrients at a modest cost in calories. Vegetables are the lowest calorie foods of all and most people will automatically turn to them as fill-up food. Plenty of raw or lightly-cooked vegetables and fresh citrus fruits, plus some of the protein-containing foods mentioned above, should ensure your supply of vitamins.

Some slimming 'experts' recommend that fluid intake should be reduced during dieting — but this is nonsense. There is absolutely no need to limit the amount you drink as long as any calorie-supplying drinks are included in your daily calorie total. Unsweetened black coffee and tea and water

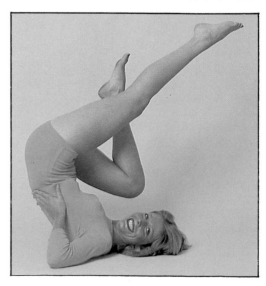

can be enjoyed freely. There are also many low-calorie soft drinks available which contain very few calories. Of course, if you weigh yourself before drinking a glass of water you will be lighter than when you weigh again afterwards as 550ml (1pint) of liquid weighs about 450g (1lb), but during the course of the day you lose that water naturally and because it contains no calories the body extracts no energy from it. It is quite natural for your body weight to fluctuate during the course of a day, and this is why you should always weigh yourself at the same time each week to accurately assess your weekly weight loss.

Stepping up your calorie output
Now for the other side of the balance. Whatever we do, we are burning up energy which is the same as using up calories. We use the least calories when we are sleeping, and more calories when we start moving. We use the most calories when we make the whole body work, or push it upwards against gravity — for instance, climbing mountains or just walking upstairs. The speed at which we perform certain activities also affects our calorie output.

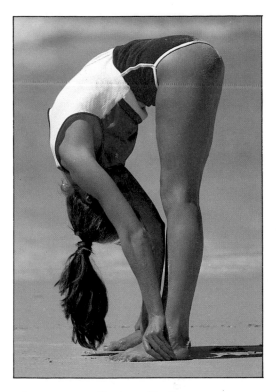

The amount of energy that is used solely to keep the body functioning, which includes pumping blood through the veins and keeping the heart beating, is called the basal metabolic rate. The amount of energy that our bodies burn up in movement and in actions, in addition to this basic bodily functioning, is called the metabolic rate. Therefore, the average woman may have a basal metabolic rate of 1,350 calories a day and if she uses up another 650 calories at the office or doing the housework, shopping and cooking, her metabolic rate will amount to 2,000 calories. Basal metabolic rate is affected by age, height and weight as well as individual differences in body functioning.

In the section called *Stepping up the calories you burn,* you will read the facts and fallacies regarding how quickly certain types of physical effort burn up energy — they may surprise you. Do you believe that you are speeding up your slimming process as you dust, or as you pound a typewriter? Does a brisk walk really help? What activity burns up the most calories? But if you hate physical exercise, do not despair because you are not unique! In fact, many scientists assert that, without our realizing it, many of us are exercise-resistant from birth and not only as a result of our socialization process. Psychiatrists studying the deep-rooted causes of unwanted weight gains have now advanced the theory that by avoiding unnecessary movement we are not being lazy so much as doing what comes naturally to us. It made sense for early Man and Woman to rest and conserve hard-won calories between bouts of necessary effort, and in the same way we are responding to the primitive survival mechanism. Varying degrees of exercise-resistance increasingly emerge as the reason why some people get fat while others remain effortlessly slim.

For many years, scientists have been looking for major differences in the basal metabolic rate between the fat and the thin. Often, apart from noticing a tendency for the metabolism of natural 'skinnies' to speed up after over-eating, researchers have been surprised at the uniformity of the rates. However, levels of physical activity that have been recorded have shown a staggering difference between overweight and slim people. On a tennis court, for instance, thin people are often found to burn up four times as many calories as do the plump players. In this case, it is not so much what you do but the way in which you do it that determines energy output. Even when it comes to the ordinary household tasks, exercise-resistant people find ways to minimize movement, and they may be quite unaware that they are doing this.

It is hard to diagnose your own exercise resistance, but if you are overweight, the evidence suggests that you and your body are almost certainly suffering from it. With a little perseverance and determination, you can cure it. Your permanent weight control depends on two factors: how many calories you expend in activity and how many you take in from food. You will find it easier to crack a surplus-weight problem for good if, besides watching your eating, you increase in every way possible your level of physical activity.

13

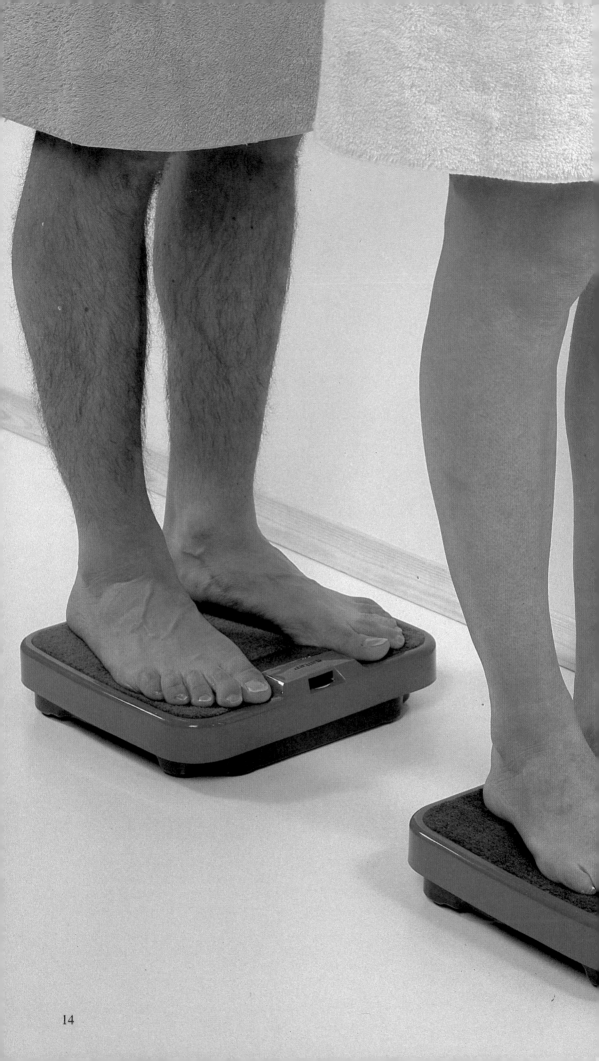

Deciding your ideal weight is not as simple as it might appear and the charts in this chapter are to be used only as a guide and not as a rigid rule. They should always be read in conjunction with an honest eye and a clear view in an unkind mirror. Not many women have a perfectly proportioned body, and if excess weight is centred on one spot, such as the thighs or the waistline, it may be necessary to reduce your weight more than a person who has the same amount of excess fat spread evenly across the body. So read on and consult, the charts overleaf to discover the ideal weight for your height and build.

What should you weigh?

The right weight for you is governed by your height, and do not take it for granted that you know this accurately. Check it carefully right now instead of relying on an approximate reference from years ago. Professor John Yudkin points out that from about the age of 25 upwards 'you could say it's downhill all the way. Over the years, we are all slowly shrinking. There's a daily height variation, too. You are slightly, but usually measurably, taller first thing in the morning than at the end of the day. Middle-aged slimmers who pinpoint a target weight from the height given on a passport taken out in their twenties, could be several pounds adrift; they have probably shrunk into a lower range. Many women who know their weight to the last ounce have never had their height accurately assessed.'

Because there is no such thing as a precise ideal weight you should use these charts only as a general guide, depending on your skeleton's spread. Thus neat, narrow body 'scaffolding' will need less cladding than a rangier bone structure. Wrist, hand and foot sizes are not a good guide to frame size, and forget about 'big' bones — it is their *spread* that matters when assessing your frame size.

Now, stand in front of a full-length mirror and take a critical look at your own figure. You are the best judge of when you are at your ideal weight. If you cannot see any ugly bulges, if your clothes fit comfortably and you can no longer grab any handfuls of fat, then you are at your target weight. Clothes sizes are not a good indication; manufacturers' sizes differ considerably and your height is also relevant. If you are small, every extra bit of weight seems to show and you may look best in a small size dress. However, taller women may fluctuate up and down on the scales without anyone but themselves noticing and will look slim in a larger size. Compare your weight with the ones given on the following charts. All heights/weights shown are minus shoes, and all weights are to the nearest 0.5kg (1lb). Weights for women and men allow 1kg (2-3lb) for light indoor clothes. Figures for girls and boys are minus clothing. For children under 17, weight is governed by height rather than by age and can be a rough indication only — an immature body grows in spurts and its proportions and shape alter constantly.

If a child appears plump, and a checkout with our chart confirms a call to action, then the emphasis should be on correcting quietly any family and personal eating habits that have caused the damage. Aim not so much at reducing the child's weight but at holding it steady. Then, as his height increases, the child will grow out of the problem.

Weigh with care

It is important to be consistent when weighing yourself. Although there is often a great temptation to leap on the scales every day, try to weigh only once a week on the same scales and at the same time of day. Hourly fluctuations in body weight can mislead you about your slimming progress, and most people are lighter first thing in the morning than in the evening.

Some women may find they weigh 1kg (2-3lb) heavier than they expect (even more, in comparatively rare cases) in the week before their menstrual period. This is due to temporary fluid retention, but such a 'gain' will disappear by the next week's weigh-in. There is no such thing as chronic fluid retention causing surplus weight in a woman who is in otherwise normal health. Plain old 'fat retention' is the problem!

Weigh yourself on good quality scales which are properly adjusted and based on a flat, rigid surface. Readings from scales based on a carpet can be misleading. Stand full-square on your scales because leaning sideways, backwards or forwards can distort the reading. However, if you *must* lean back to make yourself a little 'thinner', remember to do so every time!

Ideal weight charts

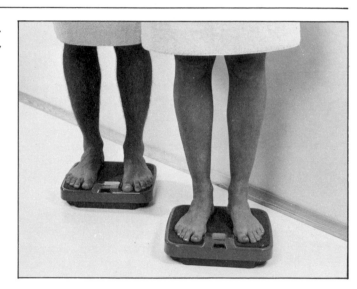

If you are a man

Height			Small frame			Medium frame			Large frame		
1.55m	5ft	1in	52.5kg	8st	4lb	56kg	8st	11lb	60.5kg	9st	7lb
1.57m	5ft	2in	54kg	8st	7lb	57.5kg	9st	1lb	62kg	9st	10lb
1.60m	5ft	3in	55.5kg	8st	10lb	59kg	9st	4lb	63.5kg	10st	0lb
1.63m	5ft	4in	57kg	8st	13lb	60.5kg	9st	7lb	65kg	10st	3lb
1.65m	5ft	5in	58kg	9st	2lb	62kg	9st	10lb	67kg	10st	7lb
1.68m	5ft	6in	60.5kg	9st	7lb	64kg	10st	1lb	68.5kg	10st	11lb
1.70m	5ft	7in	62kg	9st	10lb	66kg	10st	5lb	71kg	11st	2lb
1.73m	5ft	8in	64kg	10st	1lb	67.5kg	10st	9lb	73kg	11st	7lb
1.75m	5ft	9in	66kg	10st	5lb	69.5kg	10st	13lb	75kg	11st	11lb
1.78m	5ft	10in	67.5kg	10st	9lb	72kg	11st	4lb	77kg	12st	1lb
1.80m	5ft	11in	69.5kg	10st	13lb	73.5kg	11st	8lb	80.5kg	12st	9lb
1.83m	6ft	0in	71.5kg	11st	3lb	75.5kg	11st	12lb	81.5kg	12st	11lb
1.85m	6ft	1in	73kg	11st	7lb	77.5kg	12st	3lb	83.5kg	13st	2lb
1.88m	6ft	2in	75kg	11st	11lb	80kg	12st	8lb	85.5kg	13st	7lb
1.90m	6ft	3in	77.5kg	12st	3lb	82.5kg	13st	0lb	87.5kg	13st	11lb

If you are a woman

Height		Small frame			Medium frame			Large frame		
1.45m	4ft 9in	42kg	6st	9lb	46.5kg	7st	5lb	50kg	7st	12lb
1.47m	4ft 10in	45.5kg	7st	2lb	48kg	7st	8lb	51.5kg	8st	1lb
1.50m	4ft 11in	47kg	7st	5lb	49.5kg	7st	11lb	52.5kg	8st	4lb
1.52m	5ft 0in	47.5kg	7st	7lb	51kg	8st	0lb	54kg	8st	7lb
1.55m	5ft 1in	49.5kg	7st	11lb	52.5kg	8st	3lb	55.5kg	8st	10lb
1.57m	5ft 2in	51kg	8st	0lb	54kg	8st	7lb	57kg	8st	13lb
1.60m	5ft 3in	52kg	8st	2lb	55kg	8st	9lb	58kg	9st	2lb
1.63m	5ft 4in	53kg	8st	5lb	56.5kg	8st	12lb	60kg	9st	6lb
1.65m	5ft 5in	54kg	8st	7lb	57.5kg	9st	1lb	62kg	9st	10lb
1.68m	5ft 6in	56.5kg	8st	12lb	61kg	9st	8lb	63.5kg	10st	0lb
1.70m	5ft 7in	57.5kg	9st	1lb	61.5kg	9st	9lb	65kg	10st	3lb
1.73m	5ft 8in	59kg	9st	4lb	62.5kg	9st	12lb	67kg	10st	7lb
1.75m	5ft 9in	61kg	9st	8lb	64.5kg	10st	2lb	68kg	10st	10lb
1.78m	5ft 10in	62.5kg	9st	11lb	66kg	10st	5lb	70.5kg	11st	1lb
1.80m	5ft 11in	64kg	10st	1lb	68kg	10st	10lb	72.5kg	11st	5lb
1.83m	6ft 0in	66kg	10st	5lb	70kg	11st	0lb	74kg	11st	9lb
1.85m	6ft 1in	67.5kg	10st	9lb	71kg	11st	2lb	76kg	11st	13lb
1.88m	6ft 2in	69.5kg	10st	13lb	74kg	11st	9lb	77.5kg	12st	3lb

If you are a boy under 17

Height		Lowest			Highest			Approx. age
1.10m	3ft 7in	17kg	2st	10lb	22kg	3st	7lb	5
1.15m	3ft 9in	18kg	2st	12lb	25kg	3st	13lb	6
1.22m	4ft 0in	21kg	3st	4lb	28.5kg	4st	7lb	7
1.29m	4ft 3in	22.5kg	3st	8lb	33kg	5st	3lb	8
1.35m	4ft 5in	26kg	4st	1lb	36.5kg	5st	10lb	9
1.39m	4ft 7in	27.5kg	4st	5lb	40kg	6st	4lb	10
1.45m	4ft 9in	28.5kg	4st	7lb	43.5kg	6st	12lb	11
1.47m	4ft 10in	32kg	5st	1lb	48kg	7st	8lb	12
1.53m	5ft 0in	34kg	5st	5lb	54kg	8st	7lb	13
1.60m	5ft 3in	39kg	6st	2lb	61kg	9st	9lb	14
1.65m	5ft 5in	44.5kg	7st	0lb	62kg	9st	11lb	15
1.68m	5ft 6in	49.5kg	7st	11lb	67kg	10st	8lb	16

If you are a girl under 17

Height		Lowest			Highest			Approx. age
1.10m	3ft 7in	17kg	2st	10lb	21.5kg	3st	5lb	5
1.15m	3ft 9in	18.5kg	2st	13lb	23.5kg	3st	10lb	6
1.19m	3ft 11in	20.5kg	3st	3lb	24.5kg	3st	12lb	7
1.24m	4ft 1in	22.5kg	3st	8lb	30.5kg	4st	11lb	8
1.27m	4ft 2in	23.5kg	3st	10lb	34.5kg	5st	6lb	9
1.35m	4ft 5in	26.5kg	4st	2lb	40kg	6st	4lb	10
1.42m	4ft 8in	28kg	4st	6lb	45kg	7st	1lb	11
1.47m	4ft 10in	30kg	4st	10lb	49.5kg	7st	11lb	12
1.55m	5ft 1in	36.5kg	5st	11lb	54kg	8st	7lb	13
1.57m	5ft 2in	41.3kg	6st	7lb	55.5kg	8st	10lb	14
1.60m	5ft 3in	45.5kg	7st	2lb	57kg	9st	0lb	15
1.63m	5ft 4in	46.5kg	7st	4lb	58.5kg	9st	3lb	16

One method used by scientists for measuring excess fat is the calliper test. The flesh is pinched between callipers on four areas of the body: the arms, back, thighs and waist. These measurements are then calculated to give a good idea of how much weight could be dieted away. We measured the twelve women pictured here and show the results the calliper test revealed. Taller women always carry excess weight a lot easier than smaller women, but they may have a bigger frame which cannot be altered by dieting. Most women tend to have particular problem areas, such as the stomach or bottom, and unfortunately there is no guarantee that these problems will disappear completely when they reach their target weight. However, exercise can help to firm and tone saggy muscles.

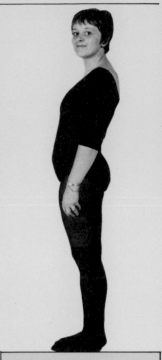

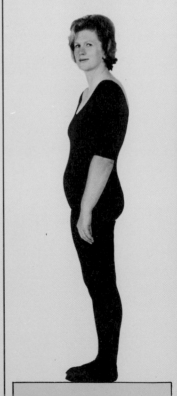

Joyce
1.52m (5ft0in)
Weighs 51.7kg (8st2lb)
Surplus 3.2kg (7lb)

Christine
1.57m (5ft2in)
Weighs 60.8kg (9st8lb)
Surplus 5kg (11lb)

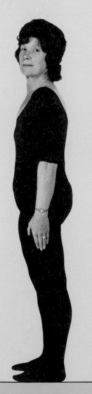

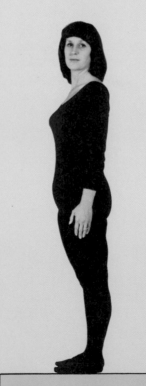

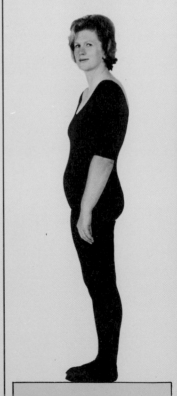

Hilda
1.68m (5ft6in)
Weighs 70.5kg (11st1½lb)
Surplus 6.3kg (1st)

Sheila
1.68m (5ft6in)
Weighs 62.4kg (9st11½lb)
Surplus 1.8kg (4lb)

Mary
1.73m (5ft8in)
Weighs 69.9kg (11st)
Surplus 9.5kg (1st7lb)

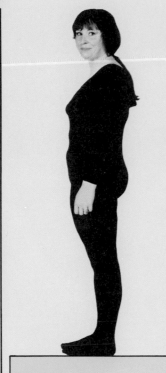
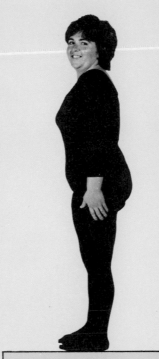
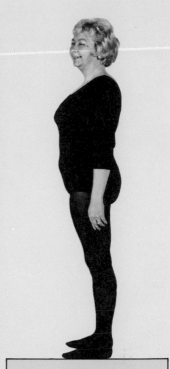

Denise
1.57m (5ft 2in)
Weighs 69.4kg (10st 13lb)
Surplus 12.7kg (2st)

Rosemary
1.60m (5ft 3in)
Weighs 79.8kg (12st 8lb)
Surplus 19.1kg (3st)

Anne
1.63m (5ft 4in)
Weighs 67.8kg (10st 9½lb)
Surplus 8.6kg (1st 5lb)

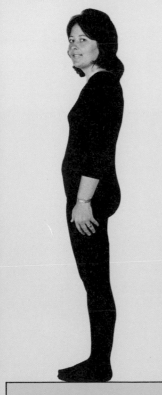
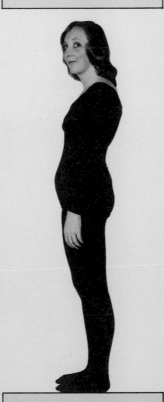
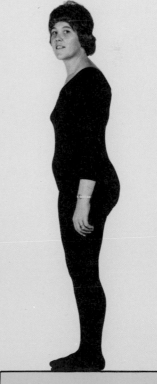

Stephanie
1.73m (5ft 8in)
Weighs 72.2kg (11st 5lb)
Surplus 2.3kg (5lb)

Margaret
1.75m (5ft 9in)
Weighs 73.2kg (11st 7½lb)
Surplus 6.3kg (1st)

Stella
1.75m (5ft 9in)
Weighs 77.8kg (12st 3½lb)
Surplus 9.5kg (1st 7lb)

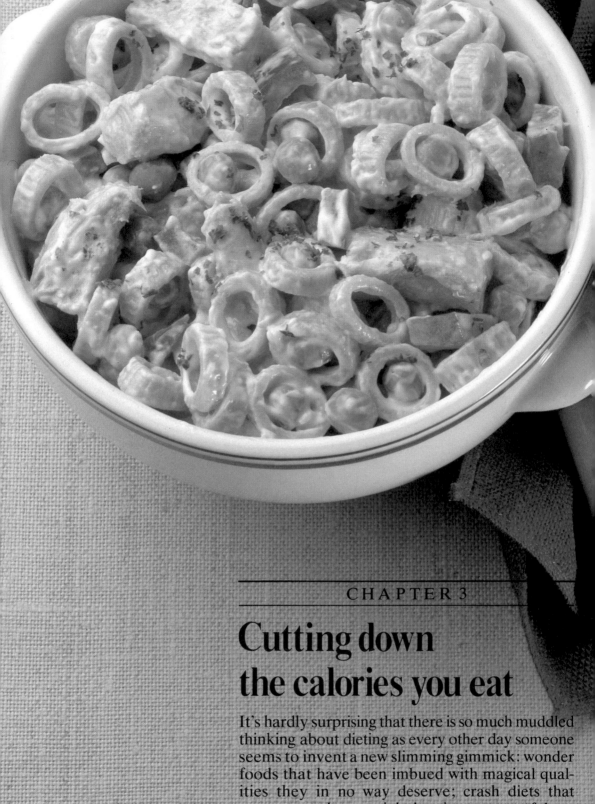

CHAPTER 3

Cutting down the calories you eat

It's hardly surprising that there is so much muddled thinking about dieting as every other day someone seems to invent a new slimming gimmick: wonder foods that have been imbued with magical qualities they in no way deserve; crash diets that guarantee a huge weight loss in a matter of days. Because losing weight is never easy, even seasoned slimmers may be willing to give these gimmicks a try just in case there is a magic answer to their weight problem.

Although crash diets may work in the short term, they fail to have any lasting effect on a weight problem. They are usually too rigid to maintain over a long period, and it is not recommended that anyone should diet for longer than a couple of weeks on an allowance of less than

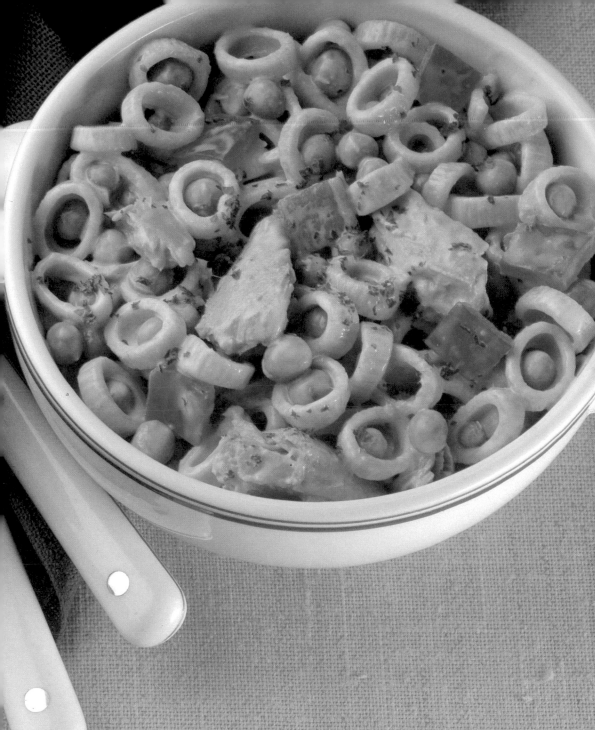

1,000 calories a day. If you do not supply your body with all the nutrients it needs, you will probably feel less active and more tired than normal. This, in turn, means that you will start using up fewer calories a day and so the crash diet eventually becomes counter-productive. All the foods that you eat, and most drinks, contain calories, and no food or drink can create a special chemical reaction in the body which will 'melt' away the unwanted fat.

The unassailable truth is that, no matter what you eat, the key to losing weight is to limit the number of calories you take in. Whether you do this by counting calories, by following a low-carbohydrate diet, a high-carbohydrate diet or a low-fat diet, the result will be the same.

Although these two dishes may look the same, the salad on the left contains 415 more calories than the special low-calorie version on the right. In order to achieve this, we used low-calorie salad dressing instead of fattening mayonnaise, and tuna in brine instead of oil. So cutting down on calories does not mean that you have to eat less. Turn to page 152 for the recipe for the low-calorie version of this delicious dish — Wholewheat Pasta and Tuna Salad.

Calorie-controlled diets

Counting every calorie is the best way to lose weight but it demands precision: all foods must be weighed and calculated and then added together to make up your daily allowance. Guess-work *won't* work. A pair of kitchen scales that weighs small amounts accurately is an essential piece of slimming equipment. You also need a jug that will measure liquids in fluid ounces or down to 25ml. Accurate measuring spoons, in either metric or imperial measurements, should be used rather than the nearest spoon that comes to hand in your cutlery drawer. Just 7g (¼oz) butter comes to 52 calories, 5ml (1 teaspoon) oil is 40 calories, and 28g (1oz) Cheddar cheese is 120 calories, so guessing by eye is not a very accurate method of determining weight. A few wrong guesses during the day and you may prevent yourself losing any weight at all. In a recent survey it was found that few people could guess accurately 28g (1oz) of hard cheese, and most of the sample cut a larger chunk from the block. The next time you cut a chunk of cheese, try guessing 28g (1oz) and then weigh it to see how well you estimated it. You will probably be very surprised.

Another disadvantage of counting calories is that you do have to write down everything you eat. It is surprisingly easy to develop a form of amnesia about those foods you do not want to remember you ate. Calorie counters tend to organize their dieting in one of two ways: some plan out their day's eating in advance, calculate their calories before they start, and keep to just those foods; others allot themselves a calorie total and deduct the calories as they eat them. The danger with the latter method, of course, is that you have to beware of being too generous with your calories early in the day in order to leave yourself an adequate calorie allowance for the evening meal.

The great advantage of counting calories is that you can eat absolutely anything you fancy as long as it does not exceed your allowance. Although most diets try to cater for differing lifestyles and tastes, it is likely that there will be at least one food you dislike, or one which is difficult to purchase. However, if you know your calories, you can substitute a food of equal calories.

If you do not wish to follow a set diet you can easily construct your own using the calorie charts at the end of this book. The best diet for you is the one you find easiest to follow and that which fits most neatly into your own lifestyle.

In addition to the calorie reference chart at the back of this book, there is a picture guide to calories in basic foods in the section called *Calories on view*. It is worth learning the calorific values of your favourite basic foods by heart; once they are memorized you will find it easier to make a diet-wise choice in restaurants or when you are away from home. You will learn which foods you must avoid and which foods are filling and satisfying for little calorie cost. Absorbing these few initial facts will not only help you to lose weight now but will also make it easier for you to stay slim.

The recipes section gives you a selection of diets which count the calories for you in various ways. Designed to fit a variety of lifestyles and patterns of eating, these diets cater for all tastes and figures. The diet-package plan does all the thinking for you. Each diet is worked out in detail from the first bite to the last crumb and is balanced carefully to give you a good supply of all the essential nutrients. As a general rule, if you are over 12.7kg (2st) overweight (see the charts in *What should you weigh?*), start off on a 1,500 calorie a day diet. However, if you have less than 6kg (1st) to lose, you will need to keep to 1,000 calories. Whether you choose 1,000, 1,250 or 1,500 calories a day, provided you eat precisely what you are told and weigh out all foods accurately, then weight loss will follow.

The low-carbohydrate diet

The low-carbohydrate diet has enjoyed popularity for many years. It is based on the theory that such sugary and starchy foods as bread and potatoes, which are high in carbohydrates, are the really bad fatteners. Provided that these foods are cut out or, at least, severely restricted, all carbohydrate-free foods, including butter, cheese and fatty meats, can be eaten freely. Many people still regard this slimming method as the only really valid diet although nutritional research has now proved that there are much more effective methods of dieting.

A low-carbohydrate diet works best for men and heavily overweight women in the early stages of their weight loss campaign. Men have a considerably higher calorie requirement than do women; and heavily overweight women have a higher calorie requirement than those who weigh only marginally more than their ideal weight. Although both will lose weight on 1,500 calories a day, many women with a modest weight problem would probably find the low-carbohydrate diet depressingly slow.

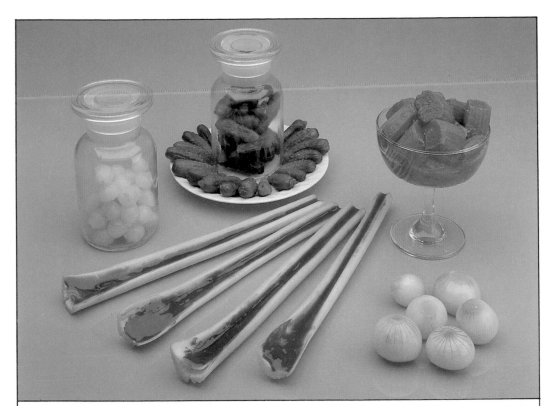

What can I eat between meals, apart from carrots, that add few calories to my daily total? Not a lot, unfortunately, apart from low-calorie vegetables. A few suggestions that might help are pictured here in the quantity it takes to supply only an insignificant 20 calories: 6 pickled onions; 20 cocktail onions; 60 small gherkins; 4 sticks of celery spread with yeast extract; or 284g (10oz) rhubarb, stewed in water and sweetened with artificial sweetener.

The average person consumes just under half his, or her, daily calories in the form of carbohydrates. The prime object of the low-carbohydrate method of dieting is to remove some of these carbohydrate-supplied calories from the daily menu, and thus sufficiently reducing the total calorie intake to a slimming level. But on the conventional low-carbohydrate method of dieting there is nothing to prevent you from cancelling out all the calories you save in sacrificing sugary and starchy foods by increasing your intake of high-protein and fatty foods. However, if you substitute a fat or protein calorie for each carbohydrate calorie, you will not shed any surplus weight at all.

By cutting out carbohydrates, dieters often eliminate the fats that are usually eaten with them, butter with bread, for example. As we are not in the habit of eating, say, three pork chops at one meal, we tend to naturally restrict our protein intake. Many of our 'extra snack' foods are high in carbohydrates and thus low-carbohydrate diets reduce food intake in that direction.

One of the reasons for the decline in popularity of this diet is that over the past 10 years, and due to new breakthroughs in nutritional research, there has been a shift of expert opinion about which types of foods should be reduced in our diets and which should be increased for good health. High-carbohydrate foods, such as cereals, pasta and root vegetables, with their valuable nutrients, play a vital part in maintaining health with their bulk and fibre content. Fibre provides the roughage that prevents constipation, and lack of fibre is thought to be connected with various disorders of the bowels. Some experts believe also that lack of fibre may lead to diabetes and possibly heart disease. So modern nutritionists have recommended that high-carbohydrate foods should be included in a diet. However, the human body requires very little fat for health and, if eaten too freely, low-carbohydrate, high-calorie fatty foods, such as butter, margarine, milk products and fatty meats, contribute to overweight and obesity-related diseases. The very bad dietary reputation of sugar has in no way improved, and most nutritionists are, if anything, even more convinced that eating a large quantity of sugar can be detrimental to good health.

One of the advantages of the low-carbohydrate diet is its very simplicity — foods containing carbohydrates can be given a unit equivalent and a wide range of 'free' foods can be eaten. Keeping to 10 carbo units a day is simpler mathematically than counting 1,500 calories. Now, with the development of the low-fat diet, it is possible to diet just as simply in a more effective and healthier way.

The low-fat diet

Fats *are* fattening, and that is why low-fat dieting has become a very successful method of losing weight. By reducing your fats intake you are indirectly controlling your calories, and by controlling the amount of fat you eat you will slim in a very healthy way.

Low-fat dieting has been greeted with unqualified support in both medical and nutritional worlds. The Royal College of Physicians, the British Cardiac Society and top nutritional experts in the United States have all recommended an overall reduction of fat in British and American diets.

In recent years, nutritionists have found a direct parallel between the percentage of

Is it necessary to weigh everything when you count calories?
The really low-calorie vegetables are the only safe exceptions. Here you see a small plate of salad vegetables (no salad dressing, of course) and a large plate. We also picture a modest serving of Brussels sprouts and a more generous one. In each case, the calories added by extra generosity are not significant enough to make any difference to daily weight loss.

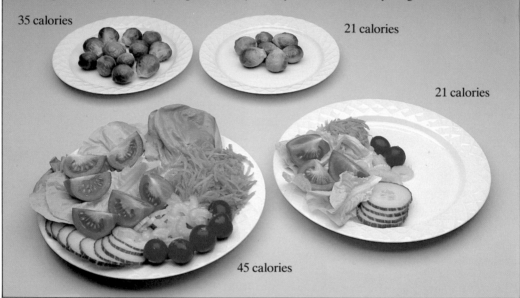

35 calories

21 calories

21 calories

45 calories

However, the look-and guess method can be deceiving in other instances. The portions in this picture do not look much different but, by helping yourself to the thicker or larger slices or portions (and counting the calories for the smaller one!), you can soar over your daily slimming calorie total. So be careful to weigh all foods before you eat them.

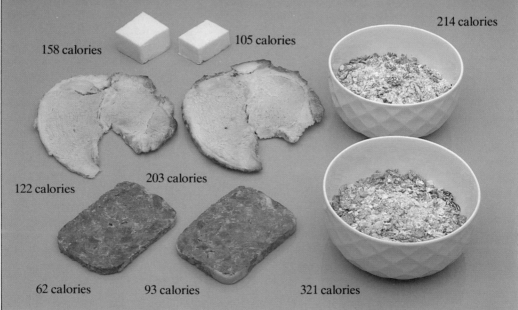

158 calories

105 calories

214 calories

122 calories

203 calories

62 calories

93 calories

321 calories

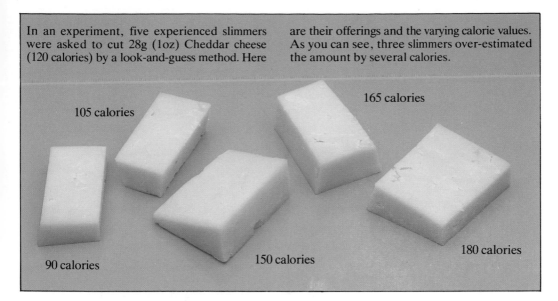

In an experiment, five experienced slimmers were asked to cut 28g (1oz) Cheddar cheese (120 calories) by a look-and-guess method. Here are their offerings and the varying calorie values. As you can see, three slimmers over-estimated the amount by several calories.

105 calories

165 calories

90 calories

150 calories

180 calories

fats in national diets and the prevalence of weight problems. In countries where the diet contains a very high percentage of fat (America, for instance), obesity has become a health problem of epidemic proportions. In countries where the diet is marginally less fatty (as in some northern European countries, for instance), the obesity problem is correspondingly less severe. But in those states where the basic diet is very low in fat (Korea, for instance, where fat accounts for only 8 per cent of daily calorie intake), obesity is extremely rare.

The most widely agreed picture of an ideal healthy diet is one that is low in fats, particularly the animal fats. Doctors looking into the causes of heart disease have found now that an important factor may be the concentration of fat-like substances in the blood stream, one of which is cholesterol. This is affected by what we eat and it is thought that reducing fat in our food can help to prevent the build-up of cholesterol in the blood. A healthy diet should contain also a generous quantity of high-fibre cereal and vegetable foods to provide some roughage. It should be low in sugar, which is just concentrated calories and can cause dental decay. It should provide a generous quantity of fruit and vegetables with their essential nutrients. Salt helps to retain fluid in the body and the recommendation is that the average diet should have a lower salt content. When you follow the new low-fat method of dieting you will automatically follow the same pattern as that recommended for good health.

The low-fat diet is very successful as a reducing diet because, by controlling the intake of fats, it also controls automatically your intake of the highest calorie foods. If you look at the calorie chart, you will see that such fats as butter and lard are even higher in calories than carbohydrate foods. You will notice also that fatty meats and cheese contain more calories than do low-fat proteins, and the lowest calorie foods of all are those that contain no fat.

An astonishing number of innocent-looking foods contain 'invisible' fats, and although it is easy to see and remove the fat from the outside of a slice of ham or a lamb chop, it is more difficult to identify fat if it is hidden in homogenized milk or hard cheese. In order to slim effectively using this method, you must be aware of the invisible fat in foods. The pioneer low-fat method, as devised by *Slimming Magazine,* allocates a fat unit number to each food according to the amount of fat it contains. Hundreds of basic foods have been analyzed to provide this information. On this diet, you are allowed up to 10 fat units a day and have access to a wide range of 'free-foods'.

This diet's popularity lies in its utter simplicity. There is no need to count every single calorie — as long as you keep to your allowance of 10 fat units each day it is unlikely that you could eat enough free-food calories to prevent you losing any weight. Switches from high-fat foods to lower-fat foods are often effortless and non-sacrificial. By changing from 75g (3oz) Cheddar cheese with your salad to 75g (3oz) roast chicken you will save 240 calories. If you switched to 75g (3oz) prawns instead, you would save another 30 calories. Fruits and vegetables are unrationed, and cereals, rice and pasta are allowed in generous quantities, so that you get the filling, healthy fibre you need.

Many slimmers are delighted by the results they have had by following this diet. Not only have they become slim but they are also staying slim, because they continue to follow some of the fat-cutting habits they learned on the diet. A low-fat diet is included in the diets section. Here we show you some examples of fattening, fat-containing foods that will make you think twice about eating them in future.

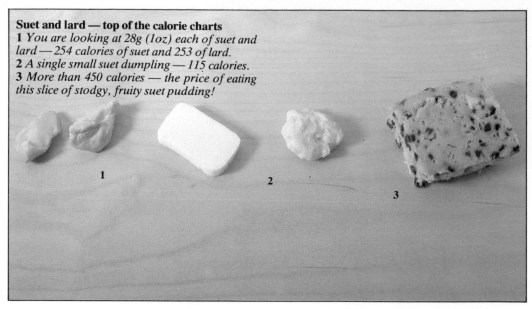

Suet and lard — top of the calorie charts
1 You are looking at 28g (1oz) each of suet and lard — 254 calories of suet and 253 of lard.
2 A single small suet dumpling — 115 calories.
3 More than 450 calories — the price of eating this slice of stodgy, fruity suet pudding!

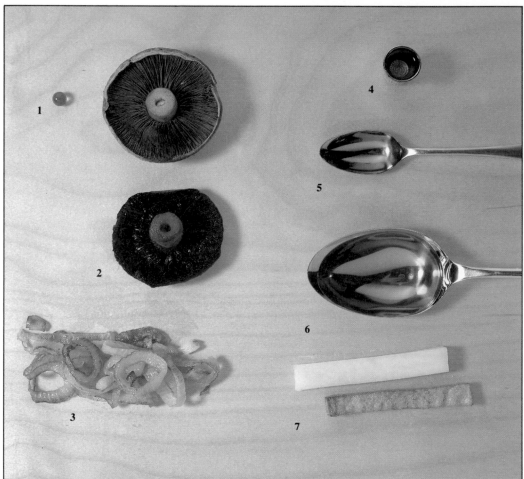

Such a little fat but what a LOT of calories
1 There are 2 calories in this tiny halibut liver oil capsule — as many as in this 14g (½oz) mushroom.
2 Soaked up by this single fried mushroom are 30 fatty calories. Simmered in stock instead of fried, an identical mushroom could cost only 2 calories.

3 This 28g (1oz) onion, 7 calories, soaks up 40 more calories by being fried.
4 Just a thimbleful of oil, yet 25 calories!
5 Just 5ml (1 teaspoon) oil, yet 40 calories!
6 Every time you add 15ml (1 tablespoon) oil, remember you are adding 120 calories to a dish.
7 Single chip, raw, costs 7 calories. Same chip after frying costs 12 calories.

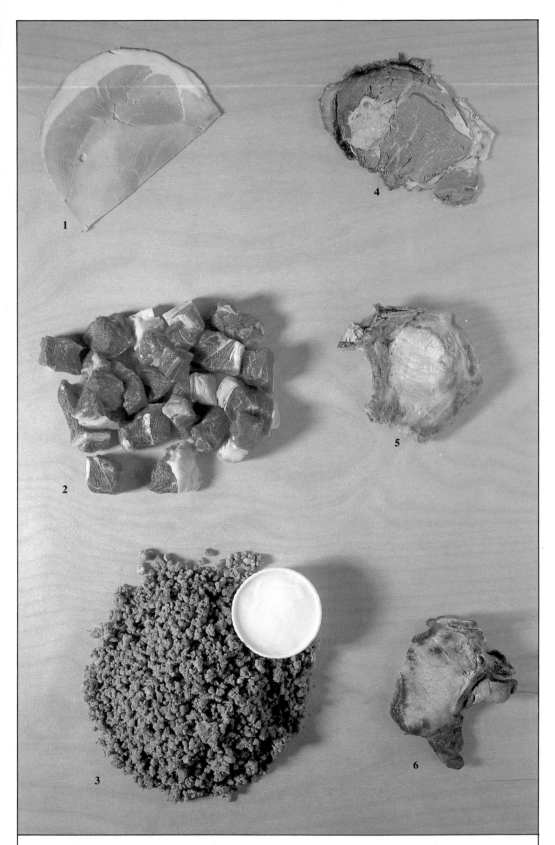

Meat-fat can make it VERY fattening
1 On this slice of ham there are 45 calories of lean meat and 35 calories in fat. Trim it off!
2 Tossed straight into the stew, this 454g (1lb) fatty stewing steak costs 960 calories. You could save 490 calories by first trimming off *all* the fat ·
3 Drained off just 454g (1lb) minced beef are the 290 calories' worth of fat you see here.

Always brown and then drain mince before further cooking.
4 On this slice of cooked roast beef you see 45 calories of lean meat and 48 calories of fat.
5 Choose chops with care. This fatty one, only moderately well grilled, costs 430 calories.
6 Same weight chop as above but leaner and thoroughly grilled to shed fat — 285 calories.

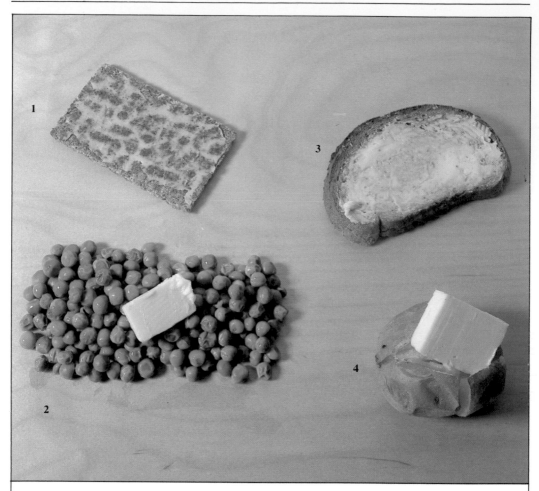

Butter and margarine
1 There are 25 calories in the sparse amount of butter you see spread on this single crispbread.
2 Just 45 calories in this portion of peas but another 70 in the butter (about one-third of an ounce) on top.

3 Lavish butterers beware! There are 100 calories in this slice of toast and 105 more in the butter on top.
4 This small baked potato costs 125 calories but you almost double the figure by adding 14g (½oz) butter.

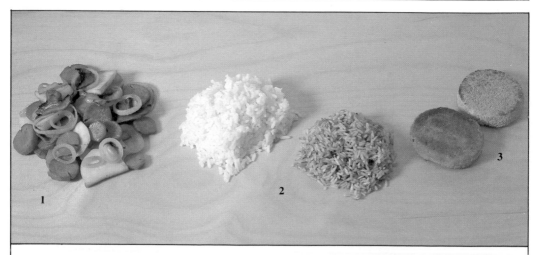

Why fry when there is no need?
1 There are 105 calories' worth of fat in this quantity of fried vegetables (an unnecessary step before being added to a casserole).
2 This 57g (2oz) portion of rice costs 206 calories

boiled — 53 more calories if you fry it first.
3 There is never any need to fry frozen fish cakes. They cost 140 calories each if you fry them but only 60 when you just grill them without fat. Much more slimming!

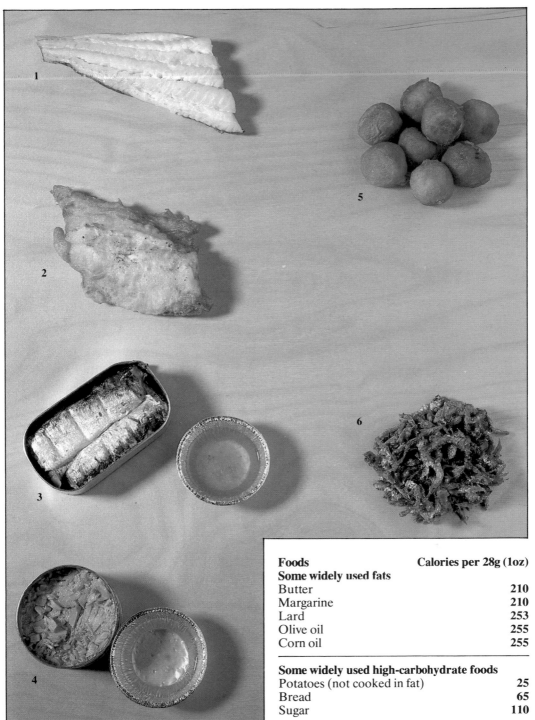

Fish without fat
1 Portion of white fish grilled without fat, only 135 calories.
2 Same amount of same fish, deep-fried in batter — 460 calories.
3 This amount of oil, drained off a can of sardines, saves 145 calories.
4 This quantity of oil, drained from one 198g (7oz) can of tuna, is 155 calories' worth.
5 Worst fish to fry: packaged fish portions, or small fish, because there is more surface area to soak up the fat. This 198g(7oz) portion of crisp, fried cod balls when deep-fried is 390 calories.
6 This 85g (3oz) portion of deep-fried whitebait has 445 calories.

Foods	Calories per 28g (1oz)
Some widely used fats	
Butter	210
Margarine	210
Lard	253
Olive oil	255
Corn oil	255
Some widely used high-carbohydrate foods	
Potatoes (not cooked in fat)	25
Bread	65
Sugar	110
Some fatty protein foods	
Roast breast of lamb	115
Cheddar cheese	120
Cream cheese	125
Some low-fat protein foods	
Cod or haddock fillet (not fried)	22
Prawns (shelled)	30
Roast chicken (skinned)	42
Some typical fatless fruit and vegetables	
Mushrooms	4
Melon	4
Cabbage	6
Brussels sprouts	7
Orange	7
Eating apple	10

29

A dozen dieting myths

1 Restricting fluids helps you lose weight
Some diets suggest that you need to restrict your fluid intake for slimming success. If you drink a lot of high-calorie liquids, then certainly they should be restricted as the body does not need these sugary drinks. However, there is no need to restrict water, black tea and coffee or any soft drinks that are labelled low-calorie. The human body has a superbly efficient control mechanism which maintains its correct liquid level and only fails when some disease or a complicated hormone disturbance occurs, in which case you need to seek medical advice. As long as you are in normal health, there is no need to worry about restricting no-calorie or low-calorie fluids in any way. Drink all you want and your body will get rid of any surplus.

2 Wine is lower in calories than spirits
It is certainly true that, gram for gram, wine is lower in calories than spirits. But it is pointless for a slimmer to compare drinks' calorific values without also considering normal quantities. In practice, a single spirit served with water or a low-calorie mixer would be about 50 calories and a glass of dry white wine would be at least half as much again. A small glass of sweet red wine would be almost double the calorie cost of a small measure of gin or whisky.

3 Low-cholesterol margarine is low in calories
Low cholesterol does not automatically imply low in calories and margarine can be just as fattening as butter. Only the special low-fat spreads contain half the calories of butter or margarine.

4 It is essential to eat breakfast every day
To our knowledge, there is no scientific proof that eating breakfast will lessen a weight problem, and there is absolutely no reason to force unwanted calories down unwilling throats. If you are accustomed to eating breakfast you may well suffer slight 'withdrawal symptoms' if you miss it. Some people report feeling weak and even dizzy. However, if you never eat breakfast there is no reason why you should not save your calories until later in the day. Many people fear that if they keep most of their calories for evening eating, they will not be able to lose weight. The scientific indications are that the calorie-burning advantage a dieter gains from spreading her calories throughout the day, rather than saving most of her food

for the evening, are modest. How much your metabolism speeds up after a meal depends on how much you eat — the larger the meal, the faster it is burned up. However, insufficient research has been done to give reliable figures but after a modest meal the increase in metabolic rate is proably around 5 per cent. A dieter who eats throughout the day is probably burning up in the region of 100 calories a day more than an evening-eater, and most breakfasts will cost you more than that.

5 Pasta, bread and potatoes are fattening
Contrary to popular belief, pasta, bread and potatoes are not high-calorie foods. What usually does the damage is the fatty sauces served traditionally with pasta, the butter spread on bread, or potatoes being chipped and fried or roasted with fat. Any food is fattening if you eat enough of it, but it is unlikely that you would eat enough pasta, bread or potato on their own to put on weight. For example, you would have to eat almost 1.40kg (3lb) cooked spaghetti to take in 1,500 calories; a normal portion is 175g (6oz).

6 Salads are always the best buy when eating out
A salad can, in fact, be an amazingly high-calorie meal. Bought versions often come covered in high-calorie mayonnaise or French dressing and portions of meat may weigh more than you guess or have a high-fat content, thus an ordinary cheese salad may amount to 600 calories. When eating out it can often pay to be calorie-wise and choose a plain beefburger — served with a plain salad and, of course, no chips!

7 Cheese need not be limited on a diet
The idea that cheese is a safe food probably stems from the low-carbohydrate diets that allow you to eat it freely. In fact, hard cheese is high in calories and should be limited carefully on any diet. Cottage and curd cheese, however, are low in calories.

8 Brown bread and sugar are more slimming than white
A small 28g (1oz) slice of wholemeal bread will cost you 61 calories; a white slice will cost only 5 calories more. So the calorie difference is not great. Wholemeal bread, however, is much higher in fibre content as it is made with wholegrain flour but do not assume that all brown bread is automatically more healthy than white bread. Many brown breads are made from white flour that has been tastefully tinted, so look for the

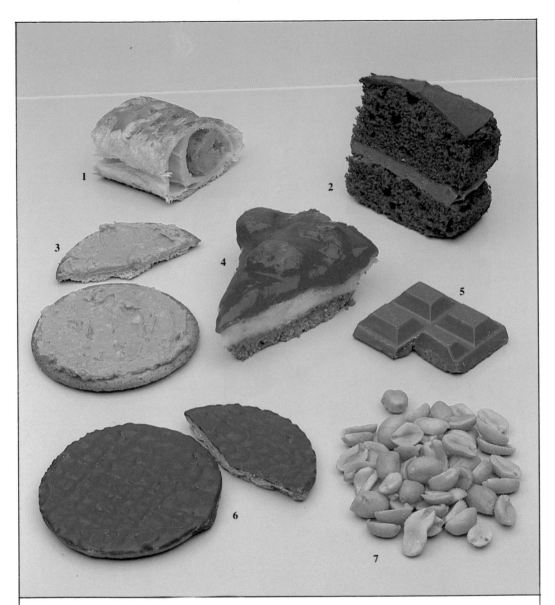

wholemeal label. Cutting down on sugar of all shades is advisable for most people, whether or not they need to slim. Although the brown sorts may look more 'natural', this does not make them nourishing, and the calories are exactly the same as for white. So buy brown bread with a high bran content.

9 Certain foods can melt away fat
Diets that suggest that foods, such as grapefruit, have special powers to dissolve body fat are nonsense. The same applies to lecithin, which is sold in pills to some

credulous slimmers who believe that so long as they swallow them they can eat what they like, thus magically preventing the body extracting every food calorie. Certainly, lecithin is an entirely natural substance which helps to emulsify fat; in other words, it breaks fat up into tiny droplets. However, the body efficiently makes all the lecithin it needs. Alas, whether it grows on a tree or comes in a bottle, no wonder food exists. When diets based on supposed wonder foods work, it is because they reduce the total number of calories consumed in a day.

Exhaustive research has failed to find any special slimming magic in a grapefruit, lecithin or any food or chemical substance.

10 You should keep to regular meal times
Although it is not essential to keep to regular strict meal times it is sometimes unavoidable because most people eat their breakfast at the same time before leaving for work, eat in their lunch hour and again when they return home in the evening. The body is programmed to a regular eating pattern and expects food at certain times of the day. If you manage to break this clock-locked habit of eating, then your ability to abstain from food when you are not really hungry increases and this, in turn, helps in overall weight control.

11 Diabetic foods are safe for slimmers
This is not always the case. If sugar is replaced by an artificial sweetener, such as Sorbitol, the product will contain as many

calories as sugar. Only if sugar is replaced by a no-calorie sweetener such as saccharin will the product be lower in calories. Diabetic lagers are usually just as high in calories, if not higher, than the ordinary sort.

12 Protein is not fattening
We all need protein, although not as much as was once believed. The average person on a Western diet usually eats about twice as much protein as he needs. Eating protein in addition to what the body needs will not make you any stronger or healthier. Certainly, protein-containing foods (none are all protein) are good for slimmers, but the calories must be counted just as with any other food. Some fatty, high-protein foods, such as cream cheese at 135 calories for 28g (1oz) and roast breast of lamb at 115 calories for 28g (1oz), need careful rationing. The lowest-calorie protein foods, such as prawns and roast chicken, are also those that contain the lowest percentage of fat.

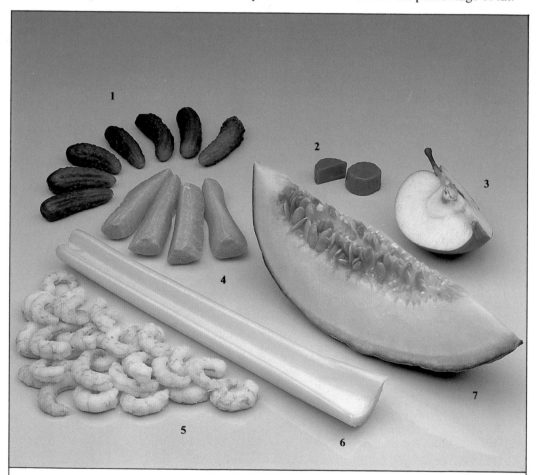

How many calories a minute?
Contrast this wide selection of foods with the fattening foods shown on the previous page. Their calorie per minute values, based on their munch-ability, are as follows:
1 Gherkins (7) — 2 calories
2 Toffees (1½) — 25 calories
3 28g (1oz) eating apple — 10 calories
4 28g (1oz) carrot — 6 calories
5 35g (1¼oz) prawns — 38 calories
6 43g (1½oz) celery — 3 calories
7 142g (5oz) melon — 20 calories

Is dry sherry less fattening than sweet sherry?
In this picture are equal calorie quantities of sweet and dry sherry (55 calories), and sweet and dry wine (75 calories), As you see, you do get a little more tor your calories by choosing the 'dry' drinks — but it's only a small saving. However, it is better to drink dry versions whenever possible both to reduce calories and curb your 'sweet tooth'.

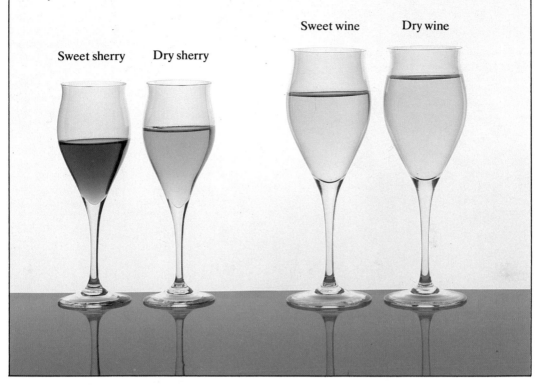

Sweet sherry   Dry sherry   Sweet wine   Dry wine

Is wine less fattening than spirits ?
Yes, if you drink the same quantity of wine as spirits. On the left, in the picture, is a bar single measure of whisky (50 calories) and the same quantity of dry white wine (only 16 calories). On the right, you can see the calories in a small 113ml (4floz) glass, and a medium 142ml (5floz) measure and a large 170ml (6 floz) measure of wine. All have more calories than a glass of spirits when you take into account the vital factors of 'normal quantity' — unless you are in the habit of pouring doubles.

Whisky   Wine

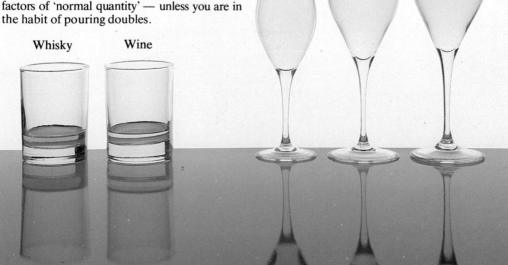

76 calories   95 calories   114 calories

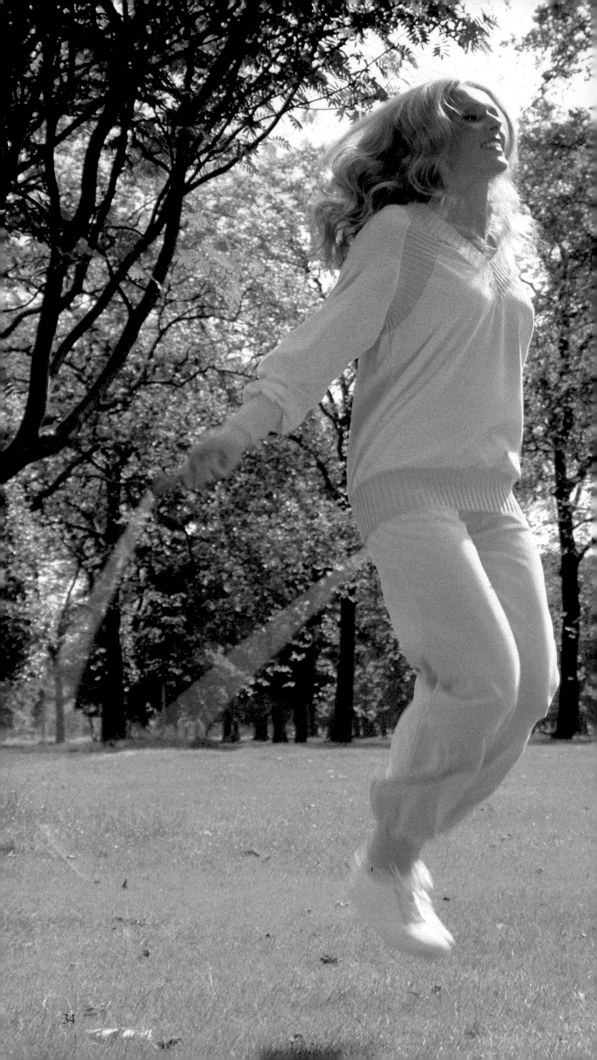

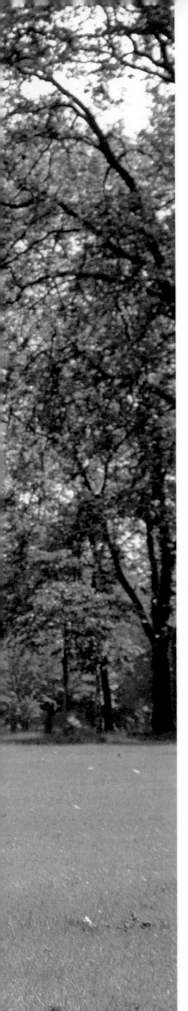

Increasing the amount of exercise you take can be an effective booster for your dieting campaign. When you are slimming, your basic aim is to eat fewer calories than your body needs each day so that it has to draw on its fatty reserves for energy. You can do this by diet alone: restricting the calories your body takes in. However, if, by extra physical activity, you also boost your body's daily calorie-output rate, you are attacking your weight problem on two fronts, by diet and exercise.

Stepping up the calories you burn

Recent research has shown that there may be many women who cannot maintain a permanently slim figure unless, besides monitoring their calorie intake, they start increasing their physical activity. The average woman burns up approximately 2,000 calories a day, of which about two thirds are used by the body for maintenance alone. We have little control over this type of calorie expenditure which forms our basal metabolic rate. For many years, scientists have been looking for major differences in metabolic rate between the fat and the thin. Often, apart from noticing a tendency for the metabolism of natural skinnies to speed up after over-eating, researchers have been surprised at the uniformity of rates. It is in the number of calories used up in activities throughout the day, however, that striking differences have been noticed.

Some people seem to be born with greater exercise resistance than others. Scientists have now discovered that variations are apparent even in young babies. Whereas there are lazy babies who lie peacefully in their cots there are also active babies, who wriggle and roll about at a rapid rate. These differences in activity levels tend to continue throughout childhood and even into adulthood. Basically, it is not so much what you do but the way in which you do it that determines energy output. Even when it comes to ordinary household tasks, exercise-resistant people will find ways to minimize movement and they may be quite unaware of their bodies' artful ploys to save calories. It is very hard to diagnose your own exercise resistance, but if you are overweight the evidence suggests that you and your figure are almost certainly suffering from it.

Physical activity is a term that embraces all bodily movement. It not only includes what we normally think of as being 'exercise', such as walking, sports and keep-fit exercises, but it also takes in shopping, climbing the stairs, and even walking across the room. In fact, every time we move we are burning up at least some calories. These days, weight control experts advocate that you should weave more total body movement into your everyday activity rather than concentrating on setting aside a period of time for special exercises. The former, they advise, is what really helps when you are aiming at lasting weight control. It is the sum total of the little movements during the course of the day that has the most significant effect on calorie expenditure and, therefore, on weight. You can observe the truth of this yourself — almost certainly among your acquaintances there will be a woman who is described as being 'full of nervous energy'. She is almost invariably lean. Watch her closely next time you visit her home. See how many times she rises from her seat to perform some task or to fetch something. Observe how brisk all her movements tend to be. It is likely, too, that your friends include at least one heavily overweight woman who swears that she does not eat a lot and cannot understand why she weighs so much — she is best observed doing housework. Although she might be coping with a busy day, see how little she actually moves in performing her household tasks, and how slowly she moves. Without being aware of it, she has devised methods of performing each task that involve a minimum of body movement. When she settles into her armchair, note her tendency to call on other people to fetch something she needs from the next room, rather than get up and fetch it herself. Most people who move a great deal are lean. Those who do not, tend to be overweight, although they may regard themselves as active people.

Even apparently young and fit people who take up some form of sport can still be exercise resistant. Some ball games, for example, offer great opportunities for being idle and standing around when you may be tricked into thinking you have exercised hard and steadily. Watch some people on a tennis court — while some players rush around the court burning up calories, others move slowly and practise only right-arm activity!

Unfortunately the whole concept of exercise breeds great resistance in many women, particularly those with a weight problem. Anyone who has been a plump child still remembers the horror of games and the humiliations of the

You can step up your general level of activity and exercise anywhere without recourse to special equipment, clothing or surroundings. Just wear some casual, loose-fitting clothing (track suits, shorts and leotards are ideal) and practise some bending and stretching exercises to loosen up and relax stiff, aching limbs and tone up sagging muscles. Details of special exercises for shaping up thighs, stomach, bottom and arms are given in Chapter 9: Getting into shape. If you prefer not to exercise alone, then seek the moral support and guidance of others and join a local gym or keep-fit and dancing classes.

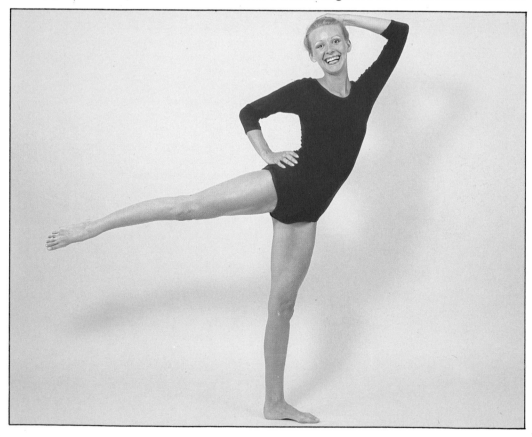

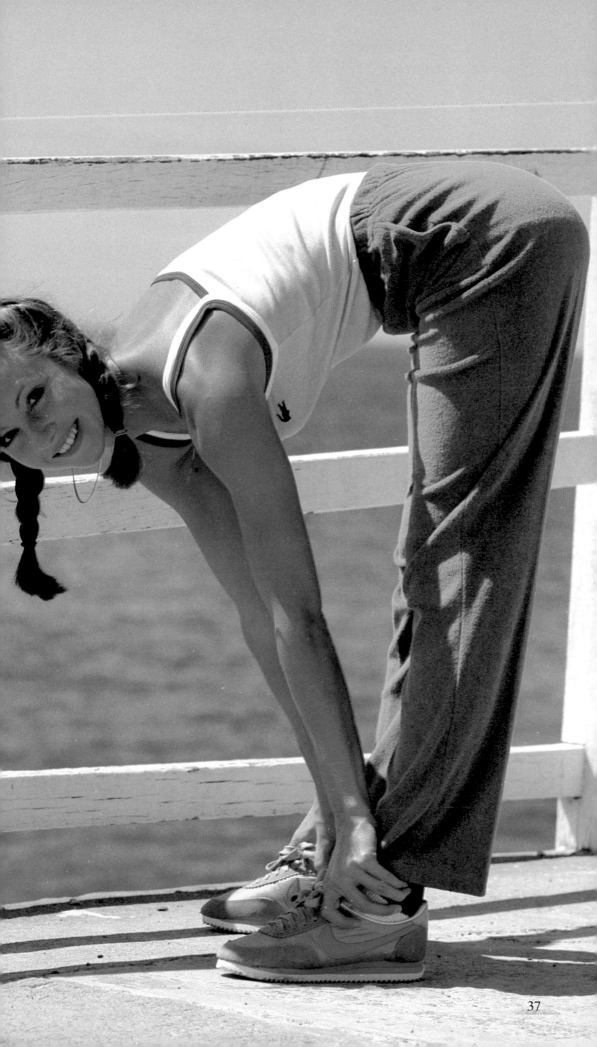

school gym. Furthermore, most of us have an in-built guilt complex about exercise which we know we ought to do, always intend to do, but never quite get round to doing. In the following pages, we outline a plan of campaign for all exercise haters.

Beating activity resistance

You can start tackling the task of increasing your daily calorie output in the simplest of ways. Begin, perhaps, by concentrating on speeding up both your movements and activities. Break your age-old habits and walk more swiftly — it will soon become habitual to you, whether you are popping out to the shops, walking to a neighbour's home or just ambling around the house.

You can also work at changing your attitude towards physical activity and exertion. Instead of cursing the fact that you must climb upstairs to fetch something, start to welcome that extra climb as an opportunity to burn a few more calories. Also, try to speed up your rate of ascent each time you go upstairs. Begin to embrace every natural opportunity to move, however small it is. This, too, will gradually become quite effortless. The 'nervous energy' person is quite unaware of the movement in her day — to her, it is effortless and natural. You, too, with a little initial effort, can become more active and less conscious of the movements you perform.

Every time we move, we are burning up at least some calories. The more parts of our bodies that we move, the more calories we burn up. Hence, moving your whole body from place to place by walking will burn up considerably more calories than simply moving one arm to iron or two hands to type. The speed at which we move also affects the number of calories we burn. The faster the movement, the greater the number of calories used. Thus brisk walking burns significantly more calories than strolling, and jogging or running burn more than a brisk walk. The third factor that affects the number of calories burned by body movement is the pull of gravity; walking upstairs or uphill will use up more calories than proceeding along level

Badminton (below) and squash (right) are good sports for burning up calories. Although badminton is a gentler game than the faster, hard-hitting squash racquets, it still involves a lot of movement on the court and stretching and reaching for the shuttlecock as it darts backwards and forwards across the net. Most sports clubs and local community centres cater for both these sports although you can, of course, rig up a badminton net in your own back garden and practise with your family and friends.

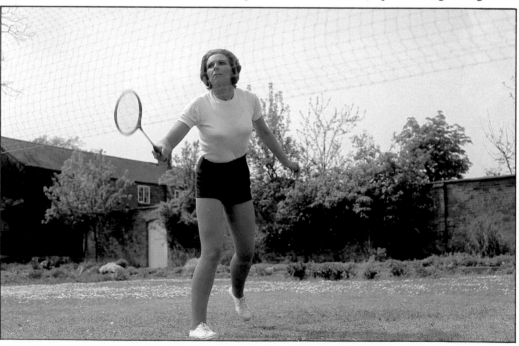

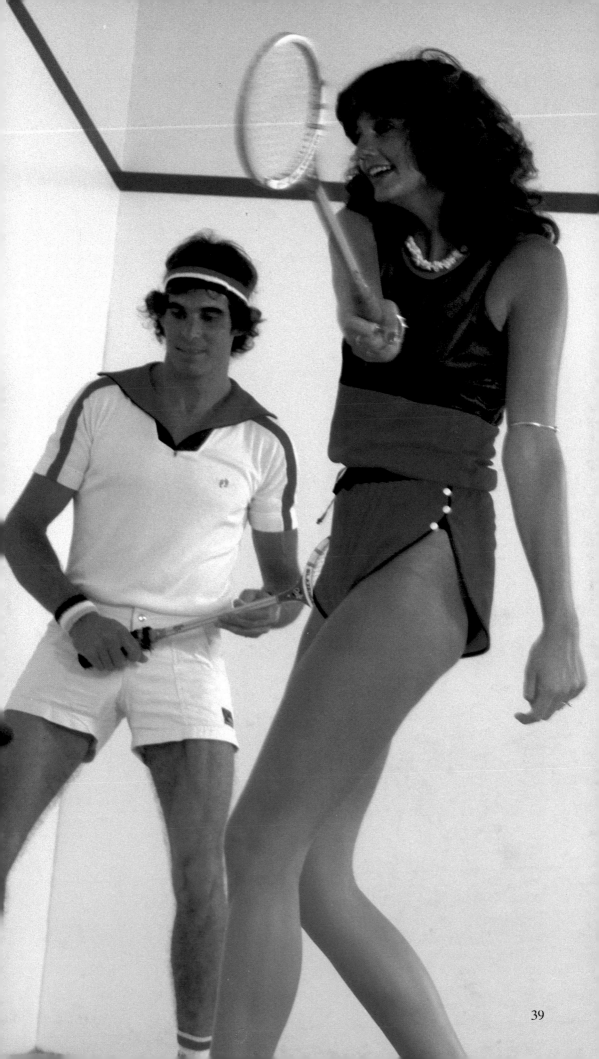

39

ground. So the activities that produce the maximum in calorie burn-up are those that involve moving the whole body, at a fast pace, in an upwards direction, such as running uphill, rushing upstairs or skipping. Climbing stairs more than usual will incorporate a great deal of high-calorie-burning activity into your routine. Resist the temptation to ask other people to fetch and carry for you, and get up and go yourself at the briskest possible pace. Before you embark on any task, consider how you can do it with the maximum amount of body movement. One bonus of being overweight is that you burn up more calories taking exercise than a slim person. This is because more calories are needed to move a heavier body.

Once you have made a start on increasing your energy output, you will soon notice the positive results. Add to it, as you go along, by introducing some deliberate exercise into your usual daily routine. Instead of driving or bussing to a regular destination like the shops or the station, walk briskly. These additional walks will supplement the increase of movement in your small daily activities and thus boost the overall calorie expenditure.

If an overweight person takes a brisk walk for 30 minutes each day for a year, it could add up to a considerable weight loss — even up to 6kg(1st) a year, in addition to the amount you lose by dieting. You could also lose that extra weight if you cycled for 20 minutes to the shops or work and then back again, five days a week. Both walking and cycling can also play a useful role in the prevention of coronary attacks. It does not matter that only your legs are being exercised — in terms of coronary circulation, exercising any part of your body affects the whole circulation of your blood. However, if you are very overweight, you should refrain from pedalling hard up enormous hills — any violent exercise is unwise for an unfit person.

Having started to think in terms of calorie output, it may be a good idea to take up some form of sporting activity that appeals to you or which you used to enjoy in the past. Remember that in order to be enjoyed, sports do not have

Walking is the simplest and easiest activity of all and a great way of burning up excess calories. Make walking an integral part of your daily routine either by going out for a special walk or by walking when you would normally drive or catch a bus. At weekends, plan a long walk in the countryside or a local park — you will find it relaxing and enjoyable.

In addition to boosting your slimming campaign, walking is a good method of alleviating boredom — an escape route from the house when you might otherwise be tempted to eat illicit, fattening snack meals.

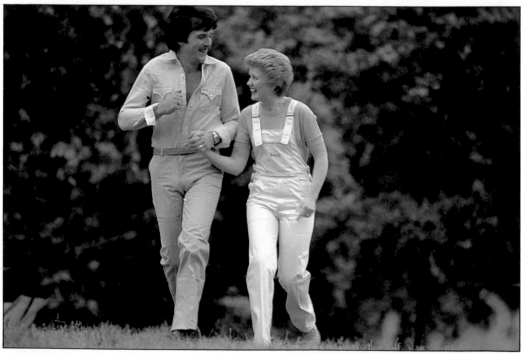

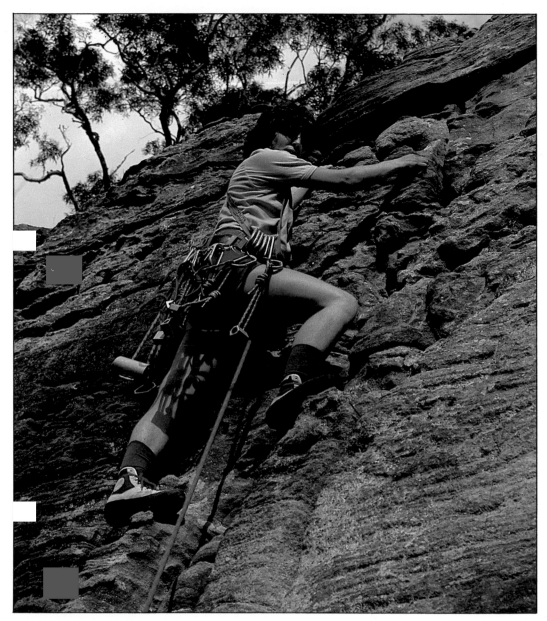

to be played or performed at a high standard. Find some like-minded friends and have a crack at tennis or badminton, for instance. It does not matter if the ball seems to spend more time on the adjacent tennis court than your own as long as you enjoy yourselves and keep active. Your twice-weekly tennis get-togethers could prove to be the enjoyable highlights of the week rather than a sacrifice as you burn up more calories to add to your total output. Not only will they add fun to your life, but they will also help to make you look and feel younger because eventually you will feel fitter and better as a result of this exercise.

If you find it difficult to exercise alone, consider joining a class to do keep-fit, taking up yoga or, if you are a little more adventurous, learning dance. Choose a group, though, that is easy to get to and meets at a convenient time, so that you are not constantly making excuses why you should not bother to turn up! Joining an exercise group has the advantage that you will certainly do your full half-hour or hour of exercise when you go along; seek out expert teachers to ensure that you are doing your exercises correctly.

There are a number of exercise machines, such as rowing machines, exercise bikes and jogging machines, on the market. These will certainly help to burn up calories, but

Rock-climbing may seem too dangerous and arduous a sport for you to take up yourself, but there are many other interesting and exciting activities that you could try — surfing, caving, parachuting, gliding and diving, to name but a few examples. Sports like these can boost your self-confidence and give you a strong sense of achievement as well as broadening your outlook and providing a means of making new friends who share your interests. However, do not attempt them on your own — always seek some expert advice and tuition.

many users report they do get rather bored using them. It is thus better and more interesting to jog around your neighbourhood, buy yourself a real bike and pedal to the nearest countryside or even hire a boat and row it down the local river. It makes more sense to increase permanently the energy used in all one's everyday activities than to get exercise only from set sessions with costly 'gadgets'.

Beware of being a perfectionist in your campaign to boost calorie output. A resolution to do a daily three-mile jog is just as doomed to disaster as a promise to eat nothing all day to compensate for the sins of yesterday. Embark gradually on your exercise programme — give yourself a plus mark every time you climb upstairs briskly when you would normally avoid it. Establish habits that, by their very nature, become effortless. Remember also that exercise can help to make you happy and improve your physical and mental well-being — another thing to motivate your campaign to become more physically active. Psychiatrists have discovered that some reasonably energetic exercise is often more effective than drugs in the treatment of depression. Try taking a very brisk walk and experience for yourself the lifting effect that it has on your spirits

Another theory holds that the higher your level of exercise the hungrier you will feel and therefore you will be tempted to eat more. It is true that if you do increase your eating you may cancel out the weight control or reduction benefits of exercise. However, research suggests that people who take regular exercise tend to find it easier to reduce their food intake on a slimming diet than do inactive people. Sitting around lethargically, feeling bored or watching television, are much greater stimulants to eating extra snacks than exercise sessions. Increasing your physical activity can play a crucial role in achieving your goal of a permanently slim figure. At the same time, it will help keep you looking young and feeling full of vitality as well as making you happy. Before you launch into your activity programme, take a look at the following guide to see exactly how many calories you will be burning up.

Horse-riding is an enjoyable and increasingly popular sport, whether you prefer a quiet hack or a more exhausting session over the jumps. Most riding stables cater for new beginners as well as advanced riders and provide instruction in the arts of horsemanship (below). Before you embark on any form of physical exercise, it is always a good idea to do a few simple warming-up exercises (opposite). These will loosen and stretch your muscles, relieving muscular tension and warming up your body in readiness for the coming exercise. In this way, you will achieve greater general suppleness and flexibility.

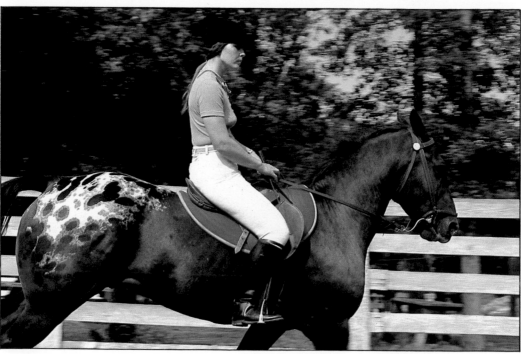

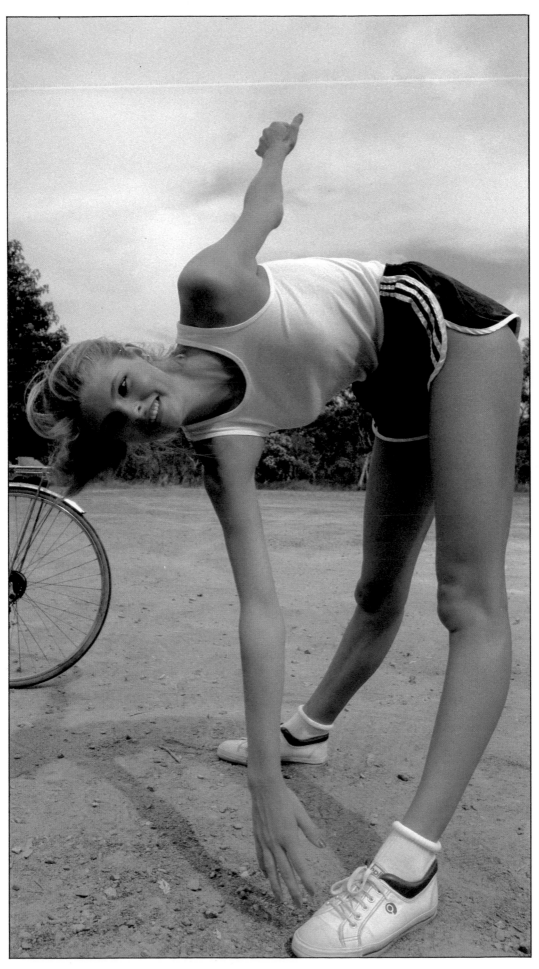

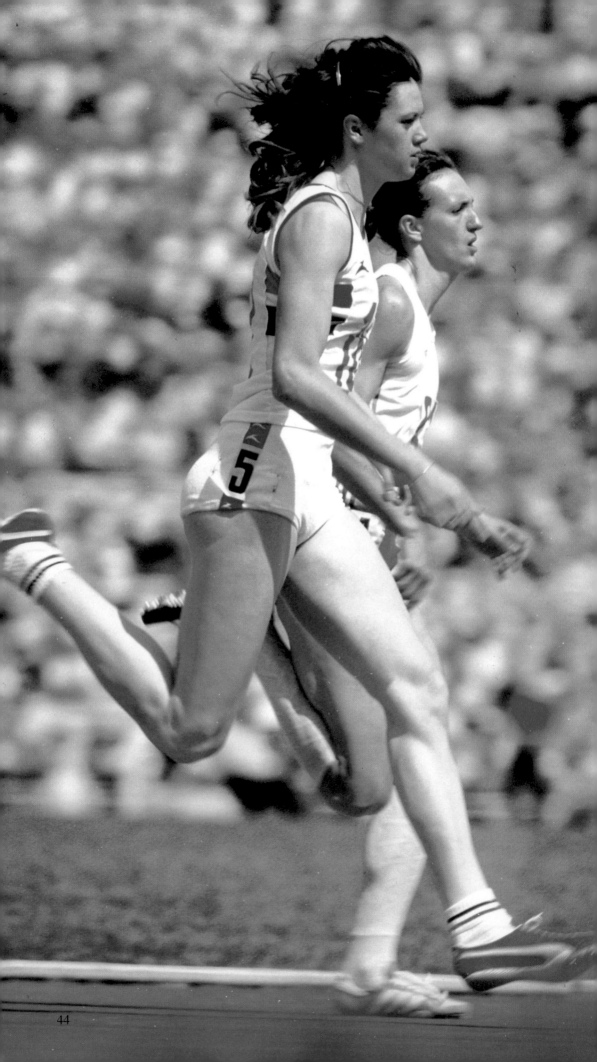

The A to Z of calorie expenditure

Even when you are sleeping or sitting down and doing nothing, your body is burning calories to keep your lungs breathing, your heart beating, your blood circulating and your body functioning generally. However, this is only the minimum number of calories you can burn. Once you start moving your body in any way, you burn more calories. The following chart shows how many calories you use up in different forms of activity.

The rate at which we burn calories while we are physically at rest is called the 'basal metabolic rate'. Scientific research has now shown that the average woman burns up calories at a rate of about one calorie per minute just on body maintenance, even when resting or lying in bed. Remember, though, that this figure is an average and many people have a slower metabolic rate, burning less than one calorie per minute. Of course, thin people are often the ones who tend to have a higher metabolic rate.

However, when it comes to the extra calories burned up in physical activity, overweight people have an advantage. In walking, or in any exercise that involves moving the whole body from place to place, they burn up more calories per minute than do slim people. The reason is very simple: the heavier a body, the more energy (in the form of calories) that is needed to move it.

The calorie figures in the chart are based on the average expenditure by a woman of average weight. An average man will use up a half calorie a minute more on light exercise to one calorie more on strenuous sports. You can expect to burn up a little more in the way of calories if you are carrying extra fat, but never over-estimate! Even average normal-weight people show differences in the way they tackle various tasks and exercises; some put far more energy into them than others do. It is fairly safe to say that, no matter what weight you are, if you go about your daily activities in an unhurried way your calorie expenditure will be about average as shown in these charts. If you do things slowly and rest rather a lot between activities, it may well be lower. Alternatively if you tackle everything very energetically, moving quickly about your daily tasks, it will be higher. The figures given for a wide range of activities in the accompanying chart are for calories burned up per minute.

Calories used per minute

Archery
A pleasant pastime, but it is mostly arms-only activity plus leisurely walking   **3**

Athletics
Can be extremely strenuous for short periods of time. During training count   **7**

Badminton
Playing with average effort, you would run about a lot   **5**

Basketball
Lots of very fast running, jumping and stretching   **7**

Bedmaking
Real bends and stretches with sheets and blankets   **3**

Bends and stretches
On-the-spot exercises such as touching your toes, knee-bends, and so on   **3**

Billiards
A game that is mostly arm movement. Alas, concentration does not burn calories   **2**

Bowls
A leisurely sport with little speed, but some bending   **3**

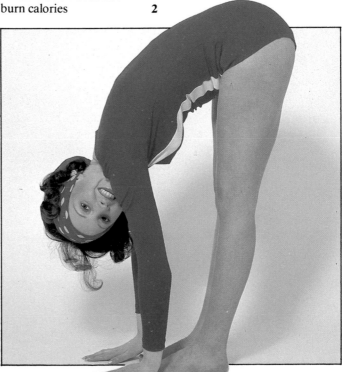

Canoeing
Paddling down the river at
3km (2 miles) an hour   3
Racing along at about 6km
(4 miles) an hour   6

Card games
Sitting and puzzling uses
few calories and you only
add the occasional flick
of the wrists   *under* 2

Circuit training
Climbing gymnasium bars,
jumping over the vaulting-
horse and other equipment,
all very strenuous
exercise   10

Cleaning
Cupboards and drawers,
mostly arm movement   *under* 2
Floors, with mop or broom
and some walking   3
Windows, if lots of bending
and stretching is involved   3

Climbing
Rock climbing and hill walking
are very strenuous and
enthusiasts keep going for
many hours. Walking up
sloping terrain   6
Tackling arduous rock
faces   *up to* 12

Cooking
Does not involve much
strenuous physical effort
and consists mostly of arm
movements   2

Cricket
If you are fielding   *under* 2
If you are batting or
bowling, the calorie output
should rise   4

Croquet
Another leisurely game that
does not demand strenuous
activity   3

Cross-country running
Marathon events can last for
three or four hours so lots of
calories are consumed   7

Cycling
At a pleasant easy pace
along the straight   5
Strenuously, enthusiastic
style   10

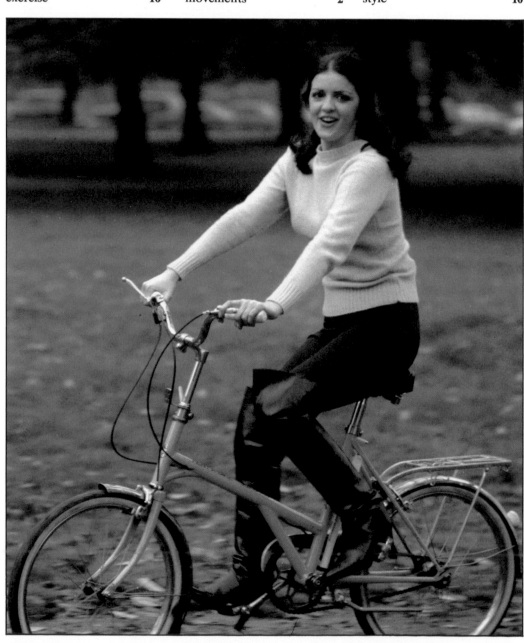

D

Dancing
Traditional ballroom, fairly
stately in style **5**
Strenuous dancing: Scottish,
country, square and disco **7**

Darts
You probably burn up more
calories walking to and from
your throwing position
on the mat than actually
throwing the darts *under* **2**

Driving a car
Through normal traffic **2**

Dusting
Just flicking the duster over
surfaces, even though you are
moving the ornaments, is
mostly arm movement. So
not a big calorie-burner **2**

F

Fishing
Sitting on the river
bank *under* **2**
Scrambling in and out of
boats and rowing to
fishing spot **3**

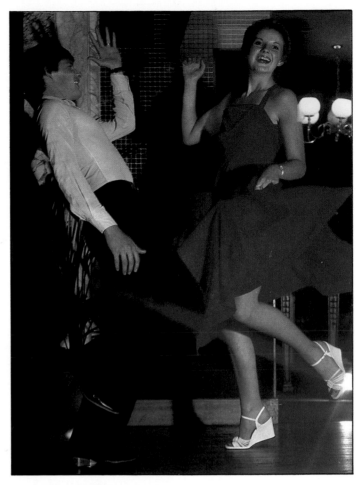

G

Gardening
Heavy work, like digging **5**
Lighter work, like weeding **4**

Golf
Some walking and effort
required, so expect to chalk
up an average calorie
expenditure of **4**

Gymnastics
The kind that demands that
you bend, stretch, jump and
so on with your whole body **5**

H

Hockey
If you stand about a lot, do
not count this as a calorie-
burner of much value. If you
play a reasonably vigorous
game, expect an average **5**

Home decorating
Lots of arm movement and
clambering up ladders **3**

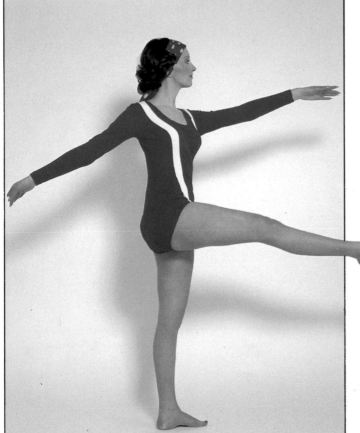

Horse riding
If you just sit on the horse while it ambles along à la pony-trekking, the horse, and not you, is getting the exercise, but if you trot, canter, gallop, you are doing well in the calorie-burning stakes **5**

I

Ice-skating
At an average pace which can be kept up for quite a while **5**

Ironing
Alas, one of those tiring jobs that does not use up many calories because the movement is mostly in the arms *under* **2**

J

Jogging
At a comfortably steady pace that can be maintained for quite a long time **6**

Judo
When you actually come to grips with your opponent a very strenuous sport **7**

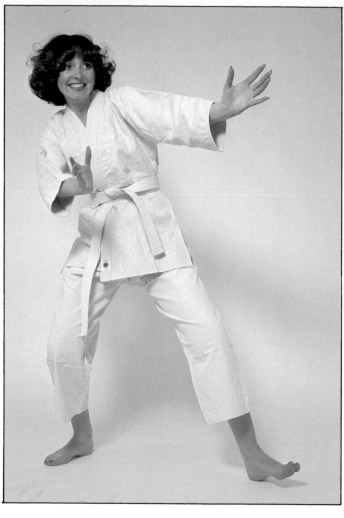

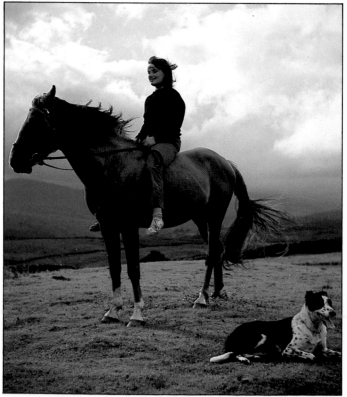

K

Knitting
Requires almost no energy however fast your needles click *under* **2**

M

Mountaineering
Not an activity anyone could tackle without being very fit. Very hard exercise for long periods *up to* **12**

Music
Playing an instrument (except drums) or conducting an orchestra **2-3**
Playing the drums **4**

N

Netball
Calorie expenditure varies a lot depending on how much you

put into it. However, a
reasonably fast game can
burn up calories speedily **6**

Polishing
Furniture polishing can
be a vigorous activity **3**
Silver polishing, etc.,
calorie output goes down **2**

Preparing vegetables
Washing, peeling, cutting
and chopping may be tiring,
but it is another standing-
still job, so not many
calories get used *under* **2**

Roller-skating
At any normal pace **3**

Rowing
Rowing lazily round a lake **4**
Competing in a race *up to* **10**

Running
Sprint-for-a-bus-style, fast
and furious **7**
Jogging — at a steady pace
that can be kept up for
quite a long time **6**
Upstairs: much higher
expenditure here because
you are moving your body
against gravity **11**

Sailing
Will vary very much with size
of boat and how much manual
work needs to be done.
Sitting holding the sail **2**
More strenuous sailing
tasks **6**

Scrubbing floors
With a will **4**

Sewing
The kind you do while you are
sitting — mending and
embroidery, for instance —
demands almost no
energy **1**
Dressmaking — cutting out
patterns and so on — does not
burn up many
calories *under* **2**

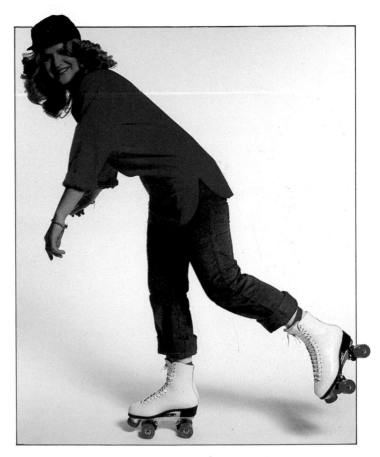

Shopping
With light load, 5kg (10lb) or
under **3**
With heavy load, over
5kg (10lb) **4+**

Sitting
Whether watching television,
pounding a typewriter or
just resting **1**

Skiing
Depends on your pace **5+**

Skipping
One of the best calorie-
burners of all **10**

Squash racquets
A very strenuous sport if
played hard **10**

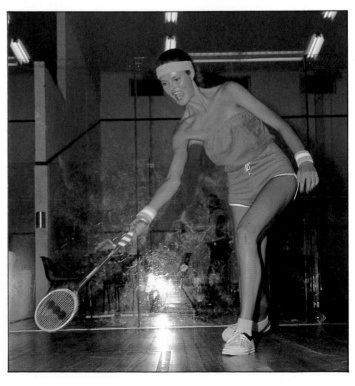

Sunbathing
You burn up no more calories
than when you are lying
in bed   **1**

Swimming
Often considered the ideal
form of exercise since
it uses all the muscles.
Gentle swimming,
easy strokes   *up to* **5**
More strenuous swimming,
the competitive kind   *up to* **10**

T

Table tennis
If you play an average game,
not too fast   **3**
If you are a demon player   **4+**

Tennis
An average game with
reasonable running
about   **4**
A hard game with a lot
of running and
retrieving   **6**

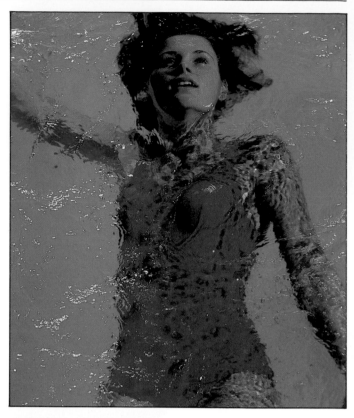

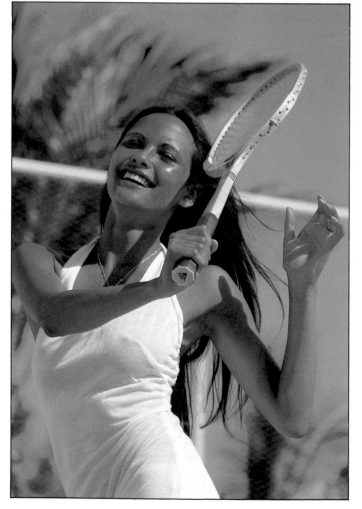

V

Vacuum cleaning
The cleaner does more work
than you do. If you move
furniture out of the way,
you will burn off more   **3**
If you do not move
furniture, you could
be using   *under* **2**

Volley ball
Moving about the court at
average speed   **4**

W

Walking
Calorie expenditure depends
on how slowly or briskly you
walk. It can be one of the
most valuable everyday
activities of all.
Strolling: ambling slowly
at an easy pace   **2-3**
Comfortable pace,
unhurried walking   **4+**
Purposeful pace: walking
quickly but comfortably   **4-5**
Walking uphill slowly   **5+**
Walking upstairs and
down again without
taking a rest   **6**
Brisk walking: quick and

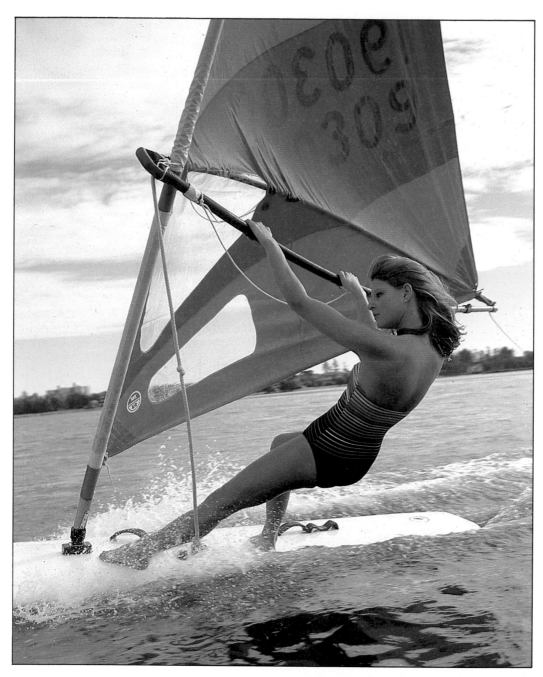

steady but enough to make
you want to stop for a
breather sometimes   **6+**

Washing
Dishes   *under* **2**
Clothes by hand. The
heavier they are, the more
calories you burn   **3**

Windsurfing
The more you fall off,
the higher your calorie
expenditure   *up to* **6**

Yoga
With average bending and
stretching   **3**

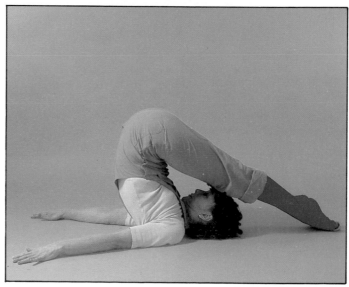

How a hard day's work can keep you fat

Many women complain that although they do not eat more than their slimmer friends, they still find it difficult to lose weight and actually gain weight. If you have experienced resentful thoughts like this it may come as a surprise to know that, as a result of modern aids, a great many of the everyday jobs we tackle around the home or at work do not rate nearly as highly in terms of calorie expenditure as we would like them to do.

In fact, any job that requires us to sit, stand or walk slowly (for example, pushing a vacuum cleaner or a supermarket trolley) uses up under two calories a minute, and one of those calories is being used by the body anyway to keep the heart beating, the blood circulating and so on! So, while you may feel worn out at the end of a busy day, your total calorie expenditure may still not be as high as the number of calories you have eaten.

In order to demonstrate this we have totalled up the calorie expenditure for two women: a housewife and an office-worker. Follow them through an average day and then cheer up, for we have devised some neat ways in which they, and you, can burn up extra calories without vowing to exercise, or making any other great changes in your way of life.

Jane is a secretary in her early twenties, who works for a big firm of accountants. She shares a flat with two other girls.

8.00am Jane wakes after 8 hours sleep during which she has burned up
480 calories

She spends 30 minutes having a shower, dressing and getting ready for work. During most of this time she is standing or sitting still rather than moving around. Her calorie expenditure averages 2 per minute.
60 calories

8.30am Jane makes toast and coffee, and chats with her flat mates while she munches. This takes 15 minutes, partly standing, mostly sitting.
20 calories

8.45am It is time for Jane to leave for work. She takes the short-cut to the station (5 minutes' walking), waits 5 minutes for the train, and her travelling time is 20 minutes. She window-shops as she strolls from the station to her office, taking nearly 15 minutes.
70 calories

9.30am From now until 1.00pm, Jane is on the telephone, taking dictation and typing. Elevenses come round on a trolley; so Jane does not leave her desk very much — only to visit other people in the office. It is a hectic morning, but not in terms of calorie expenditure. We estimate a total walking-about time of 15 minutes at 3 calories a minute; and as typing uses little more than 1 calorie a minute, we have given Jane an extra 20 calories to add to the basic 1 calorie a minute for what amounts to 195 minutes of sitting down.

260 calories

1.00pm Jane spends her lunch hour shopping for new clothes and buys a sandwich to eat at her desk. She averages 30 minutes at 3 calories a minute and the remaining half an hour at 1-2 calories. **130 calories**

2.00pm From now to 5.30pm, Jane is desk-bound again. Her work is similar to that of the morning, amounting to
260 calories

5.30pm Time to go home; Jane walks to the station fairly quickly (4 calories a minute), sits on the train for 20 minutes and takes the short-cut back to the flat again.
60 calories

6.30pm At home, Jane chats to her friends while they prepare supper. Setting the table, cooking and general preparation takes an hour. About 15 minutes walking at 3 calories a minute and 45 minutes standing at under 2 per minute.
120 calories

7.30pm There is just time for Jane to wash, change, arrange her hair and make-up before the guests arrive. A little moving about and some standing and sitting. Average expenditure: 2 calories a minute.
60 calories

8.00pm For the next 3 hours, Jane is eating, drinking and sitting. **180 calories**

11.00pm The guests leave. Jane helps with the dishes and general clearing up, burning up an average 2 calories a minute. **60 calories**

11.30pm Jane feels exhausted. She washes her face and undresses in 10 minutes, at an average 2 calories a minute. **20 calories**

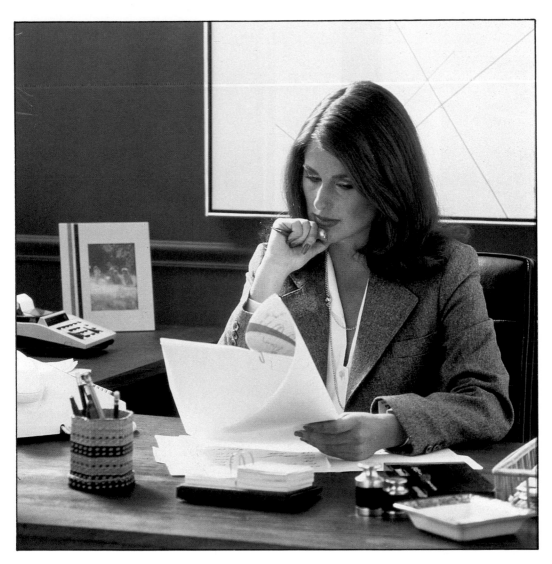

11.40pm Jane goes to bed, and reads before switching out the light. Her resting rate is 1 calorie a minute.

20 calories

12.00pm Jane falls asleep
Total expenditure: **1,800 calories**

How Jane can burn up more calories

Jane puts in a hard day's work at the office. As she has a sedentary job, it is hard for her to make any dramatic changes at work.

Here is an estimate of all the extra calories that Jane could burn up:

1 Two 20-minute walks, morning and evening, between the station and her flat equal 40 minutes at from 4 to 5 calories a minute. She will use 5 calories a minute when she is walking fast enough to have to take a breather from time to time; and 4 calories a minute when she walks at a comfortable rate of 3½ to 4 miles an hour. A healthy girl like Jane can walk at the faster pace for at least half of each 20 minutes. This way she will burn up an additional 140 calories. If she walks from the station to her office and back equally briskly, she gains another 20 minutes high-

calorie expenditure, making 50 calories extra.
2 Lunchtime walking — 20 minutes' really brisk walking-cum-jogging at an average 5 calories a minute: 90 calories extra.
3 During her day, we estimate that Jane is moving about on her feet at home and in the office for a total of 90 minutes. The average of 3 calories a minute can be increased by one calorie a minute if she moves briskly, so she burns 90 extra calories.
Total extra calories: 370

Molly is a housewife with two school-age children. Her metabolism is average, which means that her body burns one calorie a minute to function.

7.30am Molly wakes up after 8 hours' sleep at 1 calorie a minute. **480 calories** The next 45 minutes are spent dressing, washing and preparing breakfast. Walking from room to room she burns 3 calories a minute, but most of the time is spent at the wash basin or kitchen sink, and standing-still jobs are not 'hard work' (under 2 calories a minute).
90 calories

8.15am Molly sits down with the family to eat breakfast. She burns up 1 calorie a minute. **15 calories**

8.30am Having waved the family goodbye, Molly spends an hour washing dishes and tidying, Mostly standing still. Calorie expenditure **105 calories**

9.30am Bedmaking time; the family does not have continental quilts so she has to bend and stretch a great deal and burns up 2-3 calories a minute. **40 calories**

9.45am Molly spends 45 minutes cleaning the children's rooms. Although she moves around, she spends a lot of time standing while sorting out washing etc., So her average calorie expenditure works out at 2 calories per minutes. **90 calories**

10.30am Time for a quiet coffee; 15 minutes at 1 calorie a minute **15 calories**

10.45am Molly loads the washing-machine. This takes five minutes bending and lifting at 3 calories a minute **15 calories**

10.50am She spends the next 45 minutes vacuum-cleaning the carpets. She lifts light chairs out of the way but cleans around the others. As she takes the job slowly, she is spending under 2 calories a minute and burns up **75 calories**

11.35am Molly unloads the washing-machine. This takes 25 minutes because a friend rings up and the telephone chat lasts over 10 minutes. Molly feels harassed and short of time, but her total expenditure is only **35 calories**

12 noon Molly irons for 1¼ hours. Hard work, but it only takes about 1½ calories per minute. **110 calories**

1.15pm Molly has a snack lunch, then listens to the radio while she does some mending. She gives herself a whole hour to 'relax', but, as she is sitting down, she is using only 1 calorie a minute. **60 calories**

2.15pm Time for shopping before the children get back from school. Although Molly has only a few articles to buy and the supermarket is only four bus stops away, she takes the bus to the shops. She spends only 30 minutes actually walking. **60 calories**

Another 50 minutes are spent standing around (choosing foods, queueing at the check-out, chatting to a neighbour) at fractionally over 1 calorie a minute. **65 calories**

A further 10 minutes pass on the bus, standing and waiting for the bus and sitting down on it. **10 calories**

3.45pm Back home again, Molly unpacks the shopping and puts the ironing away. This takes 15 minutes. **35 calories**

4.00pm The children arrive home. Molly makes them a sandwich and joins them in a cup of tea. For the next 2 hours she can relax, chat, watch television and knit. **130 calories**

6.00pm Molly spends the next hour preparing supper, mostly standing up but interspersed with sitting down in 5 minute snatches while it is cooking. Total expenditure averages 2 calories a minute for 30 minutes, while working, and one calorie a minute for 30 minutes while sitting down. **90 calories**

7.00pm Molly eats supper and sits down afterwards, all at 1 calorie a minute. **60 calories**

8.00pm The children clear the table while Molly and her husband do the washing-up together. She cleans the stove and mops the kitchen floor — 30 minutes at an average 2 calories a minute. **60 calories**

8.30pm Molly and her husband watch television till 11.00pm — 2½ hours at 1 calorie a minute. **150 calories**

11.00pm Molly soaks in a hot bath and cleans her teeth — 1 to 2 calories a minute. **45 calories**

11.30pm Molly goes to bed.

Total expenditure **1,835 calories**

How Molly can burn up more calories

Molly hardly had an idle moment so how can she boost her energy expenditure without getting exhausted? Here are some ways that will increase calorie output *and* help her feel less tired! One of the benefits of putting more physical effort into each day's activities is that it makes you feel more cheerful and less susceptible to fatigue. Molly could increase her calorie output by taking the following advice.

1 In her hard day's work, Molly went upstairs only four times. But even by just walking upstairs, she is expending about 3 calories a minute. If you walk upstairs carrying a light load, like Molly's vacuum cleaner or a pile of

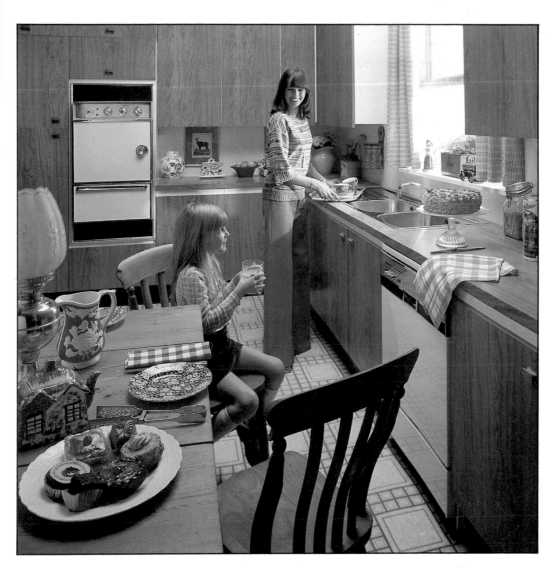

ironing, you are burning around 4 calories a minute because there is more weight to move against gravity. However, if you run upstairs, even empty-handed, then your calorie expenditure increases to 6 or more a minute. We suggest that Molly makes excuses for running upstairs as often as possible. She could make five or six fast journeys carrying a little ironing instead of one slow, ponderous ascent. All this means more work — even exhaustion you might think! Research shows that it is static standing and sitting work that causes aching backs and fatigue, not active movement. Of course, some chores use up more calories than others: for example, scrubbing floors vigorously amounts to 4 calories a minute whereas vacuum-cleaning into every corner and moving furniture is only 3 calories a minute.

2 Another simple way for Molly to increase her calorie expenditure is to do everything that requires movement with more speed and vigour. If she makes a habit of walking faster from room to room, unpacks the shopping and puts things away with vigorous bend-stretch movements, then her overall calorie expenditure will rise significantly.

3 By making shopping an opportunity for an invigorating walk (fast, easy-pace walking burns up in excess of 4 calories a minute; a brisk pace burns up 6 or more calories a minute) Molly could boost her energy output. She could vary her pace from easy to brisk, and get home feeling pleasantly refreshed instead of worn out.

Here is an estimate of the extra calories that Molly could burn up: running upstairs 12 times during the day (6 calories a minute) totals 60 calories. We estimate that Molly spends about 95 minutes of her day walking round the house from room to room. If she ambles, she burns only 3 calories a minute, but if she moves fast, she can burn up another calorie a minute making 95 calories. If Molly uses her shopping trip to walk as fast as she can, she will burn up an average 4 to 5 calories a minute. We estimate 15 minutes' fast walking (4 calories a minute) and 15 minutes' comfortable walking (3 calories a minute) totalling 105 calories. Half an hour's high-calorie-burning tasks at 4 calories a minute gives at least one extra calorie per minute: 30 calories.

Total extra calories: 290

Skip away the weight

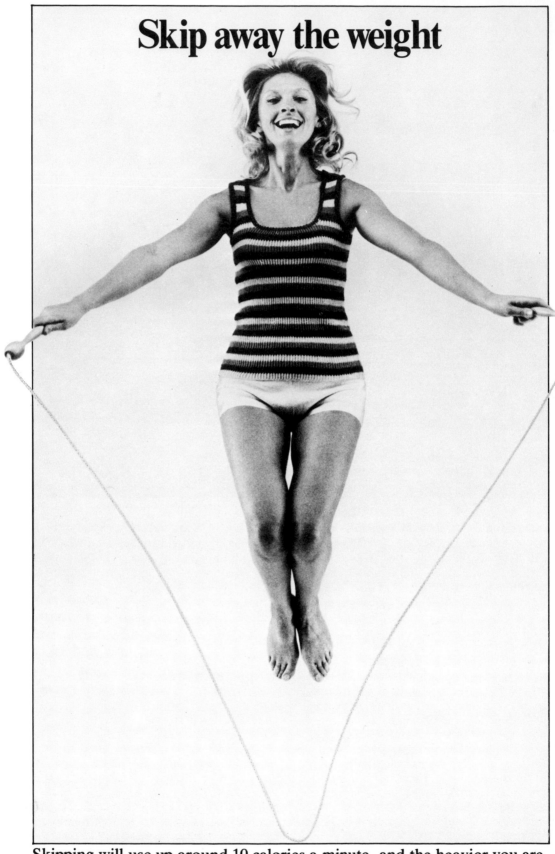

Skipping will use up around 10 calories a minute, and the heavier you are the more calories you burn. It is best to start slowly and just do about 50 skips forwards on your first day (do 25 if that is all you can manage), then add 50 skips a day until you feel able to try some of these skipping exercises.

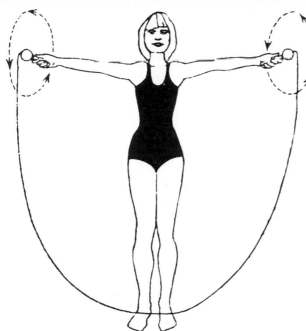

Simple backwards skip ▲

Get your skipping rope, circle handles round backwards, jump up and down with your feet together and skip. Have a long enough skipping rope so that you do not have to drop your arms to jump over it. The higher you keep your arms all the time, the better for muscle firming. It is highly unlikely that you will be able to carry on for half an hour non-stop. Our testers could not achieve this and had to take frequent short breaks. To begin with, you will probably need to break your daily half-hour stint into about three 10 minute sessions. In fact, this is advisable to help you do the exercises briskly without flagging at the end. The reason for circling the rope backwards is that, done this way, skipping is particularly effective for firming the muscles at the back of the arms, and also in giving a lift to the bosom by strengthening the muscles supporting it.

Waist-slimming skip

As well as burning up calories at the top rate, this skipping variation is designed particularly to pull in and firm slack muscles around the waist and in the 'spare-tyre' waist-to-bosom area. It is also very effective for the upper-arm flab problem. Start with six simple backward skips. Then swing both arms to the left, outstretched at shoulder level, twisting your body towards them from the waist. Now swirl the skipping rope round in the air in backwards circles as you jump up and down (just as if you were skipping) five times. Now six simple skips again, and then, arms outstretched to the right, repeat the skipping rope swirl in that direction. Make sure that you twist from the waist and that your hips are facing forwards when you do the sideways movement.
▼

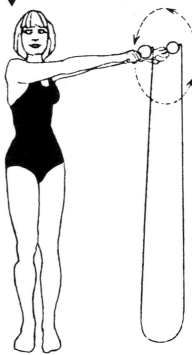

◄ Cross-over skip

If you do the simple backwards skip but cross your arms over your chest and cross the ropes on alternate jumps you make the exercise slightly more energetic — and even more beneficial for calorie-burn-up. (If you have not skipped for years you might find this difficult at first.) Unlike the other exercises, this exercise works another group of muscles supporting the bosom and across the shoulders. Therefore a good idea would be to alternate it with sessions of simple backwards skips.

The top calorie burners

How tired an activity makes you feel is often not a real indication, alas, of its effectiveness as an aid to weight control. Thus you can feel exhausted after tackling such everyday household tasks as a big pile of ironing or by typing for a long time, but, because only limited arm movement is involved, the calorie output may well disappoint you. Apart from tasks around the house like polishing silver, window cleaning or scrubbing floors, where small movements are performed vigorously, it is the amount of walking around and general body movement that really determine how many calories you burn up at home. Cooking, for instance, tends to burn up more calories than preparing vegetables because it normally involves more movement around the kitchen. Vacuum-cleaning, surprisingly, tends to burn up more calories than sweeping with a brush because of walking to and fro with the vacuum cleaner. The woman who lives in a small, well-designed home and has all the electrical equipment and gadgets she needs consequently does little physical work, and, unless she exercises regularly or has a demanding job, burns up few calories.

Likewise, a hard day of mental work does not burn up extra calories as the brain uses up only about one-fifth of a calorie a minute. However, as with some computers that use only fractionally more electric current when calculating than when idling, the busy brain uses little more energy than the idle brain. Medical experts tell us that the feeling of fatigue is partly a psychological and partly a nervous phenomenon. The brain cells get fatigued, causing a general feeling of tiredness. If we were called upon to sprint a mile, however, or to undertake any other physical task after a day's mental slog, we would perform just as efficiently as if we had spent the whole day watching television. Switching from mental to physical work often helps to stop the tired brain working and proves refreshing.

However, the form of exercise you plan to do is important. The yoga-type stretching exercises or arm-swings and toe-touches will do wonders for your muscle tone but will not necessarily burn up many calories. To increase calorie expenditure you have to move your body from point A to point B at speed. Fast walking, for example, uses up more calories than slow walking, and jogging or running will burn up almost twice as many calories as most speeds of walking.

To reach the ultimate speeds of calorie expenditure, you need to move your whole body quickly and then add another factor

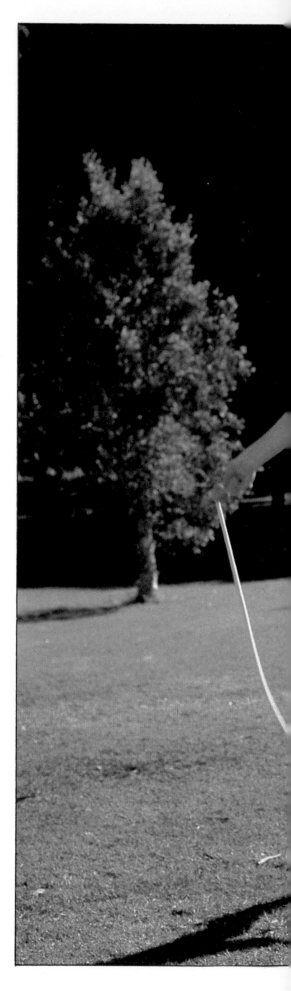

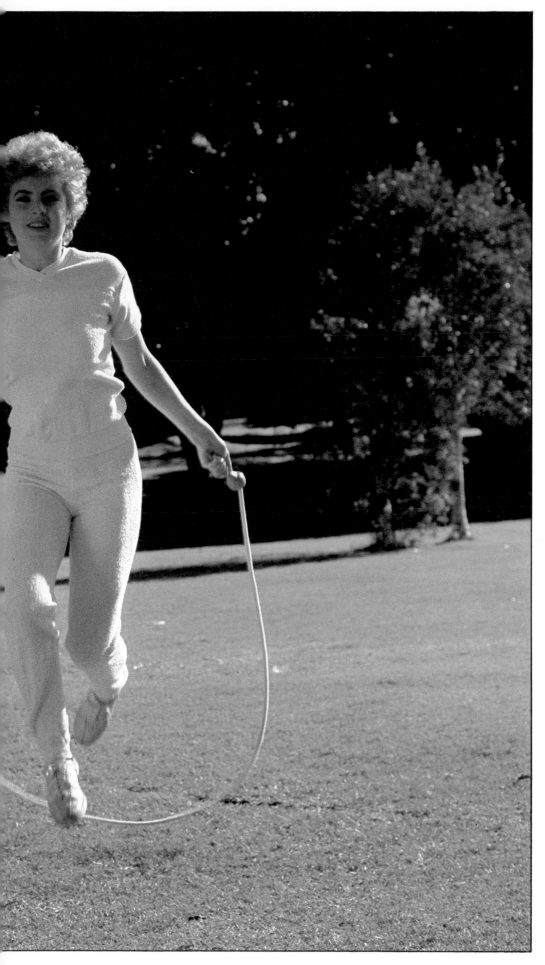

— move upwards against the pull of gravity. Hence the most slimming exercise in the world would be 'running up Mount Everest' but, lacking a handy mountain, slimmers can substitute the homely staircase. Running up and down a flight of stairs, repeatedly and briskly, is one of the best calorie-burning excercises there is. Try it for just three or four minutes and you will see exactly how taxing it can be. That is why anyone who might be a likely candidate for heart-disease (which includes anyone heavily overweight and older people) should not attempt it. By walking upstairs and downstairs repeatedly you burn up about 6 calories a minute. Run up and down and you can increase that calorie expenditure to about 11 calories a minute. The heavier you are, the more calories you are likely to burn up because you are lifting more weight. If you only have a little weight to lose, you could add to your calorie expenditure by carrying a pack on your back. We suggest as a plan of action that you start off by running up and down a flight of stairs (about 15 steps) once, then gradually build it up day by day until you reach the maximum you can do without your knees collapsing! After that, break up your indoor mountaineering into short sessions throughout the day.

The time you are likely to spend on any particular exercise has to be taken into consideration when deciding which is your best calorie burner. Check with the chart on this page to see how long you should spend exercising each day in order to lose 0.6kg (one extra pound) of surplus fat.

Ball games, such as tennis and squash, when they are played with a reasonable degree of effort, are excellent calorie burners, but if you choose them as your only form of exercise you need to ask yourself if you will be prepared to play for an hour or half an hour every day. Ten minutes' skipping each day will burn about the same number of calories as playing half an hour's squash every other day. Strenuous cycling and swimming are also high calorie burners and are worth incorporating into your exercise programme. Remember, though, to cycle up and down a few hills to get maximum burn-up, and not to spend half your swimming time just paddling around in the water.

Walking is so familiar and gentle an exercise that you may never have regarded it as a method of losing weight. Certainly, when compared with a vigorous activity like running it may appear to be of little importance, but its value should not be under-rated. You can keep going over a longer distance with greater effect than you might imagine. Also, walking is convenient as you need no special facilities, equipment or clothing.

When you walk, your body is having to use up enough calories to transfer your whole body weight from one position to another. Thus, when you walk uphill your body will burn up more calories. The faster you walk, the more calories you use, and if you walk on a rough surface, like a country track, you will use more calories than travelling on a smooth, flat footpath. If you walk either carrying a load or pushing a pram you will burn up even more calories than if you were unencumbered. As you will see from the activity chart, an hour's walk every day could burn up an extra 275 calories. If you have got out of the habit of going on long walks,

THE TOP CALORIE BURNERS

Chosen daily exercise	Minutes spent exercising	Calories burned	Days taken to lose 0.5kg (1lb)
Tennis (if played with a reasonable degree of effort which means 'keep moving')	60	300	11-12
Standard walking at a purposeful pace	60	275	12-13
Squash (played hard)	30	270	13
Cycling	60	240	14
Jogging	20	180	19
Skipping (energetically at a rate of 70 to 80 jumps a minute)	10*	140	25
Swimming (moving at a reasonably fast speed)	20	140	25
Running upstairs	10*	110	31
Floor-walking	15*	90	39

*Made up of several short sessions each day

start slowly and walk for just 10 minutes, building it up by five minutes every day until you achieve your goal. A dog, of course, can be an excellent slimming aid, particularly if it is the kind that pulls you along on the end of a leash. If your dog, however, spends most of its time dawdling around lamp-posts, it would be best to go it alone.

Exercise not only speeds up your metabolic rate while you are doing it, but it also continues to keep your metabolism working at a faster rate for some time afterwards. Of course, the longer and more vigorous each bout of exercise is, the greater the calorie-burning aftermath. As with a diet, the most successful calorie burner for you to do is the one that you can stick to and which fits easily into your lifestyle.

A simple but effective exercise that you can do sitting down watching television consists of pressing your hands together as hard as you can, for as long as you can. Then take a break for as long as you held your hands pressed together. Then press again... continue for up to an hour if you feel really strong. This exercise will increase your calorie burn-up from the normal sedentary one calorie per minute to two calories per minute.

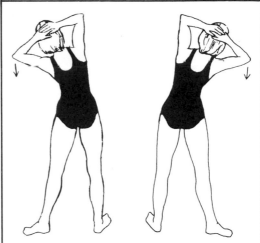

Pendulum walk

As well as burning up extra calories this exercise is a marvellous waist-whittler. It exercises those muscles at the side of the waist that can nip in the waist and make it smaller. Clasp your hands behind your head. Take three or four steps to the left, and with each step bend your body to the left from the waist. Step and bend, straighten up, step and bend, straighten — that's all there is to it. Now do it to the right, bending to the right. The bend must be sideways to give full waist-trimming benefit. Your shoulders should not twist around and must remain facing forwards. Imagine that you are moving sideways along a very narrow passage and have no room to twist your shoulders or elbows around. This exercise is also good for pulling in slack muscles which cause ugly bulges at the upper, outer side of the thighs. Do it briskly for full calorie burn-up.

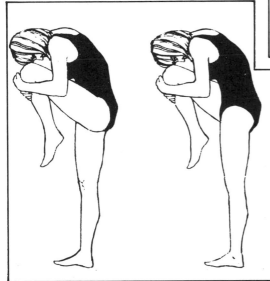

Knee to nose walk

This walking exercise is a good tummy flattener as well as a calorie burner; it is also quite hard to do incorrectly. You just walk around briskly, clasping your arms around your lower leg and bringing your nose to your knee or your knee to your nose with each step. Straighten up between each step. You might wobble a little at first until you get the hang of it. It is not advisable if you have had a slipped disc or spine troubles.

Floor-walking

Floor-walking is an exercise that you can try at home which entails your lifting and moving your whole body along the floor. Sit on the floor with legs straight in front of you. Move forwards briskly, walking on your bottom, swinging your arms backwards and forwards to help you move your body along. When you come close to a wall, go into reverse and floor-walk backwards, then go forwards again and so on for as long as you can.

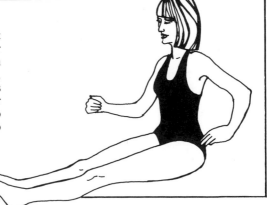

Jackie slims to become a special mum

Jackie Pedgrift, at 1.68m (5ft 6in), had always had a slight weight problem, but being a little overweight never bothered her significantly and she was a confident girl with lots of friends. The only time that she really took her weight seriously was immediately after she got married In two months her weight shot up from 63.5kg (10st) to 76 kg (12st). Frantically she dieted and lost about 9.5kg (1½st) but she resented the fact that although her husband, Roy, could eat whatever he wanted, she had to be very careful in her choice of food. When they decided to have a baby and found that Jackie could not conceive, her eating went out of control. Before long, she was a miserable 86kg (13½st) (see below), smiling only for the camera. Then some friends mentioned that they were adopting a baby and, with this new glimmer of hope, Jackie wrote to several adoption agencies. One agency asked them to go for an interview and Jackie learned that they would have to pass a medical. Suddenly she saw her size as an incredible threat, knowing that if she failed the medical because of her weight she would have lost her chance to adopt a child. She gritted her teeth and set to work. It took her six months to lose 25.5kg (4st) but she passed the medical with flying colours. When Roy took Jackie out to celebrate (right) he told her that it was lovely to live again with the attractive and happy girl he married.

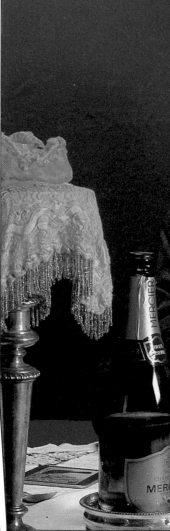

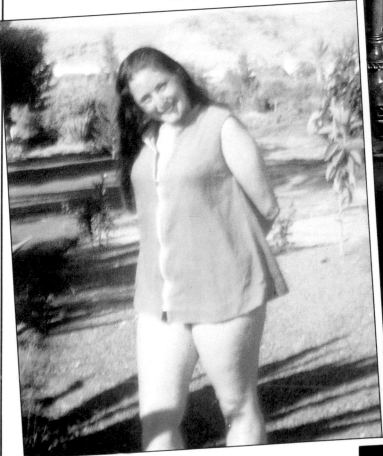

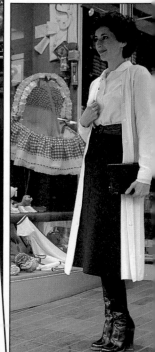

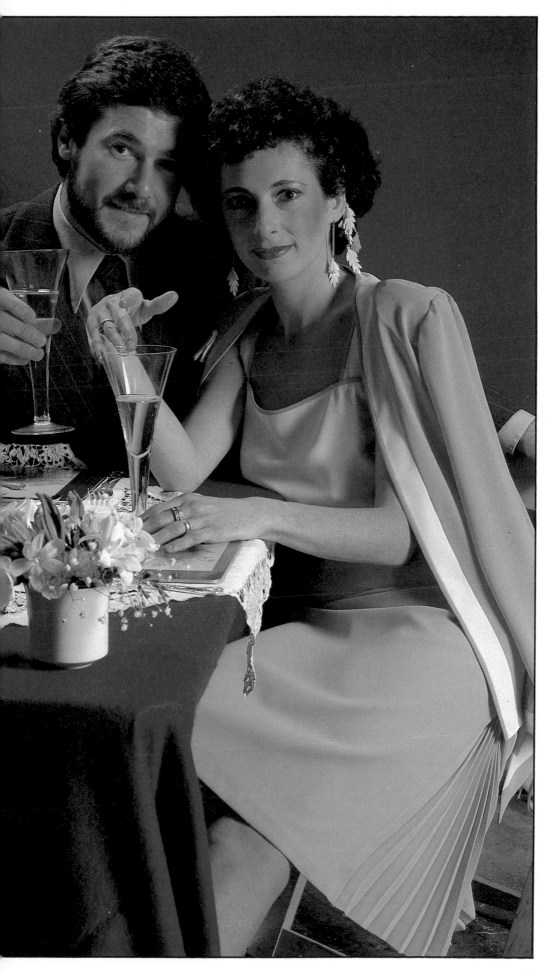

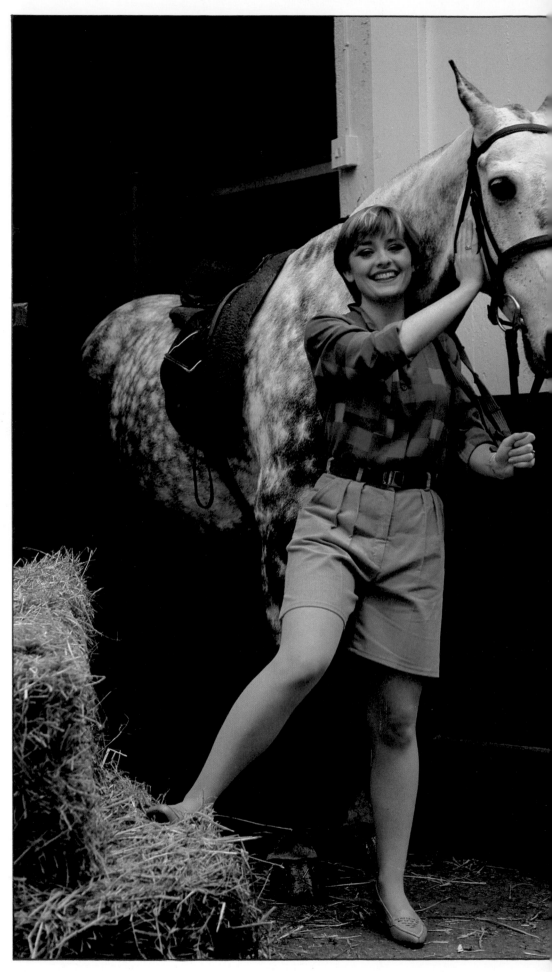

Now it's Jockey Julia

Julia Spicer had always yearned to ride and dreamed of sitting neat and elegant on the back of a beautiful grey mare, riding through lush green countryside. What kept her out of the saddle was feeling she would look so awful, bulging out of jodhpurs and jacket. At 1.60m (5ft 3in) and weighing 73kg (11½st), Julia tended to be short of courage, feeling the world was simply waiting to laugh and ridicule her at every turn. Julia's attempts at dieting consisted of starving herself for a week and consequently feeling lethargic and depressed. Then she would jog crazily for another week, hoping to run off all the surplus fat, and ached for weeks after that. Finally she had to admit she knew nothing about dieting and decided to join a slimming club where she was given a target weight of 54kg (8½st). She also set herself a very personal goal —learning to ride once she had lost her surplus weight. Dieting was not easy, and there were days when Julia longed for huge fry-ups or packets of biscuits. However, she remembered how temporary the comfort from bingeing was, and conjured up instead a picture of her slim self astride a beautiful grey mare. It took her about five months to lose just over 12.7kg (2st), and her attitude to food changed. She no longer looked to it for comfort but planned her meals carefully and enjoyed every mouthful. When she reached her target weight she immediately went along to sign on for a course of riding lessons at a local stable. Weighing in at professional jockey weight, Julia already felt like a winner.

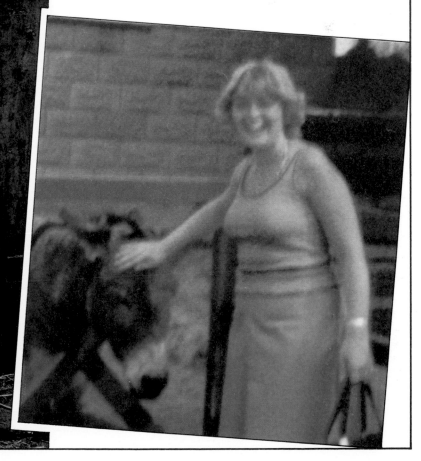

Virginia reaches for the stars

Virginia Chean had always longed to dance. When she was only four years old she begged her mother to let her have ballet lessons and saved up her pocket money to buy ballet shoes. Her mother, perhaps to spare her feelings for she was a fat child even then, would not let her join a class. The plump child turned into a well-rounded teenager and how Virginia envied the lithe girls who had gone to ballet school and who were now taking dancing examinations and winning medals. Their confidence showed in the way they moved and talked, even in the way they smiled. When she was 20, Virginia met Frank and they were married a few months later. But marriage did nothing for Virginia's figure (see below) and soon she was weighing in at 82.6kg (13st). Frank was a member of a pop group and Virginia hated the thought of accompanying him to clubs and halls where she would be on show. One day when she was in a dentist's waiting room she picked up a copy of *Slimming Magazine's* low-fat diet and decided to give it a try. In six months she was down to 66.7kg (10½st) and she then switched to calorie-counting to reach her 56.2kg (8st 12lb) target — Virginia is 1.68m (5ft 4in) tall. All the admiring comments she got gave Virginia the confidence to fulfill her ambition to take up ballet. She found a teacher who was willing to include a raw beginner of 29 years in her class and jumped in wholeheartedly. She could not have wished for a happier end to her slimming story when she was given permission to practise for a ballet examination in the famous Sadler's Wells Theatre in London, where these pictures were taken.

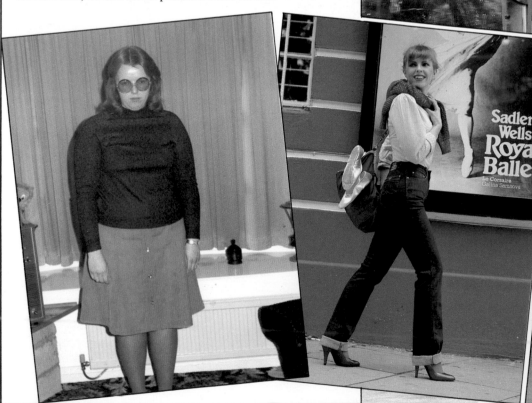

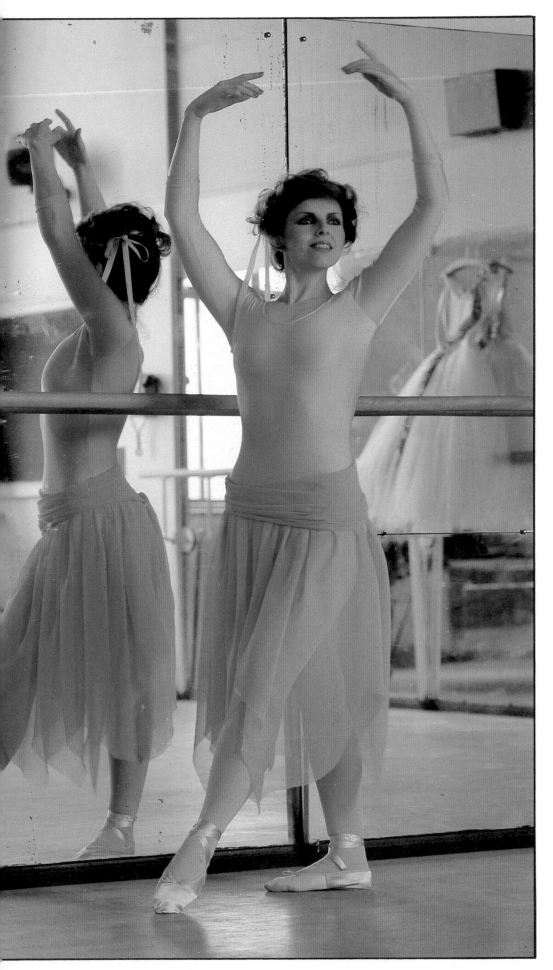

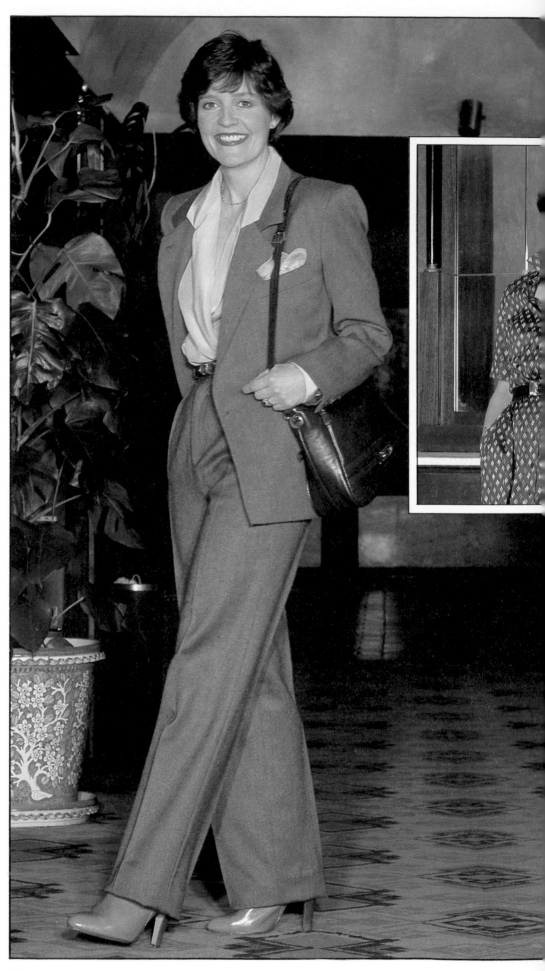

Goodbye to frumpy old Granny Rogers!

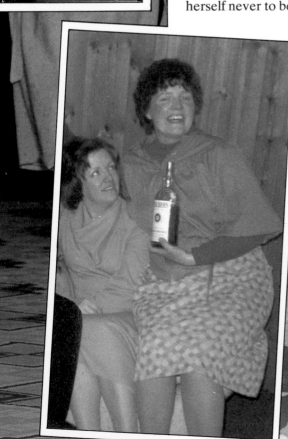

Jessie Rogers had always adored clothes, but when she was 79.5kg (12½st) she used to spend all her time admiring them on other women. While slim friends bought pretty clothes that turned heads and gave them confidence, Jessie had to wear frumpy, shapeless skirts and thick, box-like sweaters (see below). In fact, a new neighbour who moved into the same road as Jessie guessed her to be a grandmother of 47 — she was actually 27 years old! Jessie's weight problems had started with the birth of her first son and had increased with the birth of her second son. Tactless remarks about her size just drove her into the kitchen for comforting sandwiches and cakes. The crunch came when Jessie was asked to present a family gift at an aunt's silver wedding celebration, and after a fruitless search of the shops for a flattering dress to disguise her weight, she ended up in a baggy top and an old skirt that had belonged to her mother. She determined then and there to get slim and a friend suggested that they go along together to a local slimming club. When, after about five months, 1.63m (5ft4in) Jessie was down to 52.5kg (8st4lb), she went on a happy spending spree and bought all the clothes that she had wanted for years. The new Jessie (left) has more energy and enjoys many new leisure interests. She still keeps her old skirt, however, to remind her that once she filled that huge waistband and to warn herself never to become a fat grandmother again.

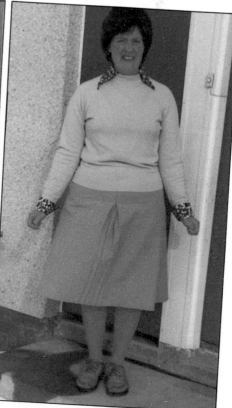

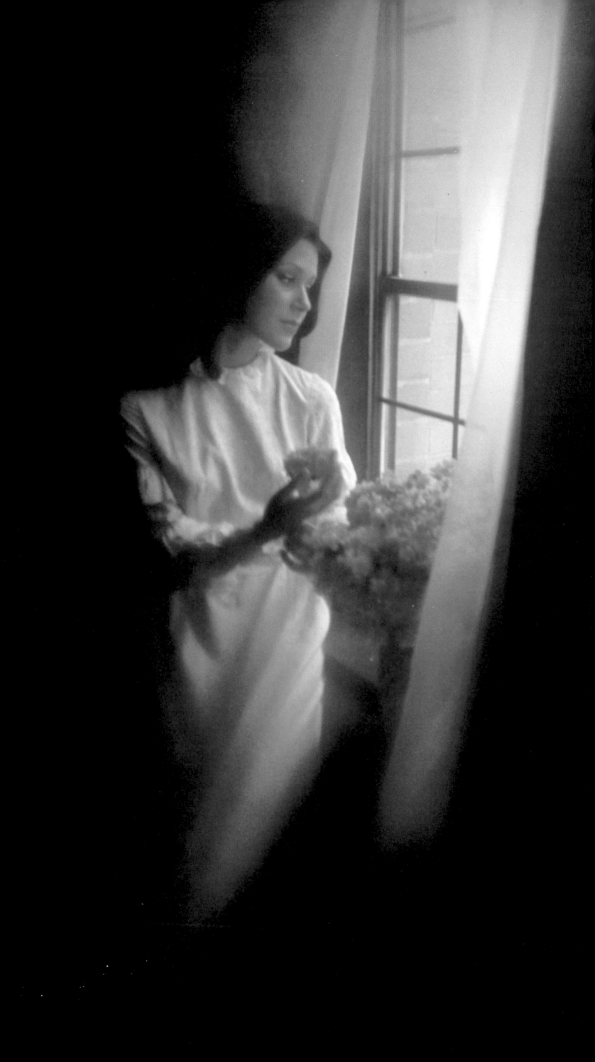

CHAPTER 5

Your mind

The success or failure of your slimming campaign depends on your mental attitude. In this chapter we discuss attitudes to dieting, to yourself, to others, to success, to failure, to sex appeal and attitudes to food itself.

Your attitude to dieting should be positive and you need to be strongly motivated to succeed. However, you need to know also how to cope with failure, for if you attempt to be perfect then you are bound to be disappointed. Slimming is not a character-building course, so make the switch from 'willpower' to 'self-control'. An example of willpower is drooling in front of the baker's shop window and resolving not to buy your favourite cake. Self-control consists of sending someone else to buy your bread while you shop in safer zones.

Lose your body hang-ups and start seeing yourself as a worthwhile person who can cope with changes in mood and in diet-breaking. A failed dieter should ask herself if she really does want to become slim or if, psychologically, she fears to change her shape and her life. The habit of eating in response to a blue mood is a difficult one to break, so be prepared to do something about it before it inevitably happens. If you have previously sabotaged your diet with sudden bouts of bingeing there are words of comfort in this section.

Your attitudes to others can also make slimming easier. Work at making friends, try to understand their reactions to your new slimmer figure and learn to be assertive in all of your relationships. Avoid putting yourself in situations where resentments about other people can build up; and, above all, learn to stop using other people as an excuse for diet-breaking.

It is hard to imagine that you could possibly have any reaction against slimming successfully, but this is not uncommon. Success means change and the loss of an excuse for delaying positive acts. Start rewarding yourself for small successes so that the road to your goal does not seem endless. The biggest potential setback to any diet is the day you break it and therefore it is essential to counteract your negative feelings of failure with some really positive thinking. Because of physiological as well as psychological changes in the few days preceding menstruation, this can be a particularly difficult time for many women, but you *can* cope with this and all the other ups and downs of dieting.

Your psychological attitude to food is, of course, vitally important during a slimming campaign. Therefore make it simple for yourself, concentrate first on resisting the calories you will not really miss, then tackle the harder task of cutting down on your favourite foods, which could damage your diet. Some foods are so dangerous that you will need to take special action against them. Remember that it is not only what you eat but also how you eat it that matters and determines the degree of success of your dieting, so learn some of the rules of eating behaviour.

Slimming is *not* easy and most of us can find dozens of reasons why it is impossible to diet during any single day. Most of these excuses must be analyzed and rejected if you are to succeed. However, a genuine few can be accepted — and should be from time to time. These excuses should be allowed, for guilt and regret are often the most destructive forces in dieting. The wrong attitudes to dieting arise from letting what you weigh govern what you say and what you do. They can stop you getting slim and staying slim, so make sure you lose them!

Attitudes to dieting

Before you begin a diet, stop and ask yourself if getting slim is one of the most important things in your life? Unless it has that major priority, the best thing you can do is just to decide not to start dieting, as a weight problem of more than modest proportions requires a major priority rating. Also there is no point in deciding to diet to please someone else — you have to do it for yourself or you will not succeed. Embarking on a slimming campaign designed to please someone close to you — a husband, in particular — is setting out on an impossible mission. Sooner or later, an apparent ingratitude, lack of understanding or lack of tact will disappoint or infuriate you into abandoning your diet, and not only your nearest and dearest can achieve this effect. When you are at your most vulnerable, any casual or uncaring remark from family or friends can bring the reaction: 'Why do I bother? After all, who really cares?' Protect yourself in advance by telling yourself now: 'I'm doing this for *me*'.

To slim successfully you will need some motivation; without it, you have no reason to exert the self-discipline that dieting inevitably involves. Self-disgust can be a major motivation for starting a diet, but if it is prolonged and excessive it may prove a serious drawback to sustained slimming. The woman who holds a low opinion of herself takes a one-sided view of her life and sees only those things that will foster her self-disgust. As one failed slimmer said: 'When I'm out shopping and see women with normal figures I get really despondent and think I shall never get to a decent weight, let alone a normal weight, and then I arrive home, put my shopping down and start to eat...' This women is so full of self-disgust that she never notices other overweight women but sees just those with 'normal' figures. This form of self-knocking is a sure road to diet-breaking.

You do need to be determined to diet, and you also need to make a lot of strong resolves. However, do not resolve *not* to cheat, even once — this is a very dangerous diet resolution because for the majority of slimmers it is a totally doomed resolution. Very few overweight people ever succeed in keeping to their diets without a single lapse for any lengthy period; this is a fact that the wise slimmer swallows right at the start. The word 'cheat' is the key to the danger. Eat one extra slice of toast and it is easy to feel that you have cheated, failed, flopped, broken your resolve and proved to yourself that you do not have the willpower that it takes to get slim. In fact, all you have done really is to eat maybe a couple of hundred extra calories, which will not put back weight or even cancel out much of the day's weight loss programme.

A common reaction is to feel so disgusted with yourself at breaking your resolve not to cheat that you carry on ploughing through, say, half a loaf of bread in a mood of defeat and utter disillusionment. It is much better, therefore, not to make any 'I'll-never-cheat' resolutions at all. Instead, decide you are going to try to diet and keep on battling on, however many slip-ups you might make on the way. Even if you had a bad day last week, you can stick to your diet this week.

When most people embark on a weight-loss programme they also make instinctively a firm resolve to embark on a character-building course. Armed with the motto 'I will be strong!', they resolve to look every food temptation straight in the plate and to resist, rejoice and feel wonderful. They do resist, they do rejoice but, because they are constantly putting their willpower to the toughest possible tests, they must eventually relapse, and then they feel terrible and give up their diet.

Try to take as much strain as possible off your willpower. Learn to separate the whole concept of character building from the idea of losing weight. There is no evidence at all to suggest that overweight people have weaker characters than do slim people. Therefore, make the switch from willpower to self-control. There is a great difference between practising self-control and trying to rely on willpower. Self-control can be learned, is realistically attainable and allows for the kind of compromises that put it within the reach of everyone. However, willpower has an all-or-nothing quality. When you try to rely on it you may either win or lose, and usually, sooner or later, you will lose.

Here is a classic situation that will have to be faced by almost every woman who is trying to shed some surplus weight. To everyone there are some tempting foods, maybe peanuts, chocolate, biscuits or cakes, that are particularly hard to resist. They are often foods that are eaten between meals, and in order to shed weight you must take positive steps to cut down these surplus calories. Using the willpower approach, you may resolve to cut out these bad foods completely. If you fail in this resolve you may well decide that you have ruined your diet and might as well continue eating in the circumstances. Thus you may end up eating several biscuits, cakes or bars of chocolate or whatever your particular downfall foods happen to be.

If you try the self-control method you will admit honestly to yourself that there are going to be times when you cannot resist a bar of chocolate or maybe a ginger biscuit. However, you will also promise yourself to make up for the damage when you succumb by cutting down on the calories for the remainder of the day. The dieter who is exercising self-control is bound to succumb to her favourite foods from time to time, but she can embark on eating them with a different mental attitude. First of all, she has never resolved not to eat these foods, only to eat less of them, so she can reach for them without a demoralizing feeling of failure and guilt. Other lines of defence are now open to her, her aim being to eat less of this food than she would normally have eaten.

If you are a person whose great temptation is cakes, then looking into the windows of your local bakery will involve a head-on confrontation with your willpower. The person who is practising self-control will take another route when out shopping so that she avoids the bakery altogether. The woman who has a favourite brand of biscuit and keeps a box of them on constant view in the kitchen is engineering the defeat of her willpower. The alternative and preferable self-control method would be to avoid buying the biscuits in the first place.

Willpower is going to a party, determined not to eat and stationing yourself in such a position that the luscious buffet is always in your sight. Self-control is planning well in advance that you will allow yourself to eat just a certain amount of the food available and then taking care to keep away from the food for the rest of the evening. Willpower is refusing the highly tempting dessert that you are offered, suffering agonies of self-deprivation as you watch others eat it and then, as a result of your ordeal, going home and eating twice as much food in secret. Self-control is accepting only a small portion of the dessert, eating it slowly and with maximum satisfaction and trying to leave at least one spoonful on the plate when you make yourself consciously realize that you have had enough to satisfy your urge for the flavour. Willpower never lasts for ever, but self-control, if learned and practised on a thoughtful step-by-step basis, can change habits gradually in a permanent way and will lead to permanent weight control.

Accept right at the start of your campaign that not every day is going to be a good day for dieting: your moods often change and problems, large and small, may arise. If you

Cycling is an effective way of getting into shape and burning up calories. Develop the habit of cycling, not driving, short distances.

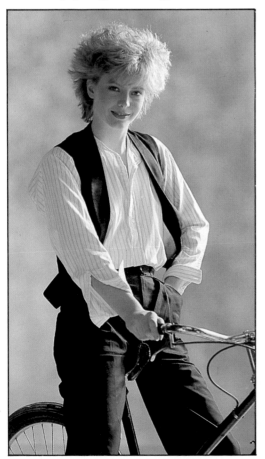

expect every day to be plain sailing you will founder at the first little ripple, let alone the storm that is bound to come along.

Attitudes to success
It is hard to imagine that you could possibly ever have any reaction against the idea of getting slim. However, this is a common experience, particularly among those women who have been very heavily overweight.

The fact is that, unpleasant as it may be in so many ways, there are actually some benefits in being overweight. It can be used as a convenient excuse for delaying positive acts that demand some effort. For instance, the bored overweight housewife who has been saying for years that she must get a job always adds: 'As soon as I lose this weight'. Now, as she sees the first positive signs that she is getting slim, she has to face the fact that she is also losing her reason for delaying taking a step which, understandably, she views with a certain amount of hesitation.

A woman who has been sufficiently overweight to have lost even her femininity to some extent may become suddenly aware that she now has to make the effort to be feminine. Often, as her size decreases, the first compliment she receives reawakens a long forgotten feeling — that of regarding herself as an attractive woman. Over the years she may have opted out of making the effort to be feminine, not specifically in the sexual sense but in her social role and in her appearance. Her relationships with other women have developed on a comfortable, non-competitive basis, and thus her change in weight is likely to transform the basis of these relationships. Most of us like to be noticed, and some surplus weight can attract attention, even though it may be of the least welcome kind. Very often, such fears are vague and not much thought about, but they can lead to sufficient conflict to make a slimming effort fizzle out.

There are many people who will say that they seem to have a weight-loss barrier and claim that they can never slim below a certain weight. That barrier will often be located at a weight at which they have ceased to be heavily overweight and are just approaching becoming slim. There can be many straight-forward dieting reasons, of course, for this barrier: for example, sometimes a stricter diet might be needed for continued weight loss at this late stage. However, the fear of getting slim can be a major factor in creating this barrier, and some people are not really aware of what it is that is preventing them from reaching their goal.

A fear of change is not an unusual human trait and it may be particularly strong among many overweight people. There is a general feeling that however bad the present may be, the future is still an unknown quantity and may be even worse. We know how most people respond to us, what to do when we go to work, in our social situations and with our families. Even though change might indicate a positive improvement in one's life, there is a basic unknown quality about it that makes many people fear to take the risk of making changes.

Any feeling of success tends to encourage further success whereas a feeling of failure encourages further failure. There are many things for which you can both reward and congratulate yourself when you are dieting, apart from the tangible achievement of a good weight loss in only one week. Reward yourself when you keep to your planned eating programme for a day. If you break your diet you can still award yourself some points if you do succeed in limiting your 'mis-eating' to a modest quantity, but do not be reckless — get back quickly to your diet. Your self-esteem and satisfaction will be increased further if you do succeed in correcting your mistakes by cutting down a little on the next day's calorie ration or by increasing your exercise output. In fact, it is often a good idea to draw up a positive contract with yourself with a daily points system, based not on total perfection but on partial success. It might read:

3 points for keeping meticulously to your diet or calorie allowance for the day.

2 points if you do eat something extra but succeed in limiting this.

1 point for completing any other item in your total slimming programme (your daily physical exercises; getting out of the house when you may get bored and eat).

There is a great psychological reward in watching the points accumulate, and this way, even if you do not score the full points, you can at least record some success in supporting behaviour.

Think of some ways in which you can give yourself tangible rewards for progress at regular intervals. Thus you could promise yourself that every time you score a certain amount of points you will allow yourself some kind of treat or self-indulgence (other than food) like buying a new dress or taking a trip to see an old friend.

Persistent triers inevitably succeed in reaching their goal but perfectionists may become disillusioned and fail in the attempt because no human beings are perfect.

Attitudes to failure

The biggest potential setback is the day on which you break your diet, and this usually happens when you succumb to negative reactions about your ability to diet and your hopes of success. It is essential to counteract these reactions with some really positive thinking. The most positive and encouraging approach of all is to think that if you have managed even to stick to a diet for a single day, you have the ability to become slim. If you think rationally about it, slimming is simply a matter of dieting for one day at a time and linking those days together.

When you feel you have 'let yourself down', dwell instead on the days when you were successful — all the positive days. Remind yourself that tomorrow is another day and resolve to make it a good day. There are many more days ahead on which you can do better, and it is a luxuriously positive thought to savour the endless chances which we all have to keep on trying again. Another big potential setback is the week in which you find that you have not lost as much weight as you had hoped for. This can produce such destructive negative reactions that you may not feel that it is worth carrying on. Therefore, it is essential to accept that weekly weight losses do tend to fluctuate during dieting and to appreciate the very positive achievement of shedding any weight, however little. It is a good, positive ploy to look at the amount lost in the form of food. Imagine yourself minus the same weight of lard or butter and you can see that it is still a worthwhile little chunk to have lost. Learn to look at the positive side of even the smallest loss.

Everyone has to expect failure and must learn how to cope with it — whether it is a brief failure or a longer one which will be reflected on the scales. Basically, it is a very sound idea to aim for a weight loss that allows for a modest degree of failure.

Fear of failure can play a useful role in motivating a slimmer to keep to her diet. Obviously the overweight person with no fears at all about the personal consequences of remaining overweight is unlikely to succeed in losing weight. If an overweight woman is contented with herself as she is and decides to have a go at dieting because someone else has suggested it, or because it seems a sensible thing to do, she is unlikely to summon up sufficient determination to overcome the continual temptations that will arise during any slimming programme.

Strong and excessive fear, however, can interfere with judgement and may often lead to dieting downfall. The dieter who fears that a slimming campaign is her 'last chance' and is, therefore, terrified of failing, will tend to see any slight deviation from her diet programme as an irreparable disaster. This, in turn, may trigger off the responses developed to deal with high anxiety in the past, namely eating.

For many women, a bad weight loss may correspond with premenstrual tension and during this time, temporary fluid retention will often cause the scales to register little, if any, apparent weight loss. When in a premenstrual mood, plus disappointment at an apparently poor weight loss, many women are in a dangerously ready-to-cheat mood.

One out of three women is said to experience a strong craving for food about three or four days before menstruation. This could be the reason why many women find that a diet campaign comes unstuck after the first three weeks. No one fully understands why these biological and psychological eating urges happen, and there is no real medical cure. Food cravings vary: some women may have an intense craving for a particular food while others may have an urge to eat anything and everything they see. Arm yourself against this difficult time of the month by recognizing the problem and being prepared. Keep a note of your period dates and of the days when you may experience some strong premenstrual eating urges. A comforting thought is that premenstrual tension does not last long and so you are unlikely to become overweight from over-eating during those few days in a month.

The after-effects of over-eating at this time are the real cause of weight gain or diet collapse. You may feel so shattered by the amount you have eaten that you carry on over-eating for comfort. You may even decide that there is no point in persisting with your diet. This is nonsense; calm down and get the problem into perspective.

There are various ways in which you can limit the extent to which you add on the calories at this time. If your premenstrual cravings lead to an urge to eat biscuits that you cannot resist, the solution may be to substitute them for one of your meals. If you eat a packet of biscuits instead of lunch, it will cost you fewer calories than eating lunch *and* biscuits. By substituting craved foods for meals you do not want particularly, you may not lose weight but it is unlikely that you will gain any. You will not become malnourished from eating biscuits or chocolates instead of nutritious meals for just three or four days every month. No nutrients are required on a daily basis; if you consume the right average quantity of vitamins, minerals and protein over a period of several weeks, you will not come to any harm.

Other methods of coping with this very hazardous time are to try banking extra calories by reducing calorie intake below your usual allowance on easier days at another time of the month and to ensure that you are kept occupied and away from food as much as possible. Accept that dieting will not necessarily bring its own expected rewards every week and come to terms with the ups and downs of slimming. Having lost a large amount of weight in the first week and then gained a little the following week you need not feel so disappointed that you must walk straight into a cake shop as some failed slimmers do. This example emphasizes the danger of the frame of mind that may follow a temporary slimming set-back.

Sometimes a blue mood can spring directly from a slimmer's attitude to her diet. The person who views things negatively and disqualifies all her positive achievements is likely to be a ready-made candidate for disappointment even if she follows her diet 95 per cent of the time. She will look at a five per cent failure area and ignore the solid achievement. The person who tends to catastrophize events can turn a small dietary indiscretion into a major disaster, and it is precisely this twisted thinking that can create the feelings of depression and failure that make dieting more difficult. It is unrealistic to expect a 'perfect' weight loss every week, and the person who sets up this goal is doomed to disappointment with her slimming progress and herself. A natural consequence of such self-disgust is going to be depression.

If you are going to make small setbacks, frustrations and disappointments an excuse for breaking your diet, it is unlikely that you are going to get through a single day, let alone a week, without finding an excuse to give up. Most slimming bids founder and sink on the day when the dieter allows herself a let-out clause, or excuse, like 'Oh, I'm much too depressed (miserable, harassed, excited, busy) today'.

Learn from past failures and do not persist in flinging your willpower into combat against a maximum-temptation situation. If you happen to love chocolate biscuits, for instance, and buy a packet knowing your weakness, then you are setting up a situation that is tempting and potentially destructive to your dieting resolution. You may resolve to give them to the family, or only have one yourself, and your determination may hold out for a while, even for hours, but when you get tired or depressed or something goes wrong and you reach for the comforting biscuit packet you rarely end up eating only one. You might even polish off the whole packet, and the longer you have resisted, the worse the explosion will be when your willpower finally blows.

There is no such thing as total defeat in dieting when you use the self-control approach rather than relying on your willpower. It even allows for a two-steps-forwards-and-one-step-backwards approach. This means that if you do over-eat some of your favourite foods on one day, you can balance it out against the days when you resisted the temptation to do so, and thus record that your self-control is producing some obviously beneficial overall results. So there is no need to feel a total failure and suffer the demoralizing consequences. Willpower is sitting in a café and ordering coffee, then putting artificial sweetener in it, when what you really want is a cake. Self-control is having a small cake, but resolving not to have any dessert later in the evening at dinner-time.

Attitudes to yourself

Psychiatrists confirm that the woman who has a good body image and self-confidence (who confidently sees herself as reasonably attractive, even though an unbiased observer might regard her as being only moderately endowed with good looks) will indeed prove more attractive to the opposite sex than a more physically beautiful woman who is unaware of herself and tends to dwell on her flaws.

A woman with hang-ups about her figure often cannot believe that a man finds her genuinely attractive. Therefore she goes on the defensive and works at establishing herself as a 'buddy' or as 'one of the boys' when she is in male company. However, if she would prefer men to find her attractive, then this attitude is sadly self-defeating. The self-confident and assertive woman usually takes the attitude that you can win the friendship and respect of anyone regardless of looks, but no one person proves to be attractive to everyone. The woman who has major hang-ups about her figure often thinks that she is not attractive to anyone, and she usually succeeds in proving herself perfectly right, over and over again. Failures in one's person-to-person relationships, so often blamed on excess weight, are more likely to result in depression and comfort-eating than sustained dieting.

The woman with hang-ups about her weight also tends to reject any compliments, suspecting the compliment-payer of making a joke at her expense. Therefore she reacts accordingly and, whatever the compliment, usually disagrees with it quite vigorously by making some downgrading or a sarcastic comment about herself. This safety-first reaction is always a mistake because it is unnecessary and springs from insecurity. If lost for words in response to an unexpected compliment, there is one simple phrase that always fits the occasion perfectly — just 'Thank you'.

For some people, being fat is like taking an appealing puppy out for a walk. It can break down barriers, provide a talking-point and be a focus for friendly attention. Trotting out a weight problem and parading one's failures in an amusing way can provide a point of contact with others, and some fat people secretly fear to lose this social link by becoming slim.

Being a bit overweight can be a form of protection, too. It allows you to opt out of keeping up appearances; after all, if you were to achieve a more fashionable shape, then colleagues might expect more of you. They might be more critical of your clothes and appearance, for example, than they were when you were overweight. Although this may appear to be a paradox, many an overweight woman would feel quite lost without her figure problem. All that surplus tissue is a way of announcing that you are non-competitive and that others can relax in your company. Thus staying overweight may absolve you from a great deal of bother and external pressures.

Failed dieters sometimes need to ask themselves if, deep down, they really want to become slim. It may help if you discuss your feelings openly and frankly with a sympathetic and well-informed person. A slimming club is an ideal place to find this kind of help. There, you quickly lose those fears that arise from isolation and also the suspicion that you are the only overweight person in the world who wants to slim down and cannot achieve it. Association with other slimmers, who almost invariably reveal the same experiences and problems, can be highly therapeutic and positively reassuring.

You will have to face the fact that, like everybody else, there are bound to be times in life when you are going to feel mentally low, and often for no immediately obvious reason. Just as dealing with surplus weight calls for a sensible appraisal of the eating mistakes that have caused the problem, so it is wise to take stock at those times when life seems both unusually hard and dismal. Whatever the problem, it needs attention. We all need to pause occasionally to re-consider our goals and also the best way of achieving them. The person who perceives the world in terms of black and white is not taking a very mature view of people and events; life is much more complicated than that! It is easy to get into the habit of magnifying the slightest mishap or backward step into a major disaster if your life lacks sufficient interests, hobbies and satisfaction.

Too many people are brought up to look for and analyze the bad things rather than the good things in themselves, yet they are entitled to take their share of praise as well as that of blame. This is not conceit; on the contrary, it is a vital part of our self-respect. Cultivating a balanced outlook and a proper self-regard can help to prevent blue moods and periods of depression which may lead to 'comfort eating'.

The habit of eating in response to a mood, especially depression, is difficult to break. You certainly will not beat it if your only plan is to sit down and tell yourself over and over again that you are not going to eat, while watching the clock creep by. Action has got to be your best line of defence. Therefore, plan to keep busy. There are two kinds of possible activities: those that we enjoy doing (hobbies, recreational and leisure pursuits); and those that are not enjoyable because they are tough or tedious but challenging enough to give us a sense of achievement afterwards.

Feeling deflated does not last for ever, and it will end all the quicker if you stop indulging in self-pity and realise that you are only human and unable to resist every little food temptation you encounter. If you can respond to such moods with some form of physical activity rather than eating, then you are over your first hurdle. However, be kind to yourself if you do fail occasionally and seek solace in the cake or biscuit tin. The important thing is to see a binge as a momentary lapse and no more.

When you have put a very big effort into slimming it is extremely demoralizing to find your progress sabotaged by sudden bouts of over-eating. Binge eaters often assume that they are exceptional, although, in fact, many slimmers seem prone to such lapses. However, binges' consequences may often be magnified by a slimmer out of all proportion to their actual effects.

Of course, food eaten during a binge is not going to help a slimming campaign, but the actual weight gain resulting from this kind of occasional indulgence will be very small and not really a tragic increase. Look at it coolly and you will soon realize that it can be lost again by getting back on the diet. However, this may be easier said than done; a slimmer who has been on a binge may feel weighed down by far more than the actual gain. She may see her lapse also as a definite moral defeat, and a serious and shaming departure from a reasonable standard of acceptable behaviour. This sense of failure may create tension which, in turn, can lead to further binge eating. Soon an attitude of resignation may set in also, summed up by such thoughts as: 'Oh, what's the use of trying to diet when I am obviously going to stay fat?' So what can be done? The most important thing is to be calm and examine the problem realistically. There are some slimmers who find it impossible to eliminate the occasional bout of over-eating, and therefore they should accept this, without guilt, and adjust their slimming programme accordingly. It is not a perfect situation, but what person, whether dieting or not, is

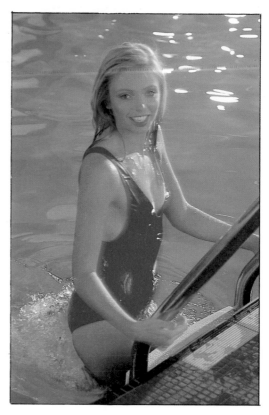

One of the best forms of exercise, swimming can help you in your dieting campaign and increase your confidence about your body image.

perfect? Note only that periods of strict dieting interspersed with the occasional eating binge can add up to a slower way of losing weight, but still a perfectly acceptable one. You are taking a longer route, but you should still achieve your ultimate aim of being slim. However, if binges occur so often that they are not only slowing down your slimming rate but are cancelling out any weight loss completely, then the situation is different and you have to look more critically at yourself.

When describing binges, slimmers often attribute a sort of mystical quality to them, as though the binge suddenly descends from the sky in a way that is both unavoidable and irresistible. 'Something takes over,' is how they often describe it, 'and I find myself eating'. This may well be how the situation appears in retrospect but certainly it is not the way in which such behaviour sequences happen. A binge does not appear 'out of the blue'; it is always triggered off by physical, emotional or social factors and there are advance warning signals which you must learn to recognize. Thus you may find that diet-breaking is usually triggered off by acute boredom, a dull and rainy day, a quarrel or premenstrual tension, to name but a few common examples. Anticipating trouble means that you can side-step any hazardous situations instead of walking into them. An obvious avoidance strategy is to take up some activity that is incompatible with eating when the signals switch to danger. Instead of raiding the larder, you could decide to do some reading or sewing or typing. Another good tactic, which has proved particularly effective since most binges take place at home, is going out for a brisk walk. This may sound too simple but it really does work for many binge-prone slimmers. It automatically prevents the binge starting, removes the slimmer from the source of food, involves beneficial exercise and allows for the passing of time.

People often make things difficult for themselves by taking decisions in situations involving high risk. For instance, deciding whether or not to go on a binge when you are standing beside a pantry full of food is clearly not weighting the scales in your favour! Getting away from the source of temptation obviously reduces the chances of a binge decision being made. Remember, too, that the feelings and situations that signal a likely binge are not permanent. Like lethargy or anger, these sensations wax and wane. Just allowing time for a binge urge to pass you safely by may be among your best counter-measures. Remove yourself from food and give your feelings time to change.

Besides representing a departure from normal consumption, a binge may also take the form of a somewhat violent interaction with food — an impulse not just to over-eat but also to cram it into your mouth and gulp it down almost fiercely. The hidden objective of a binge for many slimmers is not to eat but rather to participate in an intense confrontation with food, the source of so many of their recent sufferings. If, on reflection, you feel that this could be true for you, go ahead next time and 'interact' with your binge food. Attack it, hurl it in the dustbin, crush it, jump up and down on it — do anything except eat it. You might think that this is a waste, but food is more harmfully disposed of if it ends up stored as ugly and unhealthy surplus fat on you.

Attitudes to others

People are sociable by nature and tend to live in association with each other. Clustering together as a family or group can be traced back to the survival instinct in primitive man and such instincts go deep. Beyond the urge to feel the warmth or presence of fellow creatures, there is a great need also to communicate with them.

One of the reasons why being alone so often leads to loneliness is that many people have a tendency to consider feeling solitary as a very bad thing and, even worse, as a consequence of perceiving themselves as unattractive and unlovable. However, being alone is something we all have to experience at some time in our lives. If you have no solo interests and a circle of supportive friends you are storing up trouble for the future, even if you now enjoy a gregarious existence. Similarly, you are taking great risks if you concentrate all your emotional resources on a relationship with just one particular person — a lover, life partner, or best friend. If the people you rely on to counter your loneliness cannot, for some reason, be there when you need them most, then you are sunk. In human relationships, we need to spread our roots wide and it is worth making the effort to keep in touch, and to show care and concern for worthy friends. Friendships, like good marriages, do need to be nurtured. Working at your friendships includes sounding genuinely pleased when the telephone rings and a friend is on the line, even though you might be watching your favourite T.V. programme.

Contrast the person who moves about her locality exchanging a cheery word with a shopkeeper or neighbour with the person who goes silently about her business. Often the silent person is very lonely and would welcome friendly contact. However, if she does not initiate conversation and does not respond to friendly approaches, then people are not likely to persevere in their friendly overtures towards her. If you really want friendships and affection, you need to be prepared to take the risk of an occasional snub or, indeed, of looking foolish.

You may find that when you do succeed in losing weight, your family and friends are less than thrilled. Your behaviour and your perception of your own body-image may change drastically as a result of your new-found confidence and may make other people, even old friends, nervous. Losing weight can, in some cases, also effect a personality transformation and may thus change the equilibrium of a close personal relationship. Your steady partner in the relationship is capable of change, too, but often there is a time lag. Although you are ready and prepared for the change you have instigated, it may take a little time, subtle perseverance and tact to encourage your partner to respond in the way you would like. Be aware also of the highly popular power-game of people persuading their friends to abandon their diets. In a steady relationship, do not imagine that if you give in just once to the attractions of a forbidden food that this will be regarded as a special circumstance. On the contrary, if you refuse food at first but accept it at the third time of asking, then your tempters will realize that if they are persistent you will succumb again on the next occasion food is offered. Learn to be assertive and to refuse food that you do not really want. If you are talked into something against your real wishes, then face the fact that you will resent it. Unexpressed anger and resentment can very soon build up many different inner stresses which will not help your mental well-being; and if they lead also to additional eating, they will not help your figure, either.

'No' is one of the most useful and essential words in our vocabulary. If you are over-weight, then probably you have a tendency to go along with other people's plans and wishes. You are the giver, the nice person who finds it hard to refuse anyone but, of course, there is nothing wrong with being agreeable for the right reasons — it can be both positive and pleasurable. However, it can go sour on you if you say 'Yes' when you secretly want to say 'No'. The next step is to start brooding about it and building up hostilities and from there on it is a very short step to the biscuit tin. Your relation-ships with other people play a key part in weight control and it is possible to change your personal relationships by learning to be a more assertive person.

For the person who is very sensitive about being overweight, then the tendency to be agreeable has often developed as a defence mechanism and psychological protection policy. This policy of always being a nice person is doomed to failure on many counts because if people really want to hurt you, they will do so regardless of your good nature.

If you are in a situation where you feel that someone is taking advantage of you, react at once and say so. The longer you wait before speaking out, the more your tensions build up and the more difficult it becomes to resolve the situation without hostility. For example, if a friend suggests that you go to see a film with her when you are longing to see a different one, it is better to say 'No' and talk about the problem in the open than to spend an unenjoyable evening and come home with a smouldering feeling of resentment towards your friend.

Resentment can be a powerful comfort-eating trigger, especially for women with families, who spend many of their evenings washing up the dishes after the evening meal, or doing their household chores after a hard day at the office. For most women these are dreary tasks, and they may feel resentful that although the rest of the family have settled down to watch television, they still cannot relax. In these situations, there is a strong temptation to eat a few spoonfuls of the left-over dessert or nibble at a biscuit, just to comfort and reward yourself a little.

Probably the worst and most dangerous excuse for breaking your diet is to lamely blame someone else or an external situation over which you claim to have no control. Be prepared for tempting situations and avoid them at all costs. Research on overweight people shows that those who put the cause of their problem squarely where it belongs and admit honestly that they have been eating too much, are more likely to succeed in getting slim than those who cite other people or such uncontrollable factors as 'glands', 'fluid-retention' or 'the menopause' as the cause. Similarly, those women who find continual excuses in outside circum-stances, such as 'It's impossible in my job' or 'My husband won't co-operate', stand an equally small chance of success.

Attitudes to sex appeal
There are men who are sexually attracted to the kind of cushiony Rubens-style figure generally considered to be overweight by today's standards; and there are also men who are positively turned off by any excess weight. However, both these groups are probably minorities. Surveys show that the average man of today prefers the slimmer figure, but a woman's weight or shape is just one of the many factors that add up to that elusive quality known as sex appeal.

What is sex appeal and is it something that you can acquire? Overweight wall-flowers can blossom into slimmer women and may become considerably more attrac-tive to men, although this does not result from weight loss alone.

What is it that initially draws a person to somebody of the opposite sex? All of us, when we first meet a person, make an instantaneous judgement as to whether it is someone we want to approach or to move away from. The woman who looks attractive is much more likely to draw people into conversation than an unattractive woman. An important factor in this interaction is self-esteem. A woman who does not consider herself to be appealing will signal this to others. If she suffers from a lack of self-esteem because she feels that body weight is all-important, she may allow this to influence her behaviour. Thus when approached by anyone, a woman with a weight hang-up may shrink back or act in a somewhat apathetic way, which signals that she does not want to be friendly and to leave her alone. On the other hand, she might strike a self-protective 'just a good pal' or 'one of the boys' pose in order to emphasize that she does not wish to be considered as a sexually attractive woman in men's eyes. All aspects of appearance, including body weight, will play a major part in initial attraction between people, but what happens afterwards is based much more on behaviour than physical appearance.

A lack of grooming, or clothes that are chosen to divert rather than attract attention, usually send out negative signals. Although no one would expect a normally heavily overweight woman to suddenly wear skin-tight, figure-hugging dresses, little step-by-step changes, perhaps only in her accessories at first, can encourage and also emphasize changes in her self-perception. They can bring a rewarding feedback from other people which will encourage further diet efforts. In fact, clothes can make all kinds of sexual statements. Those that make an over-brazen statement may not bring a newly slim woman, inexperienced in dressing to be attractive, the reaction she is seeking. If she chooses a slinky dress with a plunging neckline she may well be offended with the reactions she receives from enthusiastically appreciative men and honestly wonder what she has done to create such an impression. Usually the most sexually attractive clothes are outfits that emphasize some attractive aspects of the body but only hint at others; clothes that have been chosen with care, and reveal that their wearer considers herself to be worth caring about.

Sometimes, a slimming success makes a woman feel so much better about her appearance and in herself that her behaviour will change automatically as a result. Most people, however, who are accustomed to being overweight find that their body-image, the way they imagine they look, takes longer to change than their actual weight. Thus it is common for a woman to continue to see herself as fat for several weeks or even up to a year after she has become slim. If a slim woman still sees herself as a fat person, she may well continue to fail to behave as an attractive woman.

In addition to the danger of not changing one's self-perception, there is also a danger of changing it too radically and for the wrong reason — reassurance. Flirtatiousness plays an important part in sex appeal, but it should not be confused with over-eagerness to please. Women who have become used to being overweight and succeed in their slimming campaign may lean towards promiscuity. Often this is a passing phase that works itself out as the woman re-establishes her true self-confidence. We all need reassurance from other people in order to confirm our own self-esteem, but the woman who has regarded herself as sexually unattractive may fall into the trap of seeking very positive, rather than subtle, reassurance. A woman of average self-assurance reaps her reassurance subconsciously from the signals she receives about her own sex appeal. Thus if a man takes the trouble to approach her or talk to her, she will see it as an indication of his interest. However, the woman who has had her self-image distorted by years of being overweight may lack the self-assurance to be reassured by such signals. There is a danger that she will feel sexually unattractive unless every man she dates makes sexual advances towards her.

Weight loss cannot always succeed in changing a marriage which is in a shaky state, and it is dangerous for a woman to slim in order to please and satisfy one person — even though that person may be her husband. His reaction to her new figure may not fulfil her expectations, and one of the reasons why many women regain weight is that they were shedding it only to please someone else and not themselves. A husband may feel that now his wife is much slimmer she will be more attractive to other men and this fear may cause him to react in a slightly hostile way.

We all establish patterns in everything we do in life and these tend to persist if we do not make positive attempts to alter them. If sex has become a routine activity, changes of frequency, intensity and variety will not 'just happen' as a result of becoming slim. Losing weight can help a woman to enjoy a more active sex life, but it does not automatically guarantee it.

It is unwise to slim solely in order to increase your sexual attractions. Sex is important in life but it is not the only source of deep pleasure and satisfaction. If you shed surplus weight it will help to increase your self-esteem and confidence, and as these increase and your weight reduces, you cannot fail to become more attractive to the opposite sex. Remember also, however, that extra self-esteem opens up many other paths to excitement and fulfilment — like doing all those things you never had the confidence to do in your overweight past.

Attitudes to food

What do you do when food is the foremost thing in your mind, when you are craving to eat something but cannot because you know that your slimming diet does not allow it?

First of all, try to analyze why you are yearning to eat a particular food at a given moment. Often, you may only be seeking a release from some kind of emotional tension — anger, frustration or depression. Try to assess what is bothering you and consider if there is any way in which you can release this pent-up emotion other than by eating. If you have faced up to your depression or moodiness in the past, then you will know from experience that 'getting it off your chest' always helps. If you can have a good chat, or even a moan, to someone else, in person or by telephone, you may release some of those pent-up emotions and find that food becomes more resistible. If there is no one available to talk to, sit down and write about your feelings — it can be a surprisingly good outlet. Another excellent form of release from pent-up emotions is any form of energetic physical activity. If you can force yourself out of the lethargy of a bad moment it will help a great deal.

These are actions that can help to get food off your mind, but sometimes it can also be helpful to deliberately let your mind dwell on the food... but in a different way. Recreate in your mind the feeling that you usually experience after over-indulging in your temptation food, probably one of being fat, bloated and guilty. If you can, fantasize about this negative after-effect, then try imagining putting the food aside and feeling really good and proud of yourself.

Research suggests that there are two types of slimmers: those who find it best not to eat any of their favourite foods while dieting, fearing that once they start they cannot stop; and others who are able to satisfy their desires with controlled amounts. If you count yourself among the second group of slimmers the best solution is to plan a small amount of a favourite food into your calorie allowance. If you let the eating of pleasurable foods occur, or happen by accident, you are missing out on the pleasure of anticipation — and will feel deprived of that pleasure. To get greater pleasure from less, always eat slowly while sitting down, rather than grab and gobble food standing up. Even a biscuit should be divided into small pieces and savoured slowly, bite by bite.

For some people, the psychological urge to eat at what they consider to be 'snack' times — mid-morning, mid-afternoon and late evening — is more compelling than the desire to eat at socially determined meal times. You are much more likely to succeed in controlling your weight if, instead of always trying to fight your strongest eating urges, you concentrate on resisting the calories you find easiest to resist. Experimenting with a new more flexible approach to eating pays dividends in weight control.

Our ability to control our own behaviour tends to be at its peak when we feel well rested, vigorous and in good health. For most of us, the first hours of the day are the most shining hours of weight-control resolve. In the latter part of the day, when we are feeling more fatigued, strong dieting resolves tend to collapse. The evening, in particular, is when many people, both overweight and slim, turn to eating fattening snacks.

If you are in the habit of nibbling in the evenings it is unrealistic to plan your evening without a snack — you will inevitably fail.

Plan, instead, to save some of your daily calories for at least one evening nibble, and this will give you something to look forward to. If the snack is a planned part of your diet you will not feel guilty about surrendering to an illicit food and you will enjoy this treat all the more when it happens.

When realistically planning your daily dieting, keep in mind not only the fact that you will be tempted to eat in the evening, but also what you will be tempted to eat. It may depend on which particularly tempting foods are in your house on any particular day. If there is half a delicious cheesecake in the refrigerator, do you think honestly that your strong resolve in the morning not to eat any of it will last through the evening? It is more likely that at some time during the evening, feeling a strong urge to eat that cheesecake, you will go into the kitchen in search of a slimming crispbread or fruit to quell the cheesecake craving. When this fails to work, you may succumb guiltily to a big slice of cheesecake.

Some foods, which you buy, bring home and then put away in the kitchen, are so tempting that almost inevitably your will-power will crumble and you will eat them eventually. These foods, which explode all normal food controls for nearly everyone, can be referred to as 'time bombs'. Time bombs will sit in your kitchen cupboard tick...tick...ticking away until eventually your willpower explodes. They are more dangerous than favourite foods because they are bought and stored in diet-breaking amounts, and you will be tempted to eat the lot. Time bombs are usually foods that require no preparation and can be grabbed and eaten without cooking. This is why chips, although a very tempting food for many people, do not fall into this category. They have to be prepared and cooked, and this factor acts as a brake. Usually people only succumb to temptation if they are faced with such a food in an instantly available form — when they are passing a fish and chip shop, for instance. Similarly, chocolate mousse might well be one of your favourite foods but it would not carry the danger of a time bomb because it either needs defrosting or, if home-made, requires a certain amount of preparation. Essentially a time bomb is a readily available food that does not have to be eaten with a knife, fork or spoon.

One of the sound rules of eating control is to learn to store tempting foods out of sight, so that you are not reminded constantly of them as you walk into the kitchen or open a cupboard door. However, this is not the case with time bombs. Even behind doors and inside boxes and tins, they still signal their presence to you.

Tempting foods can be tackled in many different ways in your calorie reduction programme. Serve up only a small quantity, eat it slowly, take a break before you have some more — work towards quantity reduction slowly. However, these tactics do not work with time bombs; nor does telling yourself that you are never going to have that food again. The willpower explosion that will follow this resolve is almost as inevitable as the one that takes place when you bring the food into the kitchen.

Time bomb tactics may differ depending on the particular food. With some foods — cheesecake, for instance — the best answer might lie in deciding to eat only that particular food outside the home when circumstances make it very difficult to binge without embarrassment. Thus you might order a single slice of cheesecake as dessert after a restaurant meal. Bread, which seems to be a time bomb for many women, presents different problems and calls for new tactics. If only certain types of bread tempt you irresistibly, then you should buy less tempting and smaller loaves, which will be eaten quickly by your family and friends.

If snack-type foods, such as chocolate biscuits or salted nuts, happen to be your great temptation, then do not bring them back home at all. The single woman has an advantage here in that she does not have to bring any of her time bombs home but she should guard against another diet danger. Single women with weight problems often keep the kitchen practically empty as a dieting aid, but this can be as hazardous as keeping time bombs around. At a bad moment there can be such a strong temptation to eat something nice that a slimmer may even resort to rushing out to a restaurant or shop and gobbling large quantities of high-calorie foods. So keep some foods you really like available (preferably in small quantities if they are high in calories) but keep those foods you love and find irresistible at a distance. A survey of people's time bombs showed that the most popular ones were (in order): bread, chocolates, cheese, chocolate biscuits, cream sponge cake, nuts, cheesecake, cream and sweets. Write down your own time bombs and face up to the fact that these foods are irresistible, then start working out a less hazardous route to slimming success.

Studies of human behaviour in relationship to food have shown that early influences from cradle days and childhood can play an important part in dictating future eating patterns. The child rewarded or consoled by 'sweeties' or other sweet foods will often continue to seek this kind of comfort or reward later in adulthood.

It is possible that there are some physio-logical as well as psychological factors that make it difficult for some of us to sleep unless we have been fed. This may be a remaining vestige of what happens in early infancy when babies who wake up, are made comfortable and fed and then drop off to sleep again immediately after finishing their milk. Our earliest experience of life is that sleep follows food. If you cannot sleep without a small snack first, then experiment to find the foods with the least calories that have the desired effect. For instance, if you normally have a full mug of milky drink, try pouring just half a mug for a few nights and sip it slowly. You might discover that this will achieve the desired effect while reducing your calorie intake.

For scientific reasons, calories eaten in the evening can be marginally more fattening than those consumed during the earlier, more active hours. However, in determining the rate of weight loss, when you eat is of minor importance compared to how much you eat in total during the day. If you keep to the correct number of calories you will shed surplus weight even if you eat every single one during the evening.

Eating behaviour is an important part of controlling your calorie intake, so here are some basic rules:

1 Never eat standing up. A great deal of surplus food is eaten standing at the fridge door, or in the kitchen while preparing meals or even clearing up dishes. People who are used to eating between meals find that this habit is very hard to break. Start by making a firm rule that you will never eat anything, anywhere, unless you are sitting at a table and the food — even a biscuit or an apple — is first placed on a plate. By going to the trouble of getting out a plate, going to a table and sitting down, you are not nibbling food in a mindless way but you are giving yourself time to make a choice: 'Shall I eat it or shan't I eat it? Shall I eat it all?' Sometimes, of course, you may feel that you cannot resist eating this particular snack, but on other occasions your brake controls will triumph and you will start to experience the rewards of being in control of yourself.

2 Never eat while reading, watching television or listening to the radio. This, in fact, is one of the worst things you can do. When your mind is distracted you get less mileage out of each morsel of food and need even more food to get satisfaction. You may even realize at the end of a television programme that you have not tasted the food at all. Self-control is being able to make choices from moment to moment. Unless your mind is fully involved you cannot be in full control of your actions and eating.

3 Try to avoid eating when alone. People invariably eat more when they eat by themselves. Most overweight people eat most of their excess calories when they are alone; the same applies to between-meal snacks. For many people, a single resolve not to eat anything unless in the company of at least one other person could, in itself, result in gradual weight loss.

4 Slow down before you even start a meal. The process of eating in a slower, more controlled way starts even before you reach the table. If you can prove that you have enough control to approach a meal in a slow and leisurely way, you will find that you begin to gain confidence in yourself. Always set the table in a formal way, even for one — never be tempted just to grab a tray. When you seat yourself at the table pause for a moment before eating. Tension often leads to fast and excessive eating, so relax.

5 Do not place your full meal on the plate. Your spontaneous reaction is likely to be to clear your plate, however large the quantity. Leave part of your meal in the serving dish or oven, and after you have eaten your portion stop and consider whether you need to continue. You could save the food for later when you really do feel like eating it and might otherwise turn to a snack.

6 Deliberately slow down your eating rate. Put a portion of food in your mouth, then place the knife and fork back on the plate. Concentrate on the food you are eating now, rather than on the next mouthful. Chew it slowly, noticing all the taste sensations in the food; do not wash the taste of food away. Notice your feeling of fullness and try to stop when you are beginning to feel satisfied, not when you are full. By eating each mouthful very slowly you are getting maximum mileage out of it; you are thinking about it and giving yourself time to consider whether you need to continue eating.

7 Many people are in the habit of saving the best on the plate for last. *Don't* — eat the best first because if you save it up to the end, you will have to make room for it, however full you feel. If you eat it first, you may leave some of the other foods, thus lowering your calorie intake at the meal. Do not feel obliged to eat everything on the plate, and try to shed the feeling, instilled from childhood, that if you are going to have some pudding you must eat up your dinner first. If you know that you will not be able to resist a dessert, you can still leave some of your main course. It is often necessary to be a little wasteful in order to learn the habits of food control.

8 Plan ahead how you will dispose of any leftovers, otherwise you may find yourself nibbling them. Are there enough of them to provide another meal? If you decide to allocate them for lunch tomorrow, then set them aside for that purpose. If leftovers are identified in your mind with being reserved for a special purpose you are less likely to nibble them as snacks. If you suspect that you will eat them mindlessly between meals, then give them away or throw them away immediately. Do not feel guilty about 'waste'. Think of this as a special situation.

9 If you find that you cannot resist nibbling leftovers after a meal you could ask other people to clear away the foods and do the washing-up, at least for the duration of your dieting. This may be impossible if you live alone or have an unhelpful family. Scrape the leftover food from plates straight into the bin after dinner and leave the washing-up until the stronger-willed hours of the following morning. A dishwasher would be an ideal solution to this problem, especially if you are a busy working woman.

10 If you are in the habit of 'nibbling' while preparing dinner try to prepare as much as possible of the evening meal immediately after lunch, instead of later when you are more hungry and thus more likely to eat. Alternatively, if you are out at work during the day, prepare meals in advance at the weekend and store them in the freezer until you need them. In this way, you can reheat them without preparation in the evening.

11 Faced with a dinner party at someone else's home, eat only a modest number of calories during the day so that you can safely accept at least moderate portions of whatever your hostess has to offer. If your hostess has worked hard to prepare an attractive meal, your refusal to eat certain dishes may infuriate her, and the likelihood is that if you go home starving you will cook yourself a compensation supper!

12 Put temptation in little packs. Once you have opened a packet of peanuts, crisps or biscuits it is very hard to stop eating them. It is best, therefore, to buy tempting foods in the smallest packs available.

13 If you are fortunate enough to have a family who are concerned about your weight problem, it is wise to explain that any snacks they make for themselves should be eaten out of your sight.

14 Prepare your shopping list when you are not hungry, and shop when you are not hungry. That way, you could find yourself considerably less vulnerable to the urge of impulse-buying the 'high-temptation' foods which you are trying not to eat.

15 It has been proved medically that the more we concentrate on pain, the more we feel it. The same goes for hunger, or what we may perceive as hunger. Do not sit around thinking about the food you are trying not to eat. Do something positive instead that will take your mind off it.

Lesley's not a loser any more !

Lesley Monk was trapped for years in a drearily plump prison. Now when she hears people telling a shy, chubby teenager that her weight problem is only 'puppy-fat' and will soon disappear, she feels furious. It was when she was 15 years old that Lesley first noticed that nobody liked a 82.5kg (13st) fat girl, however amiable. At 18 she was heavier still and felt so fat and ugly that she married the first man to take an interest in her. The marriage was a disaster and her dieting attempts always failed, too. It was not until after her second marriage and the birth of her third child that Lesley — pictured below at height 1.68m (5ft 6in) and nearly 108kg (17st) — found the determination to change her shape and her life. After losing 9.5kg (1½st) on her own, Lesley joined a slimming club for additional support and encouragement. The weight rolled off and in only six months she had reached her target weight of 60.5kg (9½st) (right). Feeling younger and fitter and, at 29 years old, more confident for the first time in her life, Leslie won *Slimming Magazine's* 1981 prize for the U.K. Slimmer of the Year.

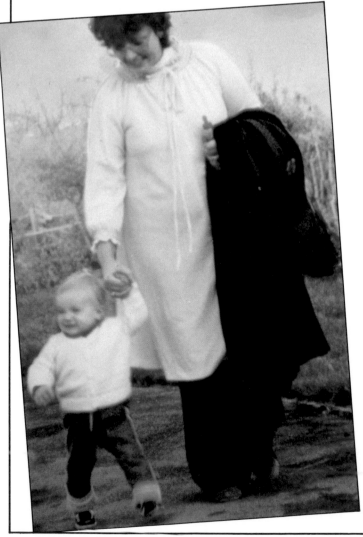

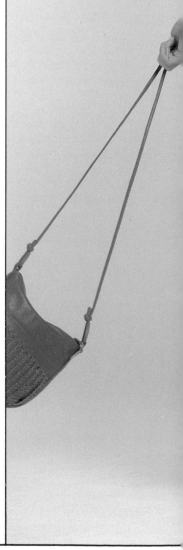

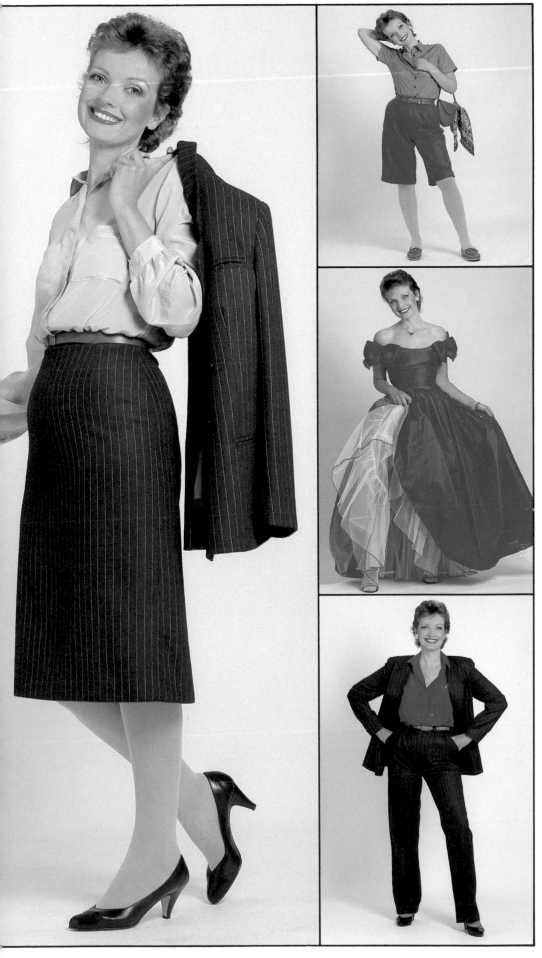

Astrid's dancing dream comes true

When 15 years-old Astrid Longhurst told a careers officer that she wanted to become a dancer and appear on television, the woman discounted the idea immediately and suggested secretarial training instead. No wonder, for Astrid (below) then weighed 95.5kg (15st). All her friends thought it a great joke that Astrid believed she could become a big star one day. However, Astrid was determined to become a dancer, even though her ballet class usually left her feeling exhausted. She eventually managed to diet off 13kg (2st) which gave her the confidence to audition for a well-known stage academy. It was like a slap in the face when the principal rejected her, saying that she thought Astrid was too heavy to keep up with the demanding schedule of work. However, when the sharpness of disappointment had softened a little, Astrid began to diet again and persevered until she had lost over 32kg (5st). Then she returned to the stage school for a second audition. This time, the principal told Astrid that she had lost so much weight that she could see her potential and was willing to accept her. At 19 years old and 1.68m (5ft6in) and 60.5kg (9½st), Astrid's dream to become a dancer came true and she even got her wish to appear on television after she became the runner-up to *Slimming Magazine's* U.K. Slimmer of the Year.

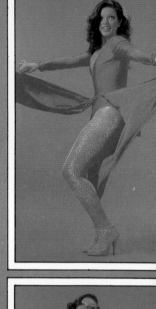

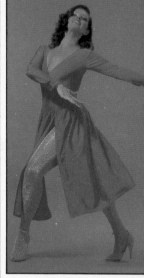

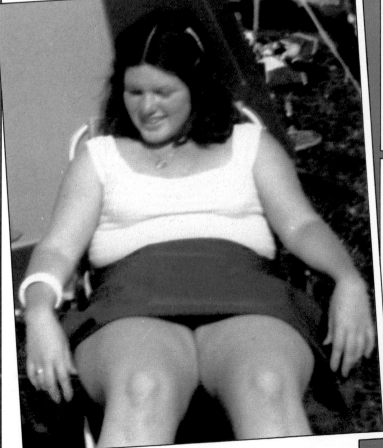

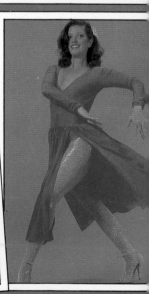

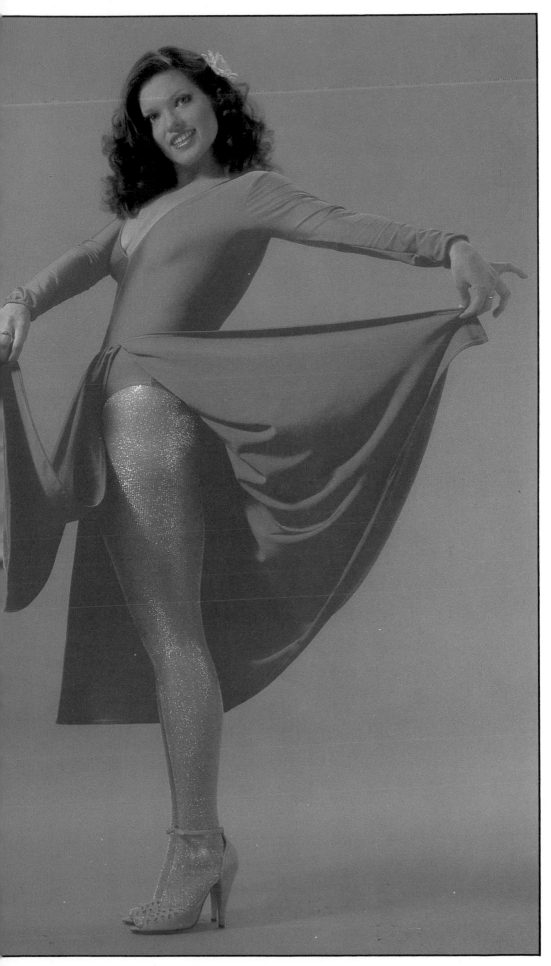

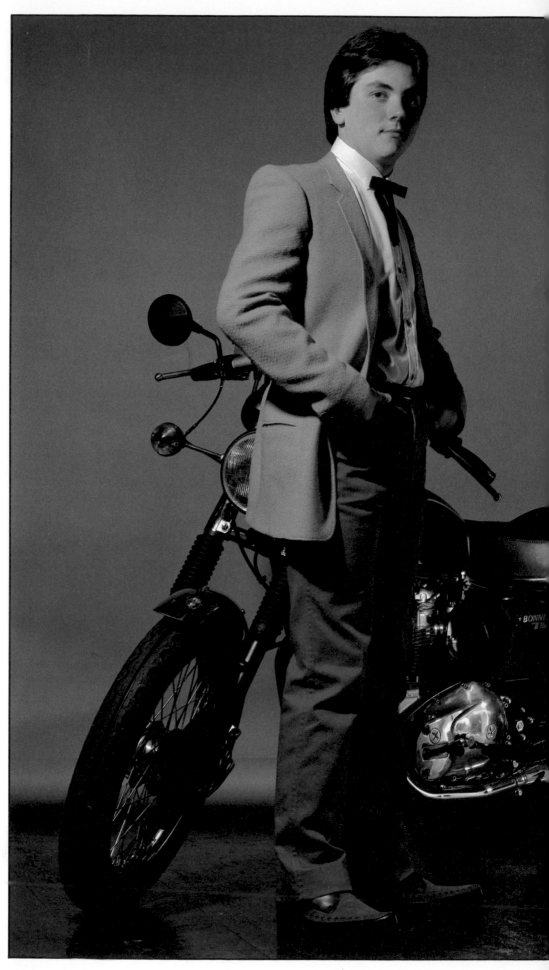

No more teasing teenager Terry

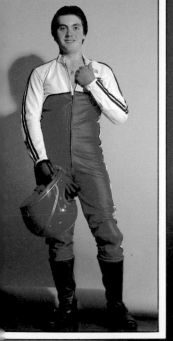

At 1.78m (5ft 10in), teenager Terry Pearce topped 108kg (17st) which is why he would allow himself to be photographed (below) only when half-hidden by his beloved motorcycle. Terry had always been big and was 95.5kg (15st) before he was 16 years old.

His first bike was a tiny moped and he now realizes how comical he must have looked perched on top of it. In comparison with his friends, he was really massive but their teasing was always friendly. When he became apprenticed to an electrical firm, however, he had to put up with such cruel pranks as being shut in a box while his workmates blew in cigarette smoke and joked about fat pigs and smoked ham! He also found that he was accident-prone and one day over-balanced in an attic, shot through a bedroom ceiling and was only saved thanks to his enormous stomach when he got stuck half-way! Terry never dared to ask a girl out for a date, and it was only after a holiday when he saw his friends chatting with girls that he finally felt tired of being fat, miserable and left out of things. No one believed that he would succeed at dieting, but Terry was desperately determined to lose weight. After losing 13kg (2st) he asked a girl for a date and could not believe his luck when she agreed. That event made him even more determined to reach his target weight. Terry finds that he dresses and looks more stylish now that he is 32kg (5st) lighter (see left). At 19 years old, he went to a discotheque for the first time ever and his girlfriend asked him jokingly where he had been hiding all his life. Terry knew the answer to that question — he had been trapped in his own unwanted fat.

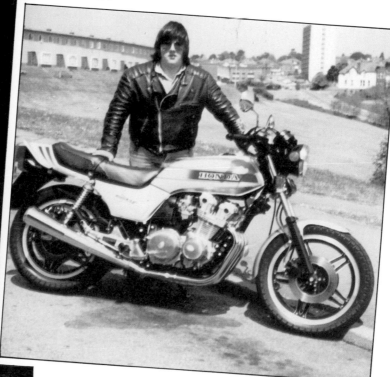

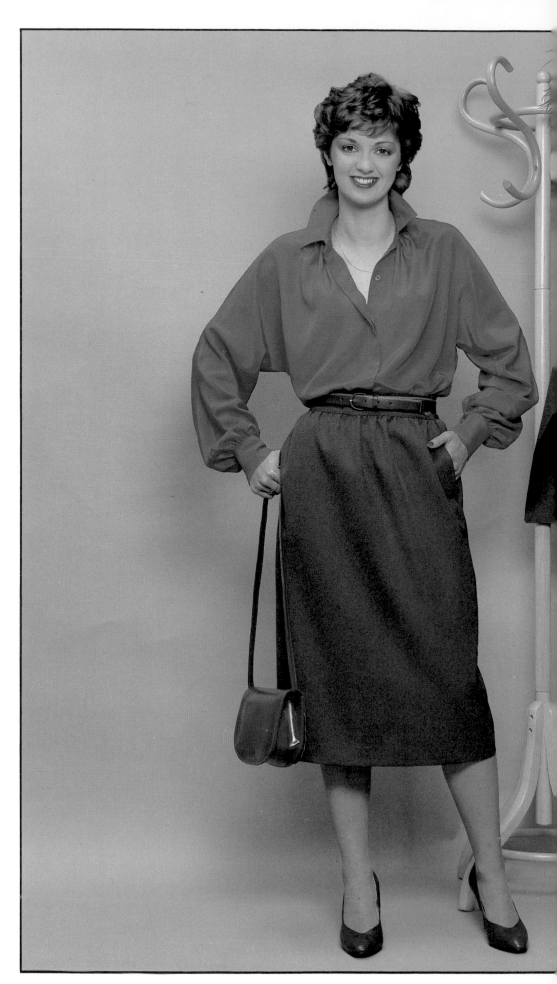

Sandra was insulted into slimming

At sixteen, Sandra had already learned that most boys prefer slim girls. Fat girls are treated as one of the boys and either teased or ignored. When she left school she thought the teasing would be all behind her, but taking a job selling toys and jokes proved to be a mistake. Other sales assistants saw Sandra as the biggest joke of all and life was one big round of funny noses and squeaky cushions, nudges and winks and very pointed remarks about big Humpty Dumpties. When Sandra first encountered Bryan she was just a head in a photograph to him. His cousin played Cupid and insisted that Sandra send her photograph to Bryan who was in the navy. Sandra daydreamed a little about meeting Seaman Bryan Morris. She could not imagine, though, what a tall, dark, slim sailor would see in a short 1.63m (5ft4in), fat 82.6kg (13st) podge like her. Boys rarely dated her and she worried that this would lead to yet another let-down. After corresponding for some time, Bryan wrote to say that he was coming home and would call round to meet Sandra. Although Sandra was very nervous about the meeting, they got on well together and eventually became engaged. The crunch came on her wedding day, for as Sandra stepped out of the limousine a passing man caught sight of her and shouted to Bryan: 'You're not going to try lifting her over the threshold, are you? You'll break both arms.' Sandra remembered that remark when she reached 88.9kg (14st) after the birth of Rachel. However, *Slimming Magazine* supplied the final incentive she needed to prove all the insults wrong. Sandra started to diet and within a fortnight she was into a satisfying routine and a steady weight loss. When she reached a slender 54kg (8½st) Sandra wished that she could meet that insulting passer-by again and show him her wonderful transformation.

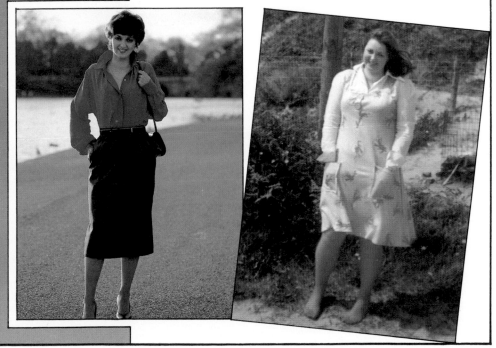

When you can see precisely one calorie — as you can 45 times in the foods pictured on these pages — it is surprising how much easier it becomes to assess the number of calories you are eating. So here's looking at you, calorie...

One calorie

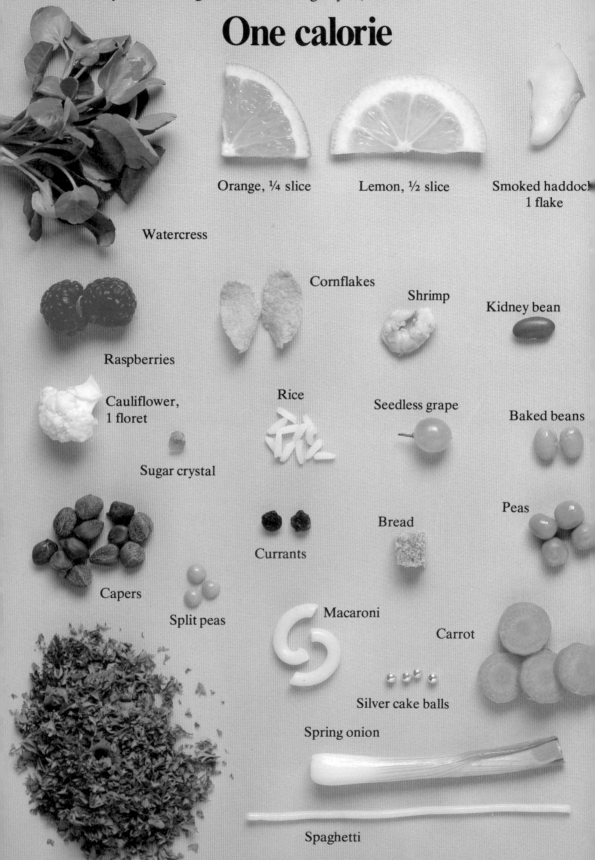

Orange, ¼ slice

Lemon, ½ slice

Smoked haddock 1 flake

Watercress

Cornflakes

Shrimp

Kidney bean

Raspberries

Cauliflower, 1 floret

Rice

Seedless grape

Baked beans

Sugar crystal

Peas

Currants

Bread

Capers

Split peas

Macaroni

Carrot

Silver cake balls

Spring onion

Spaghetti

Parsley

CHAPTER 6

Calories on view

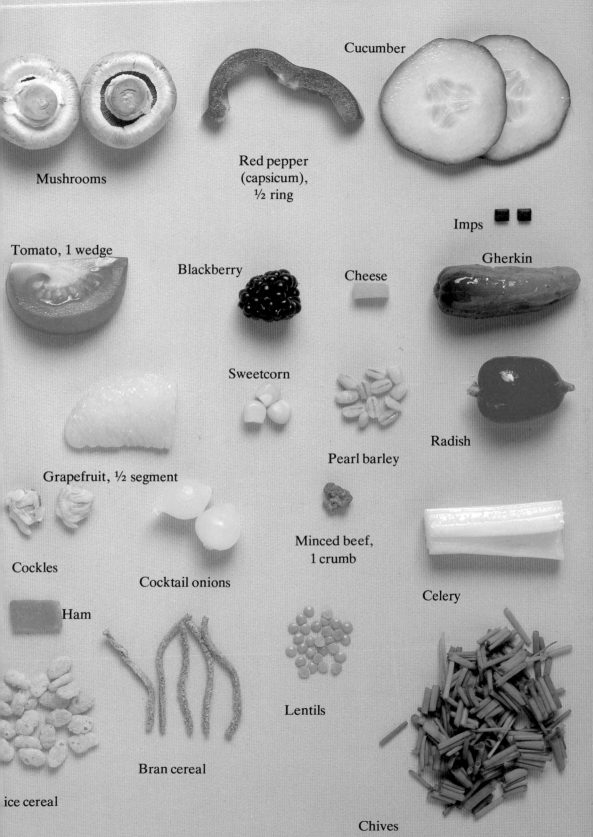

Cucumber

Mushrooms

Red pepper
(capsicum),
½ ring

Imps

Tomato, 1 wedge

Blackberry

Cheese

Gherkin

Sweetcorn

Radish

Pearl barley

Grapefruit, ½ segment

Minced beef,
1 crumb

Cockles

Cocktail onions

Celery

Ham

Lentils

Bran cereal

ice cereal

Chives

The nothing foods

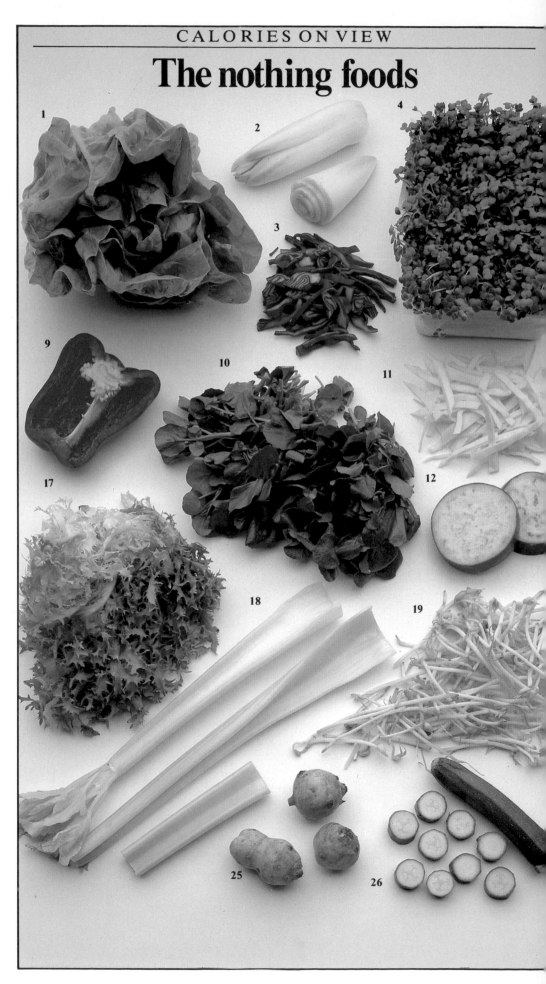

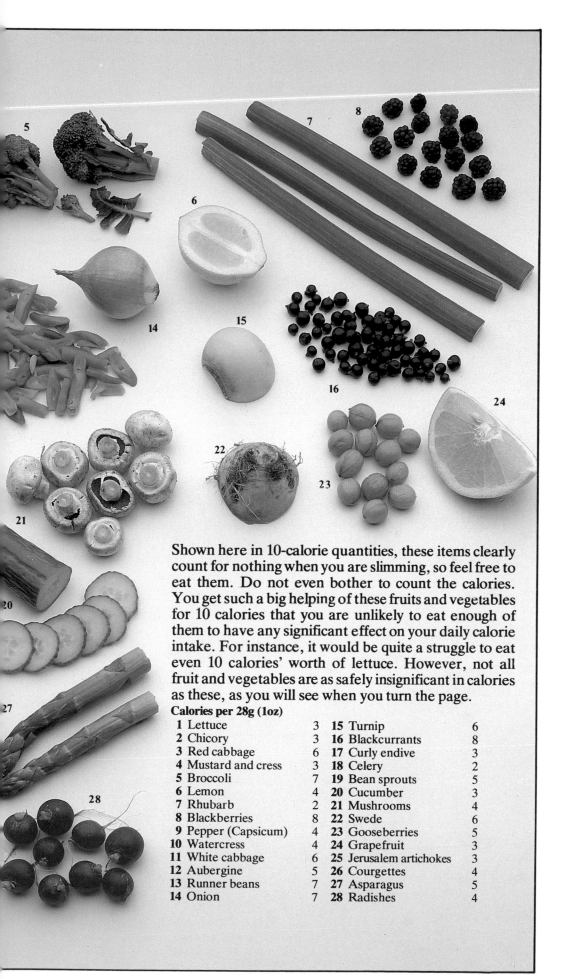

Shown here in 10-calorie quantities, these items clearly count for nothing when you are slimming, so feel free to eat them. Do not even bother to count the calories. You get such a big helping of these fruits and vegetables for 10 calories that you are unlikely to eat enough of them to have any significant effect on your daily calorie intake. For instance, it would be quite a struggle to eat even 10 calories' worth of lettuce. However, not all fruit and vegetables are as safely insignificant in calories as these, as you will see when you turn the page.

Calories per 28g (1oz)

1 Lettuce	3	15 Turnip	6
2 Chicory	3	16 Blackcurrants	8
3 Red cabbage	6	17 Curly endive	3
4 Mustard and cress	3	18 Celery	2
5 Broccoli	7	19 Bean sprouts	5
6 Lemon	4	20 Cucumber	3
7 Rhubarb	2	21 Mushrooms	4
8 Blackberries	8	22 Swede	6
9 Pepper (Capsicum)	4	23 Gooseberries	5
10 Watercress	4	24 Grapefruit	3
11 White cabbage	6	25 Jerusalem artichokes	3
12 Aubergine	5	26 Courgettes	4
13 Runner beans	7	27 Asparagus	5
14 Onion	7	28 Radishes	4

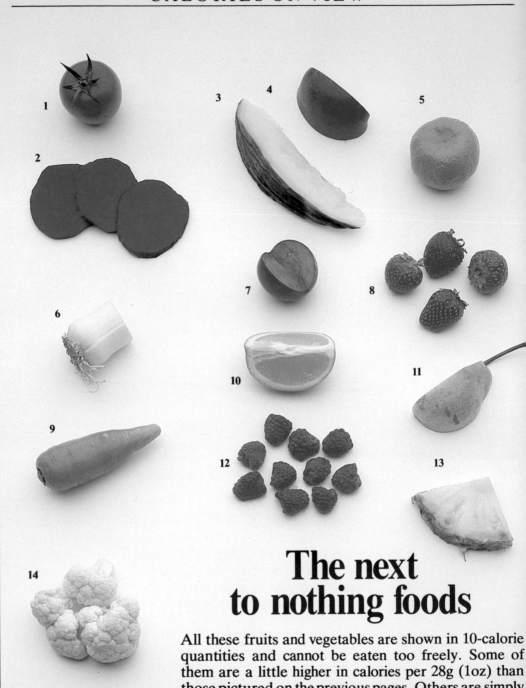

The next to nothing foods

All these fruits and vegetables are shown in 10-calorie quantities and cannot be eaten too freely. Some of them are a little higher in calories per 28g (1oz) than those pictured on the previous pages. Others are simply less bulky so that you would tend to eat more as a normal portion. Although you can still afford to eat generous quantities, a hefty helping would supply a significant number of calories, so it is wise to weigh and measure them and count the calories into your daily total. Precisely 10 calories' worth of each one are pictured here.

Calories per 28g (1oz)			
1 Tomato	4	8 Strawberries	7
2 Beetroot	8	9 Carrot	6
3 Melon	4	10 Orange	7
4 Apple	10	11 Pear	8
5 Mandarin orange	5	12 Raspberries	7
6 Leek	9	13 Pineapple	13
7 Plum	10	14 Cauliflower	4
		15 Brussels sprouts	7

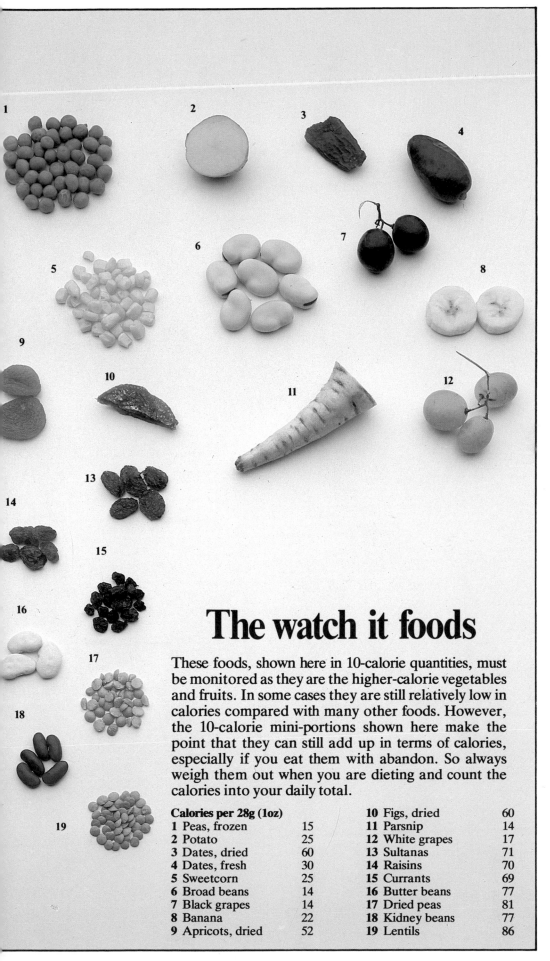

The watch it foods

These foods, shown here in 10-calorie quantities, must be monitored as they are the higher-calorie vegetables and fruits. In some cases they are still relatively low in calories compared with many other foods. However, the 10-calorie mini-portions shown here make the point that they can still add up in terms of calories, especially if you eat them with abandon. So always weigh them out when you are dieting and count the calories into your daily total.

Calories per 28g (1oz)			
1 Peas, frozen	15	10 Figs, dried	60
2 Potato	25	11 Parsnip	14
3 Dates, dried	60	12 White grapes	17
4 Dates, fresh	30	13 Sultanas	71
5 Sweetcorn	25	14 Raisins	70
6 Broad beans	14	15 Currants	69
7 Black grapes	14	16 Butter beans	77
8 Banana	22	17 Dried peas	81
9 Apricots, dried	52	18 Kidney beans	77
		19 Lentils	86

Calories by the spoonful

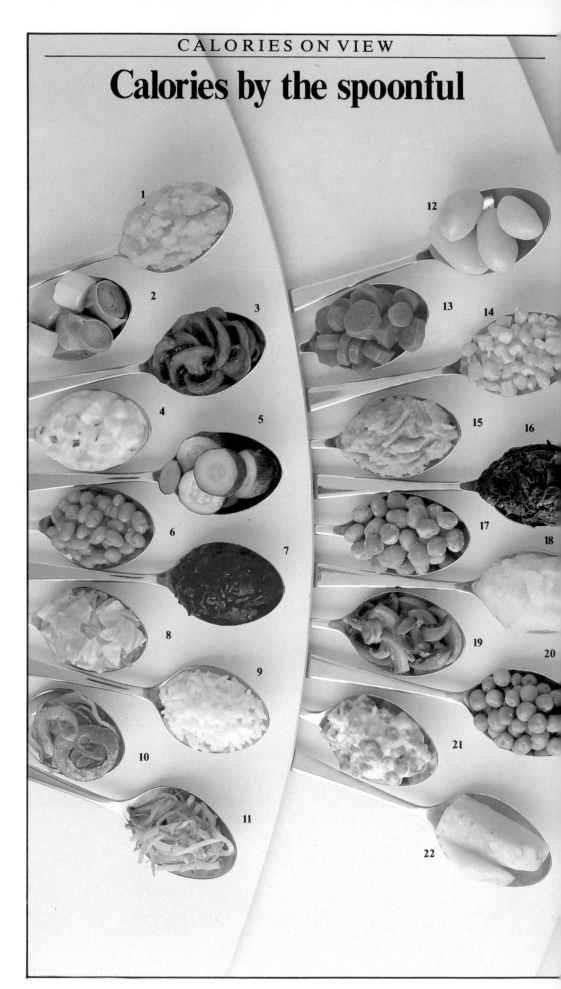

Spooning out vegetables to accompany meat and fish dishes is easy if you know their calorie values by the spoonful. Our at-a-glance picture guide shows you the number of calories per rounded tablespoon of some common foods.

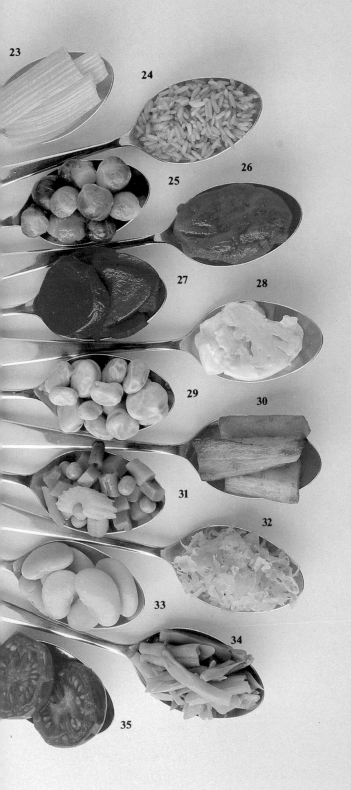

1	Swede, mashed	8
2	Leeks, boiled	7
3	Mushrooms, fried	40
4	Potato salad, canned	50
5	Courgettes	3
6	Baked beans	20
7	Pickled cabbage	3
8	Cabbage	2
9	Rice, boiled	20
10	Onions, fried	25
11	Bean sprouts, boiled	3
12	New potatoes	25
13	Carrots	5
14	Sweetcorn	20
15	Pease pudding	65
16	Spinach	10
17	Dried peas	30
18	Turnip, mashed	4
19	Mushrooms, stewed	2
20	Peas	15
21	Vegetable salad	50
22	Parsnips, boiled	16
23	Celery, braised	1
24	Rice, fried	70
25	Brussels sprouts	6
26	Tomato, canned	5
27	Beetroot, pickled	10
28	Cauliflower in white sauce	25
29	Broad beans	15
30	Parsnips, roast	30
31	Mixed vegetables	11
32	Sauerkraut	4
33	Butter beans	23
34	Runner beans	5
35	Tomato, fried	35

Calories by the carton

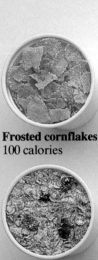

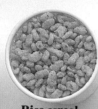

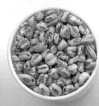

Frosted cornflakes
100 calories

Rice cereal
65 calories

Puffed wheat cereal
40 calories

Special K
90 calories

Cornflakes
90 calories

Muesli
305 calories

**Porridge
made with water**
65 calories

**Crunchy oat and
nut cereal** 320 calories

Bran cereal
130 calories

Cracklin'b
190 calories

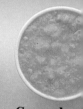

Potato, mashed
185 calories

Shredded cabbage, raw
10 calories

**Butter beans,
cooked**
125 calories

**Mashed swede
(no butter)**
30 calories

Creamed cor
155 calories

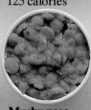

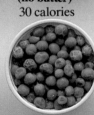

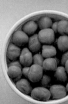

**Runner beans,
boiled** 25 calories

Broad beans, boiled
50 calories

Mushy peas
145 calories

Frozen peas, boiled
55 calories

**Processed pe
canned**
105 calories

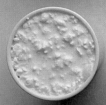

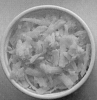

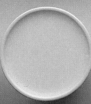

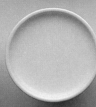

**Cottage cheese,per
113g (4oz) carton**
110 calories

**Grated Cheddar
cheese** 245 calories

Skimmed milk
60 calories

Silver top milk
110 calories

Pineapple ju
90 calories

ite rice, boiled
calories

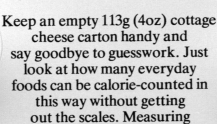

Keep an empty 113g (4oz) cottage cheese carton handy and say goodbye to guesswork. Just look at how many everyday foods can be calorie-counted in this way without getting out the scales. Measuring non-liquids, all calories are for loosely-packed cartons.

White spaghetti, boiled 130 calories

Pasta shells, boiled
135 calories

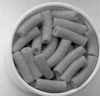

wn rice, boiled
calories

Brown spaghetti, boiled
95 calories

Brown macaroni, boiled
95 calories

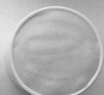

eetcorn kernels
calories

Spaghetti in tomato sauce
100 calories

Baked beans in tomato sauce
115 calories

Rice pudding, canned
155 calories

Custard made with skimmed milk
130 calories

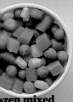
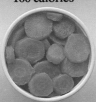

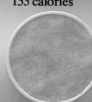
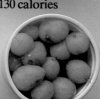

zen mixed
etables, boiled
calories

Carrots, boiled
20 calories

Tomatoes, canned
20 calories

Stewed apple (no sugar)
70 calories

Stewed gooseberries, with sugar 70 calories

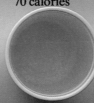

ange juice,
eetened
calories

Orange juice, unsweetened
55 calories

Apple juice
60 calories

Dry white wine
115 calories

Red wine
120 calories

How many calories in a chicken joint

The different cooking and serving methods used can determine the number of calories of the chicken joint or cooked dish in which it is used. Frying, of course, increases the calorie count, whereas poaching decreases it. It all depends on the way you cook and serve it. Here, we show you how the same chicken joint can become more or less fattening.

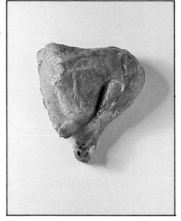

Roast it, basted with fat, and it comes to **290** calories. Without the skin it would be only **190** calories.

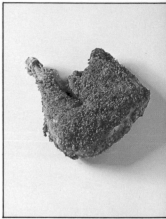

Deep-fry it, dipped in egg and breadcrumbs — **435** calories.

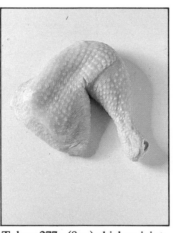

Take a 277g (8oz) chicken joint and, raw, it comes to **410** calories, including the skin. Without the skin, it would be **165** calories.

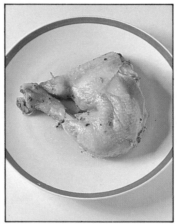

Poach it in chicken stock and then remove the skin. It comes to **165** calories.

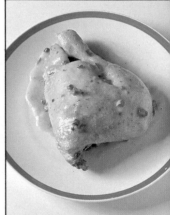

Casserole it in mushroom soup — **470** calories, which includes half of a 142g (5oz) can of condensed mushroom soup.

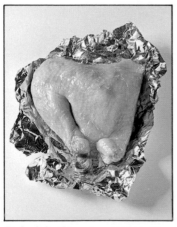

Bake it in the oven, wrapped in foil and without added fat, and you eat **340** calories. Remove the skin and it is only **195** calories.

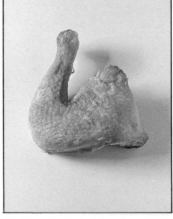

Shallow-fry it and you have **285** calories. Remove the skin and it is only **175** calories.

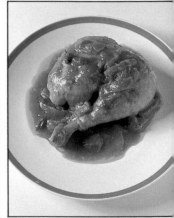

Curry the chicken joint and, with the sauce, it will amount to around **485** calories.

How many calories in a piece of fish?

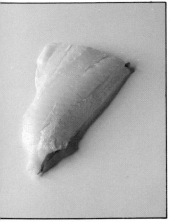

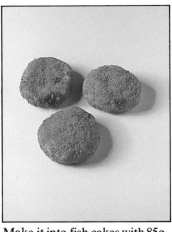

The number of calories in a piece of fish depends on how you cook and serve it. Here we take a typical white fish fillet and show how the answer varies. You will notice that if it is grilled or casseroled, the calorie count is low. However, it rises rapidly if the fish fillet is fried or served in a milk-based sauce.

Take a 170g (6oz) cod fillet and, raw, it comes to only **132** calories.

Make it into fish cakes with 85g (3oz) mashed potato, coat in egg and breadcrumbs and fry and you have **635** calories.

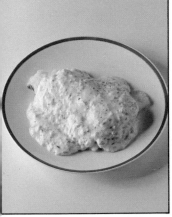

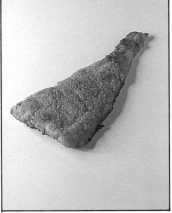

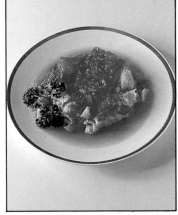

Grill it with 7g (¼oz) butter and serve in 150ml (¼pint) parsley sauce and the total amounts to **430** calories.

Coat it in egg and breadcrumbs and shallow-fry in fat or oil and you have **435** calories.

Casserole it with a small can of tomatoes and seasoning and your fish dish totals **155** calories.

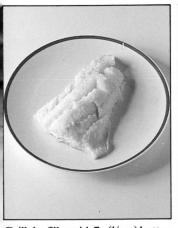

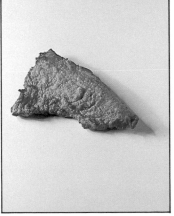

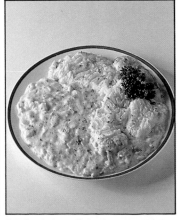

Grill the fillet with 7g (¼oz) butter on top and then you will have **185** calories.

Deep-fry your fish fillet in batter and the calorie total comes to **460** calories.

Make it into fish pie, mixed with 150ml (¼pint) cheese sauce, topped with 113g (4oz) mashed potato and the calories total **645**.

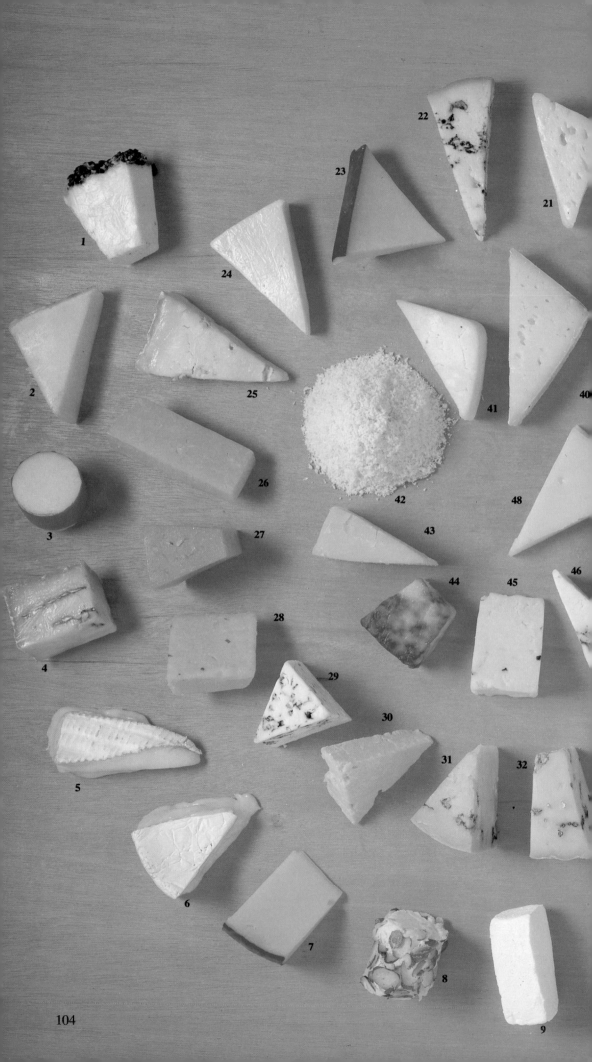

The cheese-eater's guide

Pictured here are precise 28g (1oz) portions of a selection of popular English and continental cheeses, together with their calorie values. A small piece of cheese often provides quite a lot of calories and, as you can see, it is not a 'safe' food which can be nibbled between dieting meals without counting the calorie cost.

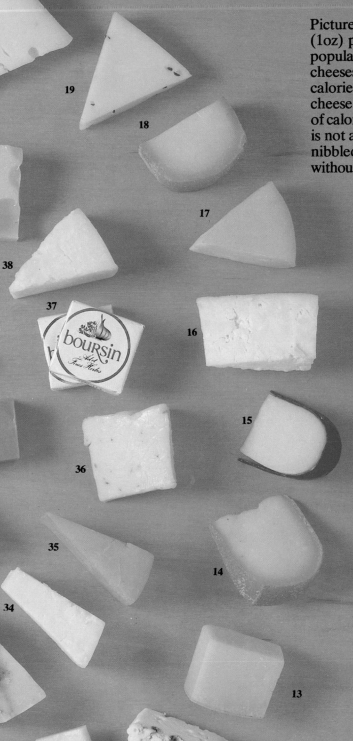

#	Cheese	Calories
1	Tôme au raisin	74
2	Bel Paese	96
3	Austrian smoked	78
4	Bresse bleu	80
5	Brie	88
6	Camembert	88
7	Edam	88
8	Orangerulle	92
9	Philadelphia	90
10	Rambol with walnuts	117
11	Jarlsberg	95
12	Roquefort	88
13	Gouda	100
14	Port salut	94
15	Babybel	97
16	White Stilton	96
17	Bonbel	102
18	St Paulin	98
19	Danbo	98
20	Danish Mozzarella	98
21	Danish Esrom	98
22	Danish Mycella	99
23	Danish Elbo	98
24	Danish Samsoe	98
25	Dolcellata	100
26	Double Gloucester	105
27	Leicester	105
28	Cotswold	105
29	Danish blue	103
30	Cheshire	110
31	Blue Cheshire	115
32	Gorgonzola	112
33	Sage Derby	112
34	Lancashire	109
35	Orkney Claymore	111
36	Ilchester	112
37	Boursin	116
38	Wensleydale	115
39	Emmenthal	113
40	Danish Havarti	117
41	Caerphilly	120
42	Parmesan	118
43	Cheddar	120
44	Red Windsor	119
45	Cheviot	120
46	Blue Stilton	131
47	Norwegian Gjeost	133
48	Gruyère	132

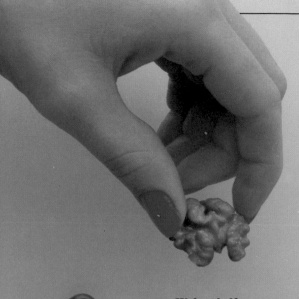

Piece of peanut brittle
50 calories

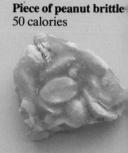

Walnut half
15 calories

Brazil nut
20 calories

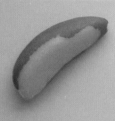

Chocolate peanut
5 calories

Sugared almond
15 calories

Triangle of nut chocolate
30 calories

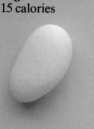

Chocolate hazelnut whirl
40 calories

Chopped mixed nuts
per 5ml (1 level teaspoon)
10 calories

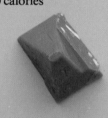

Monkey nut
10 calories

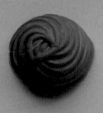

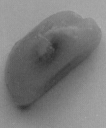

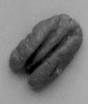

Almond
10 calories

Buttered Brazil
40 calories

Pecan nut (salted)
15 calories

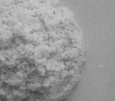

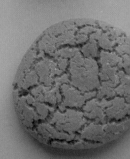

Pistachio nut
5 calories

Piece of coconut ice
110 calories

Macaroon
25 calories

Ground almonds
per 5ml (1 level teaspoon)
10 calories

The nut-eater's guide

shew nut (salted)
calories

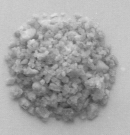

Chestnut
10 calories

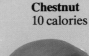

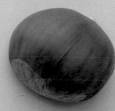

Roasted salted peanut
5 calories

Crunchy nut topping
per 5ml (1 level teaspoon)
10 calories

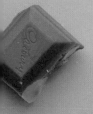

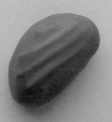

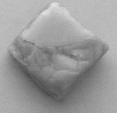

Macadamia nut
10 calories

iccated coconut
5ml (1 level teaspoon)
alories

Chocolate Brazil
55 calories

Piece of nut toffee
40 calories

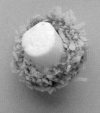

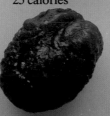

Chocolate almond
15 calories

Coconut mushroom
25 calories

are wholenut chocolate
alories

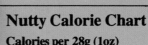

Hazelnut
5 calories

Marron glacé
45 calories

Maple Brazil
60 calories

Nutty Calorie Chart

Calories per 28g (1oz)

Almonds	160
Barcelona nuts	181
Brazil nuts	176
Cashew nuts	160
Chestnuts	48
Coconut - desiccated	172
Coconut - fresh	100
Hazelnuts	108
Monkeynuts	112
Peanut butter	175
Peanuts - roasted	168
Walnuts	149

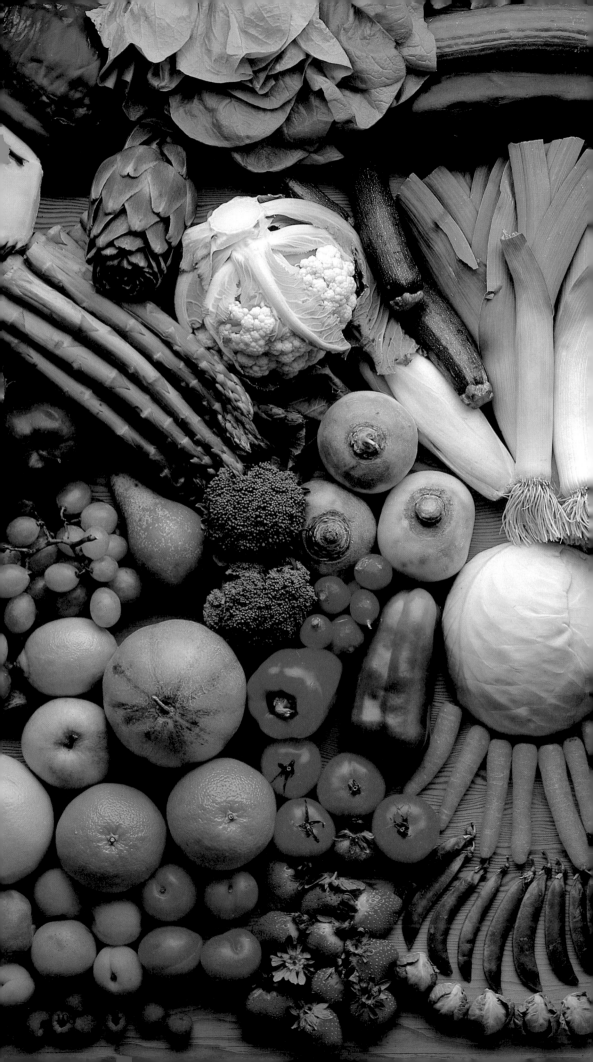

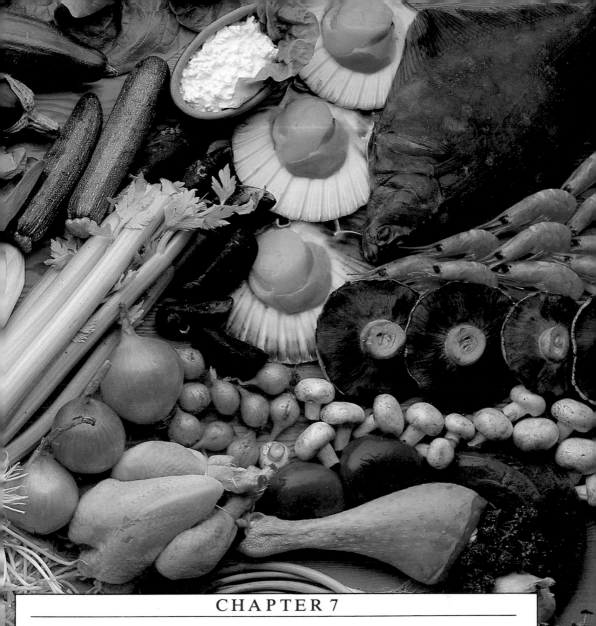

CHAPTER 7

Six diets to
suit your lifestyle

The diet that achieves the fastest weight loss is the one to which you can keep, and the diet you follow accurately is usually the one that proves easiest for you to fit into your normal lifestyle. Choose any of these six diets, keep to all the rules, and you are bound to lose weight. The *Indulgence diet* will appeal to anyone who cannot keep to a diet unless they have an occasional treat or feel deprived without an alcoholic drink or two. The *Little and often diet* will suit all nibblers and will speed up your metabolic rate fractionally. The *Do as you're told diet* guarantees success because it tells you precisely what to eat. The *Super healthy diet* includes all the foods that nutritional experts recommend for good health. The *1,000 calories diet* is ideal for anyone who has only a little weight to lose and allows you to choose your own pattern of eating. The *Low-fat diet* is based on the revolutionary method pioneered by *Slimming Magazine* which cuts calories by cutting fats. All these diets may be followed for as long as you wish to achieve your ideal weight. Read on and choose the diet that is best for you.

All foods supply us with calories, simply another word for energy, and nearly all foods contain at least some of the nutrients that restore body tissue and are essential for the maintenance of good health. In modern Western society, few people go short of calories and many are overweight as a consequence of consuming far too many calories, which are stored by the body in the form of surplus fat.

Nutritional deficiencies are not prevalent in the West as, by eating generous amounts of a variety of foods, most people take in all the nutrients they need. However, when you are trying to eat less in order to shed weight, a little more care is needed to ensure that you get an adequate supply of vitamins, minerals and protein.

Nutritional requirements are usually stated in daily terms because these happen to be the most convenient and easily understood way of expressing them. In fact, the body can store all nutrients and none is needed specifically on a daily basis. Thus, if you ate a large amount of fresh fruit and vegetables on Monday, there is no need to worry if you eat less of them on Tuesday and Wednesday. Some vitamins can be stored in the body for longer periods than others — Vitamin A, for instance, which is found mainly in dairy products and green vegetables and helps to protect the body against infection, especially the bronchial tubes and body cavities. If you have been consuming foods containing generous amounts of this vitamin, then it is unlikely that your body will run out of it. It would be difficult to choose a diet that did not contain some Vitamin A.

The body stores Vitamin C for a shorter period but it would still take several weeks, or even months, to deplete your stores and for your body to show signs of deficiency. If you eat three oranges or grapefruits, or just one can of frozen orange or grapefruit concentrate, in a week, your full Vitamin C requirement is ensured, even if you consume it all in one day.

How important is protein? If we eliminated protein from our diet completely, we would not survive for very long. Protein is the major component of human flesh and we lose tiny particles of skin all the time. This continual protein loss must be replaced in order to build up new body cells. It is not easy, however, to pinpoint the perfect daily dose. The minimum intake that will safeguard the average person from this protein deficiency has been reduced steadily over the years. As scientists' knowledge of the human body and its functioning increases, they can define its needs more accurately; but they prefer to over-estimate what a body needs rather than set the recommended dose too low. As a general rule, 300ml (½ pint) of milk and a portion of fish, meat or cheese each day will supply your minimum protein requirement. Thus, at least 10 per cent of your total daily calorie intake should consist of protein foods.

Some misguided people seem to believe that a high protein diet contains practically no calories but, like any other food substance, protein provides calories — in fact, as many as carbohydrates, compared weight for weight. You can grow as fat from eating an excess of high-protein foods as you can from consuming too much starch.

The easiest way to ensure that your diet contains all the essential nutrients is to choose one of the set diets included in this book. They have been designed to supply all the vitamins, minerals and protein you need for a healthy, and balanced diet. If you use the calorie charts at the back of the book to make up your own menus, follow the basic rule to vary meals each day, and include some fresh fruit, vegetables and protein-containing foods, such as chicken, lean meat (including liver and kidney), white fish, eggs, cottage cheese and skimmed milk in your weekly diet. Whole-grain cereal foods will provide the fibre that you need to prevent constipation and digestive problems. If you are vegetarian, be sure to include some brown rice, lentils, beans or peas in your menus — all these foods contain protein.

The following diets have been formulated to fit into a number of different lifestyles, so the best one for you is the one that you can most easily keep to. Some people, especially housewives, will find that three regular meals a day provide their best dieting method. Others may discover that dieting is easier if they follow a completely different eating pattern. In fact, altering your meal times and adopting a less rigid, or different, pattern of eating can help to achieve long-term weight control. People usually eat their three meals at regular times every day whether they feel hungry or otherwise. They may be tempted also to nibble at snacks between meals when they have a craving to eat. It is doubtful if your health will suffer if you take longer breaks between meals or change your habitual breakfast, lunch and dinner pattern.

Snack-eating urges can be enormously strong and hard to resist. Advice on weight control tends to focus on urging people to use their willpower to be strong and to resist eating what they most want to eat at times when they most want to eat it. The growing weight problems of the Western world suggest that this kind of advice has not been wholly successful. Instead of eating out of habit at times when you do not feel compelled to eat, try eating only when you really do experience a great eating urge. If you do not feel hungry at breakfast but often feel the need to eat a snack in the evening, skip breakfast and have a late snack instead.

There is a widely-held belief that food eaten in the evening is more likely to turn into surplus fat than food that is eaten earlier in the day. This seems to have arisen from the notion that if you do not exercise after eating you do not burn up the calories and they are stored by the body as fat. The truth is that the average woman uses up about one-third of her daily calorie intake in physical activity. The body burns up the remaining two-thirds during its necessary maintenance processes, which include such things as breathing, circulating the blood and keeping up body temperature. In this way, you burn up approximately one calorie a minute in order to keep alive.

After you eat a meal your metabolism does speed up for an hour or so and burns up food more quickly. If you were to eat four or five small meals throughout the day, such as the ones suggested in our *Little and often diet*, you would benefit from the four or five hours when your metabolism is working much harder to burn up calories. Moreover, if you exercise within an hour after a meal your metabolism speeds up even more. Therefore, if you were to eat during the earlier, more active part of the day, your body is more likely to be in a state of high-calorie burn-up. But is the calorie difference in eating early or late sufficiently valuable for you to change your pattern of eating? On the current evidence, it seems doubtful that the weight-losing advantages of eating often and earlier in the day are great enough to offset the late-evening willpower collapse that so often results in an illicit slice of cake or a T.V. snack. If you find that saving most of your calories for the evening is the surest way of keeping to your 1,000 or 1,500 calories target for the day, then we recommend that you continue dieting in this way. You will shed weight, however you eat those calories, whether it be early or late in the day.

When you follow one of the recommended diets, remember that there is no need to eat every single calorie each day. If you eat less food on any easy-to-diet day, you can 'bank' some of the left-over items of food for the next day, when your mood and circumstances may make it harder to keep to your allotted food allowance. Provided that your food intake averages out right, you will lose the same amount of weight, and you may even find that you do not need those extra calories tomorrow and thus manage to reduce your calorie intake even more.

If you have over 12.7kg (2st) to lose, you will shed weight on any of the following diets, but a 1,500 calories regime, such as the *Indulgence diet*, will help you to change your eating habits without feeling deprived. The amount of weight you lose will depend on how accurately you stick to the diet, how overweight you are and for how long you have been dieting. Set yourself some small weight-loss goals because you will not see enormous changes immediately. Successful weight loss takes time, patience and perseverance. Setting goals that are too large only leads to a feeling of despair if you fail to achieve them. A reasonable weight loss would be 1kg (2lb) a week, although heavily overweight people often lose more than this, particularly in the first week. Take advantage of those days when you can follow your chosen diet without temptation, and save some of your calorie allowance for the more difficult days when you slip up and have an eating binge. Remember that this does not signal the end of the diet; instead, switch to a strict 1,000 calories regime, such as the *Do as you're told diet*, for a few days to make up the damage.

When you have only a little to lose, do not expect the last stubborn flab to melt away at lightning speed. Unlike the very overweight person, who may lose 3.5kg (7lb) in the week she starts dieting, you are not likely to lose more than 1kg (2lb), maybe as little as ½kg (1lb). Aim for a steady and consistent loss; at this stage, it is best to resolve to get rid of a little fat as quickly as possible, and therefore you cannot afford the odd week of self-indulgence. Resist the temptation to jump on the scales every day, for, with a slower rate of loss, you might get the disconcerting impression that you are hardly shedding anything at all. You will need the strictest calorie control and should choose one of our 1,000 calories a day diets.

Whatever quantity of weight you want to lose, it will help to strengthen your diet with extra exercise (see the section on *Stepping up the calories you burn*). Exercise not only makes you feel better, but it also alleviates boredom and enriches your general lifestyle, which makes even a strict diet easier to follow.

Never shop on an empty stomach; go prepared with a shopping list and stick to it, no matter how tempted you are to stray from it. Never enter a food shop when you are feeling the least bit hungry.

Check your eating behaviour, too; some psychological research suggests that you should always eat in the same room, always sit down to eat, avoid eating alone and never leave the tastiest morsel of food on the plate until last!

In the introductions to each of the following diets, we describe why we believe they will help you to lose weight in the easiest and fastest way possible.

The indulgence diet
(1,500 calories)

All men and the majority of women will lose weight on this diet. It is particularly suitable if you are more than 12kg (2st) overweight and are just starting out on your weight loss campaign.

The basic daily diet, which consists of breakfast, a light meal, a main meal and a milk allowance for drinks, adds up to 1,250 calories. To this, you can add a daily 'treat' amounting to 250 calories, providing you with a daily total of 1,500 calories. So, if you sometimes crave a sweet or stodgy treat, or feel deprived without a daily alcoholic drink, this is the diet to choose. If there is a special celebration coming up, you can save up your treats and have them all at once. However, do not spend your treats with the thought that you will cut down on your allowance afterwards to compensate for these extra calories. Keep your treats for your most vulnerable moments, such as the coffee break at work, meeting friends in the pub, or for when you are sitting watching television in the evening.

As a general rule, the more overweight you are the more rapidly you will shed weight on 1,500 calories a day. If you find that your weight loss is slowing down after a time, you can speed it up again by going without your daily treat. Or you could try missing your breakfast and having your treat as a mid-morning snack. This diet allows you to indulge a little in the foods you crave most, which is why we call it the 'indulgence diet'.

Unlimited vegetables

The following vegetables are very low in calories and can be eaten freely with the light and main meals in this diet. Fats, such as butter, margarine or oil, must not be used in cooking or added before serving.

Asparagus	Jerusalem artichokes
Aubergines	Leeks
Bean sprouts	Lettuce
Beetroots	Marrow
Broccoli	Mustard and cress
Brussels sprouts	Onions
Cabbage, all kinds	Peppers (capsicums),
Carrots	green or red
Cauliflower	Radishes
Celeriac	Runner beans
Celery	Salsify
Chicory	Sea-kale
Chinese leaves	Spinach
Courgettes	Spring greens
Cucumbers	Spring onions
Endives	Swedes
Fennel	Tomatoes
French beans	Turnips
Gherkins	Watercress
Globe artichokes	

Breakfasts (200 calories)

Fruit Juice and Breakfast Cereal
150ml (¼ pint) unsweetened orange juice
25g (1oz) any breakfast cereal
5ml (1 level teaspoon) sugar
75ml (3fl oz) skimmed milk, additional to allowance

Boiled Egg and Toast
1 medium egg (size 3), boiled
1 large, thin slice wholemeal bread (40g/1½oz), toasted
7g (¼ oz) low-fat spread

Cornish Crumble: turn to the step-by-step recipe for this delicious slimming dish

Diet rules

1 You are allowed three meals a day: *one* breakfast, *one* light meal and *one* main meal. In addition, you are allowed *one* 'treat'. These meals may be eaten at any time of the day and in any order. It is advisable to keep the 'treat' for that time of the day when your willpower is at its lowest.

2 You are allowed 284ml (½pint) pasteurized milk *or* 375ml (⅔pint) semi-skimmed milk *or* 568ml (1pint) skimmed milk each day, for use in drinks of tea and coffee. Tea and coffee may be drunk freely, provided that your milk allowance is not exceeded, and that artificial sweeteners are used instead of sugar. If you really cannot exist without sugar in your tea and coffee, we have allowed a small amount as one of your daily treats. Water, including the bottled kind, and drinks labelled 'low-calorie' are unrestricted.

3 Vary your choice of meals each day to provide a balanced diet, but remember to choose only one meal from each section.

4 Plan your daily meals ahead to make sure that you have the right foods available when you need them. Buy any 'treats', but only on the day you intend to eat them.

5 If your weight loss slows down and you still have weight to lose, omit the daily 'treat'.

6 All foods must be weighed and measured accurately. Do *not* be tempted to guess, as the eye is always more generous than the scales! However, it is not necessary to weigh the low calorie vegetables (above right).

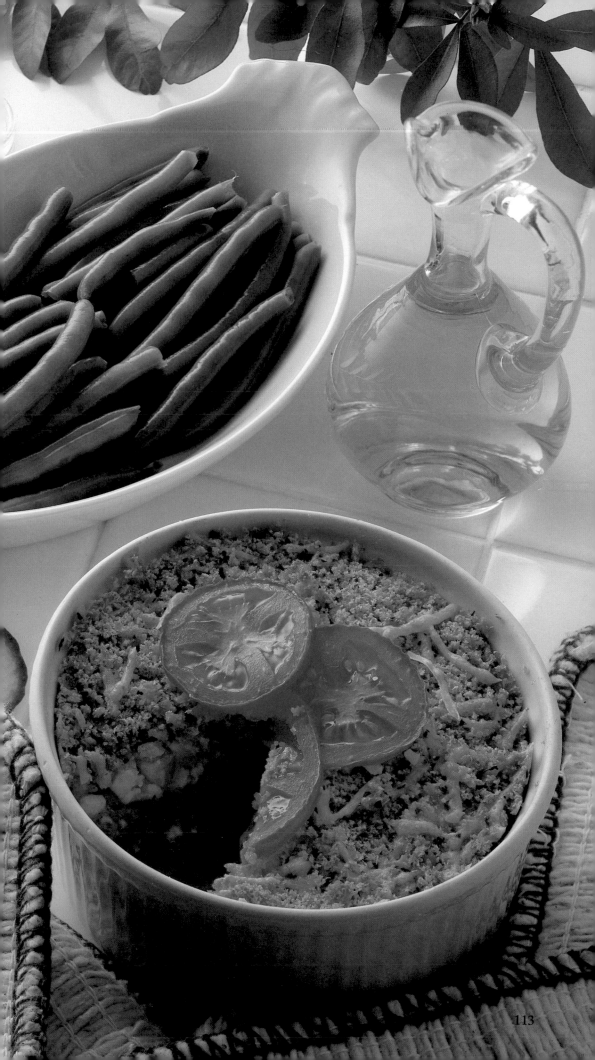

Scrambled Egg and Cheese on Toast
1 medium egg (size 3), scrambled with
50g (2 oz) cottage cheese, and served on
1 small, thin slice bread (25g/1oz), toasted

Bacon and Egg
2 rashers streaky bacon, well grilled
1 medium egg (size 3), poached
1 crispbread

Banana and Yogurt
1 medium banana (175g/6oz), sliced and
*   mixed with*
1 small carton low-fat natural yogurt and
10ml (2 level teaspoons) honey

Grapefruit, Toast and Marmalade
½ grapefruit
5ml (1 level teaspoon) sugar
2 small slices bread (25g/1oz each), toasted
10ml (2 level teaspoons) marmalade or jam

Smoked Haddock and Tomato
125g (4oz) smoked haddock (or other
*   smoked fish), poached in water*
1 tomato, sliced
1 small slice wholemeal bread (25g/1oz)
3.5g (⅛ oz) low-fat spread

Light meals (350 calories)

Note: Do not butter bread unless stated

Meat Meals
Sausage and Bacon
2 pork chipolatas (or other small sausages),
*   well grilled*
2 rashers back bacon, well grilled
2 tomatoes, grilled, without fat
1 small slice slimmers' bread

Liver Pâté and Salad Double-Decker Sandwich (Fruit)
3 small slices wholemeal bread
*   (25g/1oz each), first layer filled with*
25g (1 oz) sliced liver sausage
Slices of onion, second layer spread with
7g (¼ oz) low-fat spread and filled with
Sliced tomato and
Sliced cucumber
1 medium eating apple

Corned Beef and Coleslaw (Fruit)
75g (3 oz) sliced corned beef, served with
*   coleslaw made from*
125g (4 oz) shredded white cabbage
50g (2 oz) grated carrot
15ml (1 tablespoon) finely chopped onion
15ml (1 tablespoon) low-calorie salad cream
2 crispbreads, spread with
7g (¼oz) low-fat spread
1 small orange

Orange Juice and Bacon Sandwich
125ml (4 fl oz) unsweetened orange juice
2 small slices wholemeal bread
*   (25g/1oz each), filled with*
2 rashers back bacon, well grilled and
15ml (1 tablespoon) tomato ketchup or
*   brown sauce (optional)*

Grilled Chicken and Salad
225g (8oz) chicken joint, grilled without
*   added fat and skin removed*
Salad vegetables from list, dressed with
15ml (1 tablespoon) low-calorie salad cream
1 large, thin slice wholemeal bread
*   (40g/1½ oz), spread with*
7g (¼oz) low-fat spread

Beefburgers with Baked Beans
2 frozen beefburgers (50g/2oz each), well
*   grilled*
2 tomatoes, grilled without fat
225g (8 oz) canned baked beans

Ham Salad (Fruit)
50g (2 oz) sliced, cooked lean ham with all
*   fat removed*
30ml (2 tablespoons) piccalilli
Salad vegetables from unlimited list
1 small packet potato crisps
1 medium orange or pear

Egg Meals
Egg and Carrot Sandwich (Fruit)
2 small slices wholemeal bread
*   (25g/1 oz each), filled with*
15g (½oz) low-fat spread
1 large egg (size 2), hard-boiled
1 carrot, grated and
15ml (1 level tablespoon) low-calorie salad
*   cream*
1 large eating apple

Cheese Omelet
2 medium eggs (size 4), beaten with
30ml (2 tablespoons) water, then fried in
7g (¼oz) low-fat spread, and filled with
25g (1 oz) grated Cheddar cheese,
Salad vegetables from unlimited list
125ml (4floz) tomato juice

Florentine Eggs
2 medium eggs (size 4), poached, served on
125g (4oz) boiled, chopped spinach, coated
*   with*
Half small carton low-fat natural yogurt,
*   mixed with*
15ml (1 tablespoon) tomato ketchup,
*   covered with*
25g (1oz) grated Edam cheese, and browned
*   under grill*
Vegetables from unlimited list

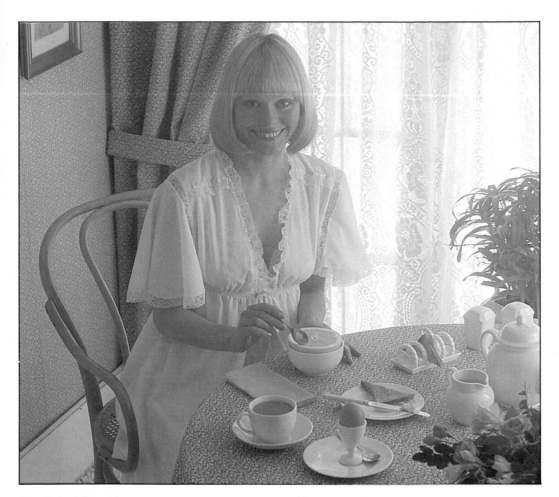

Egg Salad (Fruit)
2 medium eggs (size 4), hard-boiled
Salad vegetables from list, dressed with
30ml (2 level tablespoons) low-calorie salad
    cream
2 crispreads spread with
7g (¼oz) low-fat spread
75g (3oz) grapes

Fish meals
Fish Fingers and Baked Beans (Fruit)
4 frozen fish fingers (cod or any firm-fleshed
    white fish), grilled without fat
125g (4 oz) canned baked beans in tomato
    sauce
1 medium apple, orange or pear

Sardines on Toast
120g (4¼oz) canned sardines in tomato sauce
1 large, thin slice bread (40g/1½oz), toasted
2 tomatoes, grilled without fat.

Grilled Kipper
175g (6oz) kipper, grilled without added fat
1 small slice wholemeal bread (25g/1 oz)

Salmon Salad
99g (3½ oz) canned salmon
Salad vegetables from list, dressed with
15ml (1 tablespoon) low-calorie salad cream
1 large, slice bread (40g/1½ oz), spread with
7g (¼ oz) low-fat spread

Cheese Meals
Cheese and Pickle Toasty (Fruit)
1 large, thin slice bread (40g/1½oz), toasted
    and spread with
15ml (1 tablespoon) pickle, topped with
40g (1½ oz) grated Cheddar cheese
1 medium orange or pear

Cottage Cheese Salad (Fruit)
113g (4oz) cottage cheese
Salad vegetables from list, dressed with
l5ml (1 tablespoon) low-calorie salad cream
1 large, slice bread (40g/1½oz), spread with
7g (¼ oz) low-fat spread
1 large eating apple

Cheese and Tomato Sandwiches
2 large, thin slices wholemeal bread
    (40g/1½oz each), spread with
15ml (1 tablespoon) low-calorie salad cream,
    and filled with
40g (1½oz) Edam cheese
1 tomato, sliced, and
Sprigs of watercress

Cheesy Baked Potato (Fruit)
175g (6oz) jacket-baked potato, centre
    scooped out and mixed with
25g (1oz) grated Cheddar cheese, piled back
    in jacket and reheated
Vegetables from unlimited list
1 medium eating apple

Main meals (500 calories)

Fish and Cheese Pie

125g (4oz) haddock (or any firm-fleshed
white fish)
15ml (1 level tablespoon) cornflour
60ml (4 tablespoons) skimmed milk
60ml (4 tablespoons) dry cider or white wine
40g (1½oz) Edam cheese, grated
50g (2oz) canned pimento, drained and sliced
Dash Worcestershire sauce
Salt and pepper
175g (6oz) boiled potato mashed with
45ml (3 tablespoons) skimmed milk
1 tomato

Poach the fish, then drain and flake. Blend the cornflour with the skimmed milk and cider or wine. Heat it in a small pan until thickened, stirring continuously. Add the fish, cheese, pimento, Worcestershire sauce and seasoning. Spoon into an ovenproof dish. Spoon the mashed potato over the top. Bake at 180°C, 350°F, gas mark 4, for 30 minutes. Garnish with the sliced tomato.

Chicken Casserole with Rice (Fruit)

225g (8oz) chicken joint
1 small onion, sliced
½ small green pepper (capsicum),sliced
1 carrot, sliced
50g (2oz) button mushrooms, halved
Salt and pepper
200ml (7floz) chicken stock
5ml (1 level teaspoon) cornflour
25g (1oz) long-grain rice
75g (3oz) frozen mixed peas, sweetcorn and
peppers (capsicums)
1 large banana (198g/7oz) or 1 orange and 1
eating apple

Put all the ingredients except the cornflour in an ovenproof casserole. Cover and cook at 190°C, 375°F, gas mark 5, for 45 minutes or until the chicken is tender. Blend the cornflour with a little cold water. Stir into the casserole to thicken. Boil the rice until tender and cook the mixed vegetables, then drain and mix them together. Serve the chicken casserole with the vegetable rice, and follow with the banana or the orange and apple.

Smoked Haddock Kedgeree (Fruit)

40g (1½oz) long-grain rice
175g (6oz) smoked haddock
(or other smoked fish)
7g (¼oz) low-fat spread
Squeeze lemon juice
5ml (1 teaspoon) chopped parsley
1 medium egg (size 4),hard-boiled and sliced
1 tomato, sliced
1 large eating apple

Boil the rice until just tender, then drain. Poach the fish, then drain and flake. Mix the rice, fish, low-fat spread, lemon juice and parsley together. Serve topped with the sliced egg and tomato. Complete the meal with the apple

Baked White Fish

275ml (½pint) mushroom soup made up
from a packet
1 small, thin slice bread (25g/1oz)
175g (6oz) cod, coley, haddock
(or any firm-fleshed white fish)
1 small onion, sliced
50g (2oz) mushrooms, sliced
15ml (1 tablespoon) lemon juice
125g (4oz) frozen mixed peas, sweetcorn and
peppers (capsicums)
175g (6oz) boiled or canned new potatoes

Place the fish on a piece of foil, cover with sliced onion and mushrooms and sprinkle over the lemon juice. Wrap the foil around the fish and bake at 180°C, 350°F, gas mark 4, for about 30 minutes, or until the fish and vegetables are tender. Serve the soup and bread first, then follow with the baked fish and vegetables.

Stir Fried Chicken *(opposite)*

125g (4oz) raw chicken meat
1 small onion
1 leek, or 4 spring onions
125g (4oz) button mushrooms
125g (4oz) fresh bean sprouts
15ml (1 tablespoon) vegetable oil
15ml (1 tablespoon) soy sauce
15ml (1 tablespoon) dry sherry (optional)
Salt and pepper
1 small carton fruit yogurt

1 Cut the chicken meat into bite-sized pieces, removing all the skin.
2 Finely chop the onion, slice the leek or spring onions, and slice the mushrooms thinly. Wash the bean sprouts.
3 Heat the oil in a frying pan and add the chopped onion and sliced leek or spring onions. Fry over medium heat for about 2 minutes, stirring continuously. Add the chicken and stir-fry for about 5 minutes, until the chicken is cooked and the vegetables are tender but still crisp. Add the mushrooms and stir-fry for 2 minutes.
4 Add the bean sprouts, soy sauce and the sherry, and stir-fry briskly for another 2-3 minutes. Season with the salt and pepper.
5 Serve immediately while the dish is still hot and follow with the fruit yogurt.

Serves 1

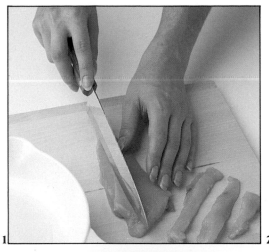

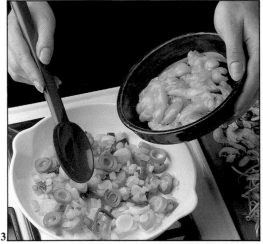

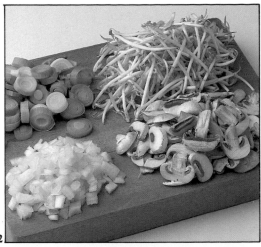

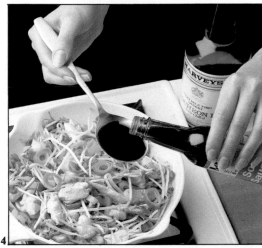

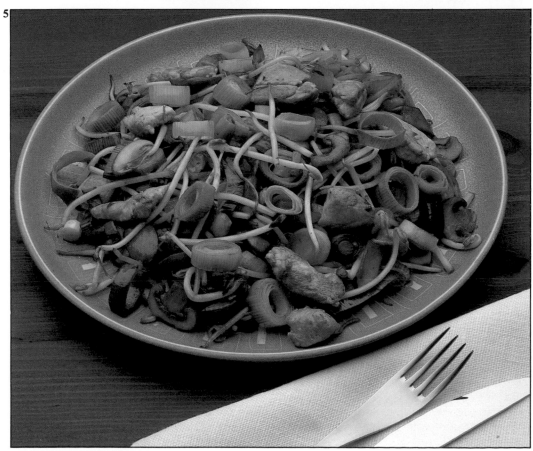

Baked Chicken and Jacket-baked Potato

225g (8oz) chicken joint
175g (6oz) potato
15g (½oz) low-fat spread
Green vegetables from unlimited list
2 crispbreads
15g (½oz) cheese spread portion

Bake the chicken wrapped in foil and the scrubbed potato at 200°C, 400°F, gas mark 6, for 45 minutes. Remove and discard the skin from the chicken joint and serve with the baked potato topped with the low-fat spread and with some green vegetables. Complete the meal with the crispbreads spread with cheese.

Roast Dinner (Ice-cream)

75g (3oz) lean roast beef or leg of lamb or
pork or 125g (4oz) roast chicken
45ml (3 tablespoons) thin, fat-free gravy
125g (4oz) roast potatoes
Boiled vegetables from unlimited list
50g (2oz) portion vanilla ice-cream

Cut off and discard any fat from the roast beef, lamb or pork or remove the skin from the chicken. Serve the roast meat with the gravy and vegetables. Complete the meal with the ice-cream.

Steak and Salad (Cheese)

125ml (4floz) unsweetened orange or
grapefruit juice
175g (6oz) steak, grilled and fat removed
Salad vegetables from unlimited list,
dressed with
15ml (1 tablespoon) oil-free French dressing
2 crispbreads
25g (1oz) Edam cheese

Serve the steak with the salad. Complete the meal with the crispbreads and cheese.

Savoury Mince (Cheese)

125g (4oz) minced beef
1 small onion, chopped
225g (8oz) canned tomatoes
50g (2oz) mushrooms, sliced
Salt and pepper
Pinch mixed herbs
50g (2oz) long-grain rice or spaghetti
1 crispbread
15g (½oz) Edam cheese or 15g (½oz)
cheese spread portion

Fry the minced beef in a pan until well browned, drain and discard the fat. Add the onion, tomatoes, mushrooms, seasoning and herbs. Cover and cook for 20 minutes. Boil the rice or spaghetti until tender and drain. Serve the savoury mince with the rice or spaghetti. Complete the meal with the crispbread and cheese.

Herring in Cider (Cheese)

175g (6oz) herring, (or any oily fish),cleaned
1 small onion, sliced
125ml (4floz) dry cider
Salad vegetables from unlimited list
2 cream cracker biscuits
25g (1oz) Cheshire or Lancashire cheese
(or any hard cheese)

Put the herring in an ovenproof dish, add the onion and cider, and cover and bake at 180°C, 350°F, gas mark 4, for 40 minutes. Serve with salad vegetables. Complete the meal with the biscuits and cheese.

Grilled Pork Chop and Apple Sauce (Fruit)

213g (7½oz) pork chop
30ml (2 tablespoons) unsweetened apple sauce
Selection of vegetables from unlimited list
1 medium orange and 1 medium pear

Grill the pork chop until well done. Serve with the apple sauce and a selection of cooked vegetables. Complete the meal with the orange and pear.

Scotch Egg Salad (Fruit)

1 Scotch egg
Salad vegetables from unlimited list,
dressed with
15ml (1 tablespoon) low-calorie salad cream
1 small slice wholemeal bread (25g/1oz),
spread with
7g (¼oz) low-fat spread
1 medium orange

Serve the Scotch egg with a selection of salad vegetables, and the low-calorie salad cream and the bread. Complete the meal with the orange.

Cheese Salad (Fruit)

50g (2oz) Cheddar cheese
Salad vegetables from unlimited list,
dressed with
15ml (1 tablespoon) low-calorie salad cream
2 small slices wholemeal bread
(25g/1oz each), spread with
15g (½oz) low-fat spread
175g (6 oz) slice melon

Serve the cheese with the salad vegetables, low-calorie salad cream and the bread. Start or complete the meal with the melon.

Bacon Steaks and Pineapple

2 bacon steaks (99g/3½oz each)
2 rings canned pineapple in natural juice
125g (4oz)frozen peas
175g (6oz) boiled or canned new potatoes

Grill the bacon steaks until they are cooked thoroughly, then top with the pineapple rings and heat through. Cook the peas and serve with the bacon steaks and potatoes.

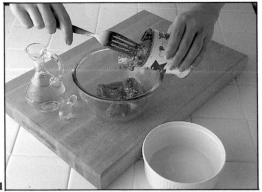
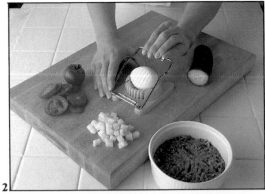
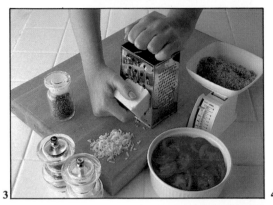
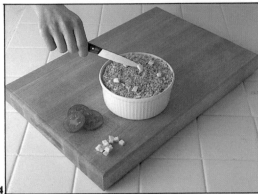
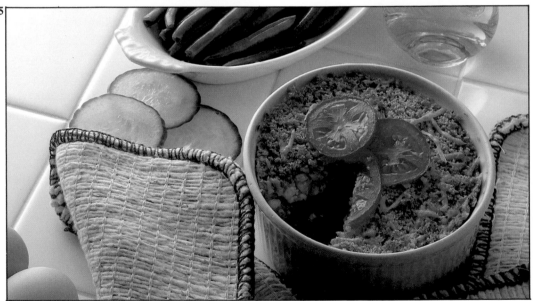

Cornish Crumble

213g (7½oz) pilchards in tomato sauce
15ml (1 tablespoon) wine vinegar
1 medium egg (size 4), hard-boiled
2.5cm (1in) piece cucumber
3 small tomatoes
25g (1oz) dry bread
25g (1oz) strong Cheddar cheese
2.5ml (½ teaspoon) dried basil
Salt and pepper
7g (¼oz) butter
225g (8oz) cooked French beans
125g (4oz) vanilla ice-cream
2 medium (170g/6oz) bananas

1 Drain off the excess tomato sauce from the pilchards and mash them with the wine vinegar. Place in an ovenproof dish.

2 Shell and chop the egg, and peel and dice the cucumber. Slice the tomatoes. Mix the egg and cucumber together and place on top of the pilchard mixture. Cover with the tomatoes, reserving 3 slices for the topping.

3 Crumb the bread in a blender and grate the cheese. Mix together with the basil and seasoning and sprinkle over the dish.

4 Dot the top with butter and arrange the reserved tomato slices on top. Bake at 180°C, 350°F, gas mark 4, for 20 minutes.

5 Serve with the French beans and follow with the ice-cream and bananas.

Serves 2

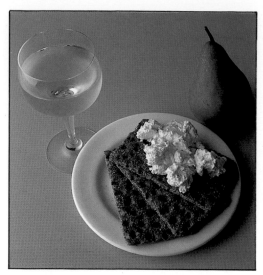

A savoury treat of fruit, cheese and wine.

Mixed Grill

125g (4oz) lamb's liver, sliced
1 lamb's kidney, halved and cored
5ml (1 teaspoon) oil
2 rashers streaky bacon
1 tomato, halved
50g (2oz) mushrooms
Green vegetables from unlimited list
1 medium eating apple

Brush the liver and kidney with the oil and grill with the bacon and tomato until the liver, kidney and tomato are cooked and the bacon is crisp. Serve with the mushrooms, poached in stock or water, and the boiled green vegetables. Complete the meal with the eating apple.

Sausage and Mash

2 large pork sausages
2 tomatoes, halved
175g (6oz) boiled potato, mashed with
45ml (3 tablespoons) skimmed milk
1 medium orange and 1 medium pear

Grill the pork sausages until well cooked, and grill the tomatoes without added fat. Serve with the mashed potato. Complete the meal with the orange and pear.

Treats (250 calories)

Choose one of these each day:

Sweet treats

5 small wholewheat biscuits
4 large wholewheat biscuits
3 chocolate wholewheat biscuits
50g (2oz) sugar (15 level 5ml teaspoons)
125g (4oz) stoned dates
125g (4oz) dried figs
100g (3½oz) currants, raisins *or* sultanas
75g (3oz) fruit flavoured pastilles or jellies
65g (2½oz) wine gums
65g (2½oz) fruit gums
65g (2½oz) boiled or clear fruit sweets

50g (2oz) nougat
50g (2oz) toffees
50g (2oz) assorted filled chocolates
50g (2oz) mint imperials
50g (2oz) popcorn
40g (1½oz) chocolate
2 chocolate covered mini Swiss rolls
1 mince pie
1 chocolate cup cake and 2 Jaffa cakes
312g (11oz) can mandarin oranges and
 25g (1oz) vanilla ice-cream
1 small carton fruit yogurt with 1 large banana
2 small whipped ice-cream cornets
1 chocolate coated ice-cream bar and
 2 medium eating apples
284ml (½pint) chocolate flavoured low-fat
 milk and 1 orange

Savoury and stodgy treats

3 cream cracker biscuits, with 25g (1oz)
 Cheddar cheese and yeast extract
2 small, thin slices bread (25g/1oz each)
 spread with 15g (½oz) low-fat spread
 or 7g (¼oz) butter and 15ml (a slightly
 rounded tablespoon) jam
3 crispbreads, 40g (1½oz) curd cheese, 1 pear
 and 1 glass dry white wine
1 Bath bun with 15g (½oz) low-fat spread
50g (2oz) piece French bread with
 15g (½oz) butter
175g (6oz) jacket-baked potato with
 15g (½oz) butter
2 slices malt loaf (25g/1oz each) spread with
 15g (½oz) low-fat spread and 10ml
 (2 level teaspoons) jam
1 small packet potato crisps, any flavour,
 with 15g (1oz) Edam cheese
50g (1¾ oz) peanuts and raisins
225g (8oz) canned baked beans, or
 213g (7½oz) canned spaghetti in tomato
 sauce on 1 large, thin slice toasted
 wholemeal bread (40g/1½oz)
70g (2½oz) piece rich fruit cake
50g (2oz) steamed sponge pudding with
 45ml (3 tablespoons) custard

Drinks

3 bottles (185ml/6½floz) Coca-Cola
2 bar measures Campari and soda water
80ml (1½pints) light or mild beer or lager
 or 550ml (1pint) home-brewed beer or
 550ml (1pint) stout
550ml (1pint) cider
3 bar measures or small schooner sherry
4 bar measures (25ml/ gill) brandy,
 whisky, gin or rum with water or
 low-calorie mixers
3 (113ml/4floz) glasses dry wine or
 2 glasses sweet wine
3 glasses dry champagne
1 cup drinking chocolate or malted bedtime
 drink made with 186ml (⅓ pint) milk
 additional to allowance and 5ml (1 level
 teaspoon) sugar

Low-fat diet

This simple method of reducing calories by cutting fats has led to a revolutionary new approach to dieting. About 40 per cent of the average person's calories comes from the fats in his or her diet — the cooking and spreading fats like oil, lard, butter and margarine, and the 'invisible' fats that lurk in foods like cheese and chocolate. A sharp decrease in fat intake will lead to an equally sharp reduction in calorie intake, and when this is sufficiently reduced the body sheds its own surplus weight.

The joy of low-fat dieting is that you have only to cut out a small quantity of food in order to save a large number of calories, because all fats are enormously high in calories. For every 28g (1oz) of fat you can eliminate from your daily meals, you reduce your calorie intake by more than 200 calories. When you follow the low-fat dieting method you will find yourself eating the same-sized meals as before, but those meals will supply considerably less calories because you have eliminated the really fattening ingredients — the fats.

It is not always obvious exactly how much fat a food contains, so the experts have devised a method by which all foods are given a simple unit count relating to their fat content.

On the following pages, you will find many food items and drinks listed with their appropriate fat units. To shed surplus weight, you may eat normal quantities of all foods with an '0' rating. Ration all foods that are given a fat unit count of 1 or more so that you do not consume more than 10 units of fat each day. Only these foods need to be accurately weighed and measured.

This is not a totally 'no-fat' diet, as a small amount of fat is necessary for good health. However, if you do not need to use up your 10 fat units a day, you can safely reduce the number to 7.

There are a few fat-free foods and drinks that contain a high sugar or alcohol content. These could easily supply surplus calories and have been given a 'fat unit equivalent' at the end of this diet section. If you wish to include these in your diet just count the equivalent fat units into your daily total of 10. However, to ensure a nutritionally balanced diet, it is advisable to allow no more than 3 equivalent fat units a day.

To achieve a speedy weight loss, be moderate in your portions of non-rationed foods, and vary the foods you eat each day to ensure that you have an adequate intake of all nutrients.

When you reach your target weight, gradually increase the number of fat units until you find the level at which you maintain your weight.

Low-fat diet menus

The following daily menus are designed to help you to plan your allowance of 7 to 10 fat units. These are made up of three meals a day plus one snack. You can eat these meals and the snack in any order you wish during the day. Most of the menus have one sandwich or salad meal which can be packed to take to work or school.

Vegetables can usually be eaten freely, as long as they have been prepared or served without added fat. All fresh raw vegetables, such as carrot sticks, cucumber slices, raw mushrooms, cauliflower florets, slices of red and green pepper (capsicums) and celery sticks, are so low in calories that they can all be nibbled freely between meals without affecting the daily calorie count significantly.

In addition to the stated food on each daily menu, you can allow yourself two pieces of fresh fruit (with the exception of fat-containing avocado pears) or a small glass of unsweetened fruit juice each day.

Use no more than 275ml (½ pint) low-fat milk (skimmed, separated or reconstituted low-fat powdered milk) for drinks each day. Where skimmed milk is listed in a day's menu, for example on breakfast cereal, this is in addition to your allowance for drinks. You can drink unlimited quantities of tea and coffee (either black or with your allowance of skimmed milk and sweetened, if necessary, with artificial sweeteners). All drinks with a negligible calorie value can be consumed freely. These include tap or bottled water, squashes, bottled and canned drinks with a 'low-calorie' label, and beefy or yeast extract drinks.

If you find it difficult to give up alcohol, you can replace the daily snack with one glass of sherry, wine, whisky, gin or vodka (with low-calorie mixers) or 275ml (½ pint) beer or cider each day. Remember that most alcoholic drinks are high in fat units.

Menu 1 *9 fat units*

Light Meal 1   *1 fat unit*
Fruit Muesli

25g (1oz) muesli, served with
1 small carton natural yogurt, and
1 orange, segmented

Light Meal 2   *2½ fat units*

Mock Pizza

1 small, thin slice white or brown bread
*   (25g/1oz)*
1 tomato, sliced
Salt and pepper
Pinch dried mixed herbs or basil
25g (1oz) Edam cheese, grated
1 stuffed olive (optional)
Salad vegetables
15ml (1 tablespoon) oil-free French dressing

Toast the bread on one side. Cover the untoasted side with the sliced tomato, and season with salt and pepper. Sprinkle with herbs and cover with the grated cheese. Arrange the sliced olive on top, if liked. Cook under a moderate grill until the cheese melts. Serve with a dressed salad.

Main Meal   *4½ fat units*

Roast Chicken and Vegetables (Fruit)

75g (3oz) roast chicken (skin removed)
Fat-free gravy
150g (5oz) roast potatoes, large chunks
Green or root vegetables
220g (7¾oz) canned fruit in low-calorie syrup
15ml (1 tablespoon) evaporated milk

Serve the chicken with the gravy and cooked vegetables. Follow with the canned fruit and evaporated milk.

Snack   *1 fat unit*

2 small plain biscuits

Menu 2   *9½ fat units*

Light Meal 1 *1½ fat units*

Fruity Cereal

50g (2oz) bran breakfast cereal, served with
125ml (4floz) skimmed milk, and
15ml (1 level teaspoon) raisins or sultanas

Light Meal 2   *4 fat units*

Cauliflower, Kidney Bean and Sausage Salad
(Fresh Fruit)

2 pork chipolatas, well grilled
125g (4oz) fresh cauliflower
75g (3oz) canned kidney beans, drained
2 or 3 spring onions
30-45ml (2-3 tablespoons) oil-free French
*   dressing*
1 eating apple or orange

Cool and slice the grilled sausages. Break the cauliflower into small pieces and place in a bowl with the kidney beans. Chop the spring onions and add them to the bowl with the sausages and dressing. Toss well and leave to stand for 30 minutes before serving. Follow with the fresh fruit.

Main Meal   *3½ fat units*

Tangy Pork with Noodles (Stewed Apple)

See step-by-step opposite page
1 small onion
50g (2oz) button mushrooms
125g (4oz) pork fillet
7g (¼oz) low-fat spread
1.25g (¼ teaspoon) dried thyme
Salt and pepper
5ml (1 teaspoon) flour
30ml (2 tablespoons) chicken stock made
*   with*
¼ chicken stock cube
30ml (2 tablespoons) lemon juice
30ml (2 tablespoons) low-fat natural yogurt
25g (1oz) noodles
1 slice lemon
Parsley to garnish
Green salad vegetables
Stewed apple sweetened with
Sugar-free sweetener
30ml (2 tablespoons) natural yogurt

1 Chop the onion finely and slice the button mushrooms. Trim off all the fat from the pork. Cut the meat into bite-sized pieces.
2 Heat the low-fat spread in a pan and sauté the onion over a very low heat until soft and translucent. Add the pork, mushrooms, dried thyme and seasoning. Cover the pan and cook for 10 minutes until tender, stirring occasionally.
3 Sieve the flour over the meat mixture in the pan. Stir well until all the flour is blended with the pan juices and cook for 1 minute. Add the chicken stock and lemon juice and bring the mixture to the boil.
4 Turn the heat down very low and gently stir in the yogurt. Heat through, stirring, taking care that the mixture does not boil, or it will curdle. Meanwhile, boil the noodles until tender.
5 Arrange the Tangy Pork mixture and the noodles on a serving dish and garnish with lemon and parsley. Serve with a green salad, and follow with the stewed apple and yogurt.
Serves 1

Snack   *½ fat unit*

Cottage Cheese Sandwich

2 small, thin slices slimmers' bread, filled
*   with*
25g (1oz) cottage cheese.

Menu 3   *10 fat units*

Light Meal 1   *3 fat units*

Grapefruit, Egg and Bread

½ grapefruit (no sugar)
1 medium egg (size 3), boiled
2 slices slimmers' bread, spread with
7g (¼oz) low-fat spread

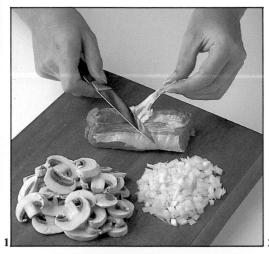

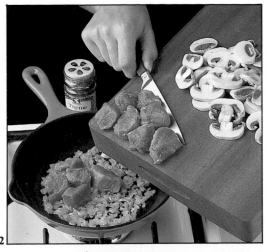

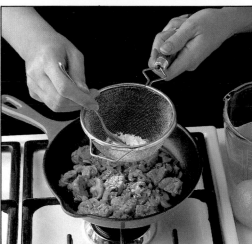

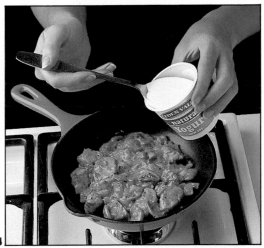

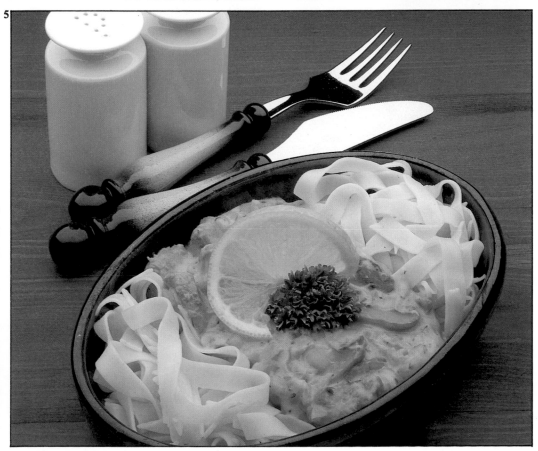

Light Meal 2   *4½ fat units*

Sausages and Beans (Fruit)

2 pork chipolata sausages, well grilled
220g (7¾oz) canned baked beans
1 eating apple

Main Meal   *2 fat units*

Fish Fillets with Vegetables

175-200g (6-7oz) cod or haddock fillets,
*   brushed with*
7g (¼oz) low-fat spread, and grilled
Boiled green vegetables

Flaked Rice with Pineapple

45ml (3 level tablespoons) flaked rice
150ml (¼pint) skimmed milk
5ml (1 level teaspoon) sugar
1 canned pineapple ring in natural juice,
*   drained*

Put the rice and milk in a small pan and then bring to the boil, stirring continuously. Simmer for 15 minutes until thickened, then stir in the sugar. Pour into a serving dish and top with the pineapple ring.

Snack   *½ fat unit*

1 round or 2 finger Rich Tea biscuits

Menu 4   *7 fat units*

Light Meal 1   *1½ fat units*

Sandwich and Juice

1 glass unsweetened fruit juice
2 small, thin slices wholemeal bread
*   (50g/2oz), spread with*
7g (¼oz) low-fat spread
Yeast extract or beefy spread

Light Meal 2   *2 fat units*

Sunshine Chicken (Yogurt)

See step-by-step opposite page

25g (1oz) long-grain rice
5ml (1 teaspoon) mixed dried vegetables
2.5ml (½ teaspoon) turmeric
10ml (4floz) water
Salt
1 fresh peach, or 2 canned peach halves
75g (3oz) cooked chicken
142g (5oz) natural low-fat yogurt
Pinch paprika
Lemon slice to garnish
1 small carton fruit yogurt

1 Place the rice, dried vegetables and the turmeric in a small saucepan. Cover with the water and add a pinch of salt and bring to the boil. Cover the pan and simmer until the water is absorbed and the rice is tender but

still firm. Add more water while the rice is cooking if necessary.

2 Meanwhile, skin, halve and stone the fresh peach (you can dip it in boiling water to loosen the skin) and chop it into bite-sized pieces (or chop up the canned peaches). Remove and discard the skin from the chicken and chop the meat into small pieces. Place the peach and the chicken in a small pan.

3 Mix in the natural yogurt and season to taste with salt and paprika. Heat the mixture through very gently over a low heat, taking care that it does not curdle.

4 Arrange the rice in an attractive border on a serving dish and pile the chicken mixture into the centre of the rice ring.

5 Sprinkle the Sunshine Chicken lightly with paprika and then garnish with a slice of lemon. Serve the Sunshine Chicken immediately while the dish is piping-hot. Follow with the carton of fruit yogurt.

Serves 1

Main Meal   *2 fat units*

Minced Beef Hotpot (Fruit)

125g (4oz) minced beef
Small piece onion, chopped
125g (4oz) canned tomatoes,
*   roughly chopped*
5ml (1 teaspoon) tomato purée
Pinch dried mixed herbs
Salt and pepper
30ml (2 tablespoons) water
1 medium potato, peeled
10ml (2 teaspoons) Worcestershire sauce
Green vegetables
1 orange or eating apple

Brown the minced beef in a non-stick pan without added fat, then drain and discard any fat and juices. Add the onion, tomatoes, tomato purée, herbs, seasoning and water to the meat. Bring to the boil, cover and simmer for 5 minutes. Meanwhile, boil the potato in lightly salted water for 5 minutes, then drain and slice thinly. Turn the meat mixture into a small ovenproof dish and top with the potato slices. Sprinkle with the Worcestershire sauce, cover and cook at 180°C, 350°F, gas mark 4, for 30 minutes. Uncover the dish and cook for a further 15 minutes until the potatoes are crisp and golden. Serve with boiled green vegetables and follow with fresh fruit.

Snack   *1½ fat units*

Cheese and Salad Sandwich

2 small, thin slices wholemeal bread
*   (50g/2oz), sandwiched with*
1 triangle cheese spread, and
Salad vegetables

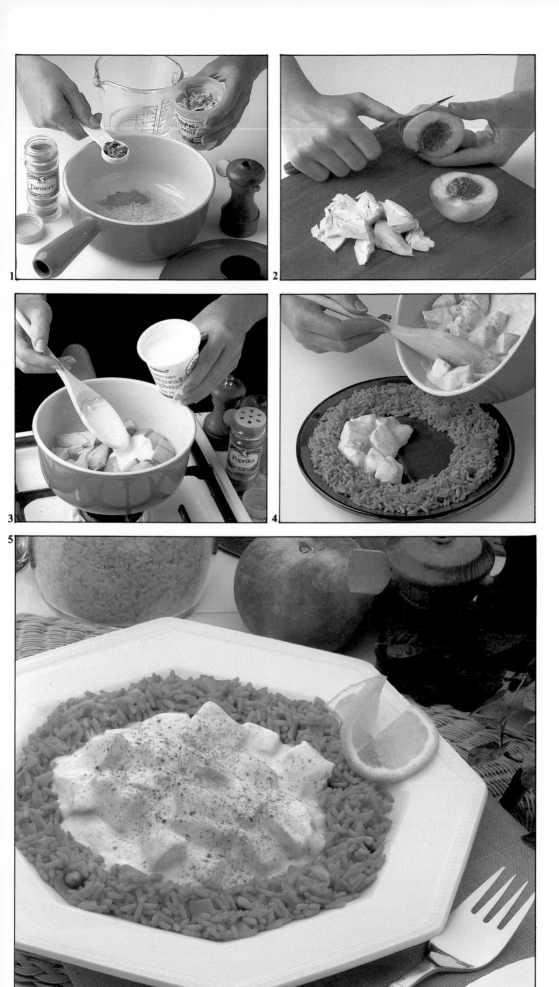

Menu 5 *8½ fat units*

Light Meal 1   *½ fat unit*
Fruit Muesli

25g (1oz) muesli, mixed with
1 banana, sliced, and
125ml (4floz) skimmed milk

Light Meal 2   *2 fat units*
Double-decker Ham Salad Sandwich (Yogurt)

3 small, thin slices white bread (75g/3oz)
Little prepared mustard
1 thin slice lean, boiled ham (25g/1oz)
7.5ml (½ tablespoon) low-calorie salad
  dressing
Little lettuce or watercress
1 tomato, sliced
Small piece cucumber, sliced
Salt and pepper
1 small carton low-fat fruit yogurt

Lightly spread one slice of bread with the mustard. Trim any fat off the ham and place on top of the bread. Cover with the second slice of bread and spread with salad dressing. Top with lettuce or watercress and slices of tomato and cucumber. Season well and top with the third slice of bread. Cut into two and serve with additional salad, if liked. Follow with the fruit yogurt.

Main Meal   *5½ fat units*
Stuffed Liver (Fruit and Ice-cream)

125g (4oz) lamb's liver (in two slices)
15ml (1 level tablespoon) sage and onion
  stuffing mix
30ml (2 tablespoons) boiling water
Salt and pepper
65ml (2½floz) dry cider
Green or root vegetables
50g (2oz) vanilla ice-cream
125g (4oz) fresh or frozen raspberries
  or strawberries

Wash the liver and place one slice in the bottom of a small, ovenproof dish. Blend the stuffing mix with the boiling water and leave to stand for 3 minutes. Spread the stuffing on the slice of liver in the dish and top with the second liver slice. Season well and add the cider. Cover the dish and cook at 180°C, 350°F, gas mark 4, for 45 minutes. Serve with boiled green or root vegetables. Follow with the ice-cream and fruit.

Snack   *½ fat unit*
Open Sandwich

1 small slice white bread (25g/1oz), spread
  with
Yeast extract or beefy spread, topped with
Sliced cucumber or mustard and cress

Menu 6 *9 fat units*

Light Meal 1   *½ fat unit*
Cereal and Fruit

Moderate portion cornflakes or bran flakes,
  served with
125ml (4floz) skimmed milk, and
5ml (1 level teaspoon) sugar, and
1 banana, sliced

Light Meal 2   *2½ fat units*
Pasta and Salmon Salad (Fruit)

25g (1oz) pasta shapes
99g (3½oz) pink salmon, drained
2 tomatoes, skinned and chopped
½ small green pepper (capsicum), deseeded
  and chopped
25g (1oz) button mushrooms, sliced
Few small gherkins, sliced
30ml (2 tablespoons) oil-free French dressing
5ml (1 teaspoon) tomato purée
5ml (1 teaspoon) lemon juice
Salt and freshly ground black pepper
Lettuce leaves
Chopped parsley
1 orange

Cook the pasta in boiling salted water until tender. Drain and rinse under cold water until cool, then drain again. Flake the salmon and place in a bowl with the pasta, tomato, pepper (capsicum), mushroom and gherkin. Mix the dressing with the tomato purée and lemon juice and pour over the salad. Toss well and season to taste with salt and pepper. Arrange on a bed of lettuce and sprinkle with chopped parsley. Follow with the orange.

Main Meal   *5 fat units*
Spanish Eggs (Pineapple and Custard)

7g (¼oz) low-fat spread
Small piece onion, finely chopped
½ small green pepper (capsicum), chopped
150g (5oz) canned tomatoes, chopped
½ clove garlic, crushed
Salt and pepper
2 medium eggs (size 3)
Boiled pasta or rice
Salad vegetables
2 rings canned pineapple in natural juice
125ml (4floz) custard made from skimmed
  milk and artificial sweetener

Melt the low-fat spread in a small pan and gently sauté the onion and pepper (capsicum) until softened. Stir in the tomatoes and garlic, cover and simmer for 10 minutes. Season to taste with salt and pepper. Meanwhile, boil the eggs for 10 minutes, then cool just enough to shell. Cut the eggs in half lengthways and arrange them, cut-side down, on a serving dish. Pour over the tomato sauce and serve with boiled pasta or rice and salad. Follow with the pineapple and custard.

Snack   *1 fat unit*
Cheesy Crispbreads

2 crispbreads, spread with
1 triangle cheese spread, topped with
Few slices tomato or cucumber

Menu 7 *9½ fat units*

Light Meal 1   *2 fat units*
Juice, Egg and Bread

1 small glass unsweetened fruit juice
1 medium egg (size 3), poached, served on
1 small, thin slice toasted white or wholemeal
*   bread (25g/1oz), unbuttered*

Light Meal 2   *3 fat units*
Corned Beef Salad (Fruit)

75g (3oz) corned beef
Pickled onion or mixed pickle
Salad vegetables
Oil-free French dressing
1 eating apple or pear

Main Meal   *4 fat units*
Kedgeree (Banana and Ice-cream)

150g (5oz) smoked haddock
150ml (¼pint) skimmed milk
50g (2oz) long-grain white or brown rice
1 medium egg (size 4), hard-boiled

Little grated lemon rind (optional)
Salt and freshly ground black pepper
5-10ml (1-2 teaspoons) chopped parsley
1 lemon wedge
50g (2oz) vanilla ice-cream
1 banana, sliced

Put the smoked haddock and skimmed milk in a small pan, bring to the boil, then cover and simmer for 15 minutes. Lift out the fish, flake with a fork and discard the skin and bones, reserving the milk in which it was cooked. Cook the rice in boiling, salted water until tender (about 15 minutes for white rice; 30 minutes for brown). Drain the rice, rinse in hot water and drain again. Shell and then chop the egg. Put 30ml (2 tablespoons) of the reserved milk in a clean pan and add the rice, flaked fish, chopped egg and lemon rind (optional). Heat gently, stirring continuously until heated through. Season to taste and stir in the chopped parsley. Turn onto a warm serving dish and garnish with the lemon wedge. Follow with the ice-cream and banana.

Snack   *½ fat unit*
Salad Sandwich

2 small slices white or wholemeal bread
*   (50g/2oz), spread with*
Yeast extract or beefy spread, and
*   sandwiched together with*
Grated carrot
Sliced cucumber
Mustard and cress

Fat unit guide

To help you devise your own menu, this guide lists basic foods.

	Fat units				
Biscuits		bread, 2 small, thin slices (57g (2oz)	½	**Breakfast cereal**	
				Per 28g (1oz), unless	
Per biscuit unless		Croissant, 64g (2½oz)	5½	**otherwise stated**	
otherwise stated		Crumpet 42g (1½oz)	½	Bran flakes	0
Cream cracker	½	Crusty roll, brown or		Cornflakes	0
Digestive (wheatmeal),		white, 57g (2oz)	½	Instant oats, per	
medium	½	Currant bread, 3 small		28g (1oz) dry weight	½
Digestive (wheatmeal),		thin slices, 85g (3oz)	1	Muesli or Swiss-style	
large	1	Dinner roll, soft, brown		cereal, per 28g (1oz)	½
Ginger biscuit	½	or white, 57g (2oz)	1½	Porridge oats, raw	1
Malted milk	½	French bread, 57g (2oz)		Rice cereals	0
Marie	½	piece	½	Shredded wheat, 2	
Morning coffee,		Malt bread, 1 small,		biscuits	½
2 biscuits	½	thin slice, 28g (1oz)	½	Wheat biscuit	
Nice	½	Slimmers' bread,		cereal, 2 biscuits	½
Osborne	½	6 slices	½		
Petit beurre	½	Soda bread, 57g (2oz)	½	**Cereal and cereal products**	
Rich tea finger,		Wheatgerm bread,		Bran, per 28g (1oz)	½
2 biscuits	½	2 small, thin slices		Flours, *see* Cooking	
Rich tea, round	½	57g (2oz)	½	ingredients	
		White bread, 3 small,		Oatmeal, raw, per	
Bread		thin slices, or 2 large,		28g (1oz)	1
Bap, 57g (2oz)	1½	thin slices, 85g (3oz)	½	Pearl barley, boiled,	
Brown or wholemeal		Wholemeal bread,		per 28g (1oz)	0
		2 small, thin slices,		Pearl barley, raw,	
		57g (2oz)	½	85g (3oz)	½

Cereals continued

Rice, *see* Pasta and Rice

Sago, raw, per 28g (1oz)	0
Tapioca, raw, per 28g (1oz)	0
Wheatgerm, per 28g (1oz)	1

Cheese

Per 28g (1oz) unless otherwise stated

Brie	2½
Caerphilly	3
Camembert	2½
Cheddar	3½
Cheese spread	2½
Cheese spread, per triangle	1
Cheshire	3
Cottage cheese, per 113g (4oz) carton	1½
Cream cheese	4½
Curd cheese	1
Danish blue	3
Double Gloucester	3
Edam	2½
Lancashire	3
Leicester	3
Parmesan, grated, per 15ml (level tablespoon)	½
Processed	2½
Skimmed milk soft cheese, per 227g (8oz) carton	½
Stilton	4
Wensleydale	3

Cooking ingredients

Wheatmeal flour (85%), 57g (2oz)	½
White flour, 113g (4oz)	½
Wholemeal flour (100%), 57g (2oz)	½
Plain white, wheatmeal and wholemeal flour, per 15ml (level tablespoon	0

Per 28g (1oz)

Arrowroot	0
Bran	½
Cornflour	0
Custard powder	0
Ground rice	0
Semolina, dry	0
Soya flour, full-fat	2½
Yeast, fresh or dried	0

Cream

Per 28g (1oz)

Clotted	5½
Double (thickened)	5
Half	1
Single	1
Soured	1
Sterilized (reduced), canned	2½
Whipping	3½

Crispbreads

Bran and brownwheat, 5 biscuits	½
Rye and wheat, 4 biscuits	½

Crisps and potato snacks

Crisps, all flavours, per 28g (1oz)	3
Potato chips, per 28g (1oz)	3

Eggs

Each

Size 6 (very small)	1½
Sizes 5, 4, 3 (small-medium)	2
Sizes 2, 1 (large)	2½
White of egg	0
Yolk of medium egg (size 3)	2
Fried egg, medium (size 3)	3

Fats

Per 28g (1oz)

Butter, all brands	8
Cooking and salad oils (vegetables, nut and fish oils)	10
Dripping	10
Lard	10
Low-fat spread	4
Margarine, all brands unless termed 'low-fat'	8
Solid vegetable oil	10
Suet, block	10
Suet, shredded	8½

Fish and shellfish

Cod, raw, steamed or poached, 198g (7oz)	½
Cod, grilled or baked, brushed with a little fat, 113g (4oz)	½
Cod, fried in batter, per 28g (1oz)	1
Cod, fish fingers, each as sold	½
Coley, raw, steamed or poached, 227g (8oz)	½
Crab, meat only, 28g (1oz)	½
Fish cakes, frozen, each, as sold	0
Haddock, raw, steamed or poached, 227g (8oz)	½
Haddock, fried in breadcrumbs, per 28g (1oz)	1
Haddock, smoked, flesh only, 142g (5oz)	½
Haddock, frozen buttered fillets, per 198g (7oz) pack	2
Halibut, raw, flesh only, 57g (2oz)	½
Halibut, steamed or poached, per 28g (1oz)	½
Herring, raw, flesh only, per 28g (1oz)	2
Herring, grilled or fried, flesh only, 28g (1oz)	1½
Herring, whole, 142g (5oz), boned and çleaned, grilled	6½
Kippers, baked or grilled without fat, flesh only, per 28g (1oz)	1
Kippers, whole, 170g (6oz) on the bone, baked or grilled without fat	3½
Kippers, frozen buttered fillets, per 170g (6oz) pack	7
Mackerel, flesh only, grilled without fat, per 28g (1oz)	1
Mackerel, kippered, fillet, per 28g (1oz)	1½
Mackerel, frozen buttered kippered fillets, per 170g (6oz) pack	8
Mackerel, smoked fillet per 28g (1oz)	2½
Mackerel, whole, 170g (6oz), boned and cleaned, grilled	6½
Pilchards, canned in tomato sauce, per 28g (1oz)	½
Plaice, steamed or poached in water, 142g (5oz)	1
Plaice, fried in breadcrumbs, per 28g (1oz)	1½
Plaice, fried in batter, per 28g (1oz)	2
Prawns, fresh or frozen, without shells, 85g (3oz)	½
Salmon, fresh, on the bone, poached or steamed, per 28g (1oz)	1

Salmon, fresh, flesh only, poached or steamed, per 28g (1oz) 1½
Salmon, pink, canned, per 99g (3½oz) can 2½
Salmon, smoked, per 28g (1oz) ½
Sardines, canned in oil, fish only, per 28g (1oz) 3
Sardines, canned in tomato sauce, per 28g (1oz) 1
Sole, fillet, raw or steamed, 113g (4oz) ½
Sprats without heads, fried, per 28g (1oz) 4
Trout, brown or river trout, flesh only, poached or steamed per 28g (1oz) ½
Trout, rainbow, whole, 170g (6oz), steamed or poached 2
Trout, smoked, fillet, per 28g (1oz) ½
Tuna in brine, per 99g (3½oz) can ½
Tuna in oil, drained of oil, per 28g (1oz) 1½
Tuna in oil, fish plus oil, per 28g (1oz) 2
Whitebait, with bones, fried, per 28g (1oz) 5

Fruit
Per 28g (1oz)
Fresh fruit with the exception of avocados 0
Avocado, flesh only 2½
Dried fruit: apricots, apples and prunes 0
Canned fruit, in natural juice, apple juice or low-calorie syrup 0

Note: It is recommended strongly that you avoid canned fruit in sugar syrup when following this diet plan.

Ice-cream
Per 28g (1oz)
Chocolate 2
Cornish dairy 2
Neapolitan 1½
Raspberry ripple 1½
Strawberry 1½
Vanilla 1½

Meat and poultry
Fresh or frozen
Per 28g (1oz) unless otherwise stated
Bacon, 1 back rasher, well grilled 1½

Bacon, 1 streaky rasher, well grilled 1
Beef, brisket, boiled, lean and fat 2½
Beef, fore rib, roast, lean only 1½
Beef, minced, raw 1½
Beef, minced (weighed raw), well fried and drained of fat ½
Beef, rump steak, raw 1½
Beef, rump steak, grilled, lean and fat 1
Beef, silverside, salted, boiled, lean only ½
Beef, sirloin, roast, lean only 1
Beef, stewing, raw or stewed, lean only 1
Beefburgers, raw, 57g (2oz) 4
Beefburgers, well grilled, 57g (2oz) raw weight 1½
Chicken, raw, meat only (no skin) ½
Chicken, roast or boiled, meat only (no skin) ½
Chicken drumstick, boiled or grilled, skin removed, average weight raw 100g (3½oz) 1
Chicken joint, baked or grilled, skin removed, average weight raw 265g (9½oz) 2
Duck, roast, meat only (no skin) 1
Gammon joint, boiled, lean only ½
Gammon rasher, grilled, lean only ½
Ham, boiled, lean only ½
Ham, smoked ½
Heart, ox, stewed ½
Kidney, raw, all types, 57g (2oz) ½
Kidney, whole lamb's kidney, raw ½
Lamb, leg, roast, lean only 1
Lamb, leg, roast, lean and fat 2
Lamb, shoulder, roast, lean only 1
Lamb, shoulder, roast, lean and fat 2½
Lamb, breast, boned, roast, lean and fat 3½
Lamb loin chop, grilled, lean only, average weight raw 113g (4oz) 2½
Liver, calves', raw ½

Liver, calves', fried 1½
Liver, chicken, raw ½
Liver, chicken, fried 1
Liver, lamb's, raw 1
Liver, lamb's, fried 1½
Liver, ox, raw or stewed 1
Liver, pig's, raw or stewed 1
Pheasant, roast, meat only 1
Pork fillet, raw, lean only, 113 (4oz) 3
Pork, leg, roast, lean only ½
Pork, leg, roast, lean and fat 2
Pork chop, grilled, weighed with bone, lean and fat 2
Pork chop, small whole 156g (5½oz), grilled and fat removed 3½
Rabbit, stewed on the bone ½
Sausage, beef chipolata (breakfast sausage), well grilled, each 1½
Sausage, beef, large, well grilled, each 3
Sausage, pork, large, (breakfast sausage), well grilled, each 3½
Tongue, lamb, stewed, fat and skin removed 2½
Tongue, ox, boiled, fat and skin removed 2½
Tripe, stewed ½
Turkey, raw, meat only, 57g (2oz) ½
Turkey, roast, meat only, skin removed 57g (2oz) ½
Veal, fillet, raw, 57g (2oz) ½
Veal, fillet, roast 1

Chilled cooked meats and delicatessen sausages
Per 28g (1oz) unless otherwise stated
Bacon and ham loaf 1½
Bierwurst 2½
Black pudding 2
Boiled ham, lean only ½
Brawn 1½
Cervelat 4
Chopped ham roll or loaf 2
Chopped pork and ham 2½
Continental liver sausage 2½
Corned beef 1
Danish salami 5½
Frankfurter 2½
Garlic sausage 2½
German salami 4
Ham sausage ½

Meats continued

Haslet	2
Honey-roast ham	½
Mortadella	3
Polish krajana	½
Polony	2
Pork luncheon meat	2½
Ox tongue	2½
Savaloy	2
Silverside of beef (lean only)	½
Smoked ham	½
Smoked ham sausage	2
Smoked turkey or turkey ham, per 57g (2oz)	½
Sweet cured turkey, per 57g (2oz)	½

Milk

Skimmed or separated, per 568ml (pint)	0
Reconstituted low-fat powdered milk, per 568ml (pint)	0
Pasteurized, per 568ml (pint)	7½
Canned evaporated milk, per 28ml (1floz)	1
Canned condensed whole milk, sweetened per 28ml (1floz)	1
Dried milk, skimmed or low-fat, per 28ml (1floz)	0
Dried milk, skimmed, per 10ml (rounded teaspoon), dry	0
Dried milk, skimmed with added vegetable fat, per 28g (1oz)	3
Dried milk, skimmed with added vegetable fat, per 10ml (rounded teaspoon), dry	½

Nuts

Shelled, per 28g (1oz)

Almonds, whole, flaked or ground	5½
Barcelona	6½
Brazil	6
Cashew, salted	4½
Chestnuts	½
Cob (hazel)	3½
Coconut, fresh	3½
Coconut, desiccated	6
Peanuts, fresh, dry-roasted or roasted and salted	5
Walnuts	5

Pasta and rice

Macaroni, raw or boiled	0
Pasta, all shapes, raw or boiled	0
Rice, white long- or short-grain, raw or boiled	0
Rice, brown, raw, per 57g (2oz)	½
Spaghetti, raw or boiled	0

Sauces, dressings, and pickles

Per 15ml (1 level tablespoon)

Apple sauce, unsweetened	0
Brown sauce	0
Capers	0
Chutney	0
Creamed horseradish sauce	½
French dressing	3
Gherkins	0
Horseradish sauce	0
Low-calorie salad dressing or cream (vinegar and oil)	1
Mint sauce	0
Mayonnaise	3½
Mustard pickle	0
Oil-free French dressing	0
Olives in brine, per 28g (1oz)	1
Pickled beetroot	0
Pickled onions	0
Pickled red cabbage	0
Salad cream	1½
Soy sauce	0
Sweet pickle	0
Tartare sauce	1
Tomato ketchup or sauce	0
Tomato purée or paste	0
Vinegar	0
Worcestershire sauce	0

Spreads

Bovril, per 5ml (level teaspoon)	0
Peanut butter, per 15ml (level tablespoon)	3
Yeast extract, per 5ml (level teaspoon)	0

Stock cubes

Beef stock cube, each	½
Chicken stock cube, each	½

Sugars

See High calorie, fat-free foods for equivalent fat units

Sweets and chocolates

See High calorie fat-free foods for equivalent fat unit values of fat-free sweets

Chocolate, milk or plain, per 28g (1oz)	3
Fudge, per 28g (1oz)	2
Marzipan sweets, per 28g (1oz)	2½
Toffees, per 28g (1oz)	1½

Yogurt

Per small carton,

Low-fat natural or fruit	½
Low-fat chocolate	1
Low-fat hazelnut	1
Low-fat muesli	½

Vegetables

All fresh vegetables are fat-free and most can be eaten freely when fresh or boiled. However, we recommend that you eat moderate portions of potatoes, cooked dried beans, peas and sweetcorn. If fat is added to vegetables during cooking or when serving, the appropriate fat units value for the amount of fat used must be added to your daily total.

Fried roast vegetables

Per 28g (1oz)

Aubergines, sliced and fried	2
Mushrooms, sliced and fried	3½
Onions, sliced and fried	3½
Potatoes, chipped and fried	1½
Potatoes, cut into thick chips and fried, per 142g (5oz) portion	7½
Potatoes, large chunks, roast, per 142g (5oz)	2½

Vegetables with added fat

Baked jacket-potato, 198g (7oz), topped with 15g (½oz) butter	4
Mashed potato with 45ml (3 tablespoons)	

pasteurized milk, per 142g (5oz) portion	½
Mashed potato with 7g (¼oz) butter, per 142g (5oz) portion	2

Dried vegetables and lentils
Per 28g (1oz)

Broad beans, dry or boiled	0
Butter beans, dry or boiled	0
Haricot beans, 85g (3oz) dry weight	½
Kidney beans, 85g (3oz) dry weight	½
Lentils, dry or boiled	0
Mung beans, dry or boiled	0
Peas, dried, 85g (3oz) dry weight	½
Peas, chick, 28g (1oz) dry weight	½
Peas, split, dry or boiled	0
Potato, instant, made up without butter	0
Soya beans, 28g (1oz) dry weight	1½

Canned vegetables

Baked beans with tomato sauce 220g (7¾oz)	½

Frozen vegetables

Baby roast potatoes, as sold, per 28g (1oz)	½
Oven chips, per 28g (1oz)	½
Potato cakes, as sold, each	½
Potato croquettes, as sold, each	½
Sauté potatoes, as sold, 113g (4oz)	½

Drinks
All drinks of negligible calorie value, for example tea and coffee without milk or sugar, and 'low-calorie' drinks and water can be consumed freely. However, the units from fat-containing drinks must be counted into your daily allowance.

Milk
Per 568ml (1pint)

Evaporated milk, full cream, diluted with water	7
Goat's	9
Homogenized	7½
Longlife or UHT	7½
Instant spray-dried skimmed milk, reconstituted	0
Instant spray-dried skimmed milk with vegetable fat, reconstituted	6
Pasteurized	7½
Semi-skimmed milk	3½
Sterilized	7½
Untreated farm milk	7½

Beverages

Cocoa, all brands, per 10ml/5g (rounded teaspoon)	½
Drinking chocolate, per 20ml/10g (2 rounded teaspoons)	½
Horlicks, per 30ml/27g (3 rounded teaspoons), recommended serving	½
Malted milk, 15g/½oz (3 heaped teaspoons)	½
Ovaltine, 14g (2 heaped teaspoons)	0

High calorie, fat-free foods and drinks

The following fat-free foods and drinks, which contain a high sugar content, have been given an equivalent fat unit value which must be counted as part of your daily allowance. We recommend that no more than 3 equivalent fat units be included each day, thus leaving 7 fat units to spend on other foods.

Dried fruits

Currants, raisins, sultanas, per 28g (1oz)	2½
Currants, raisins, sultanas, per 15ml (level tablespoon)	1
Dates with or without stones, per 28g (1oz)	2½
Figs, per 28g (1oz)	2½
Peaches, dried, per 28g (1oz)	2½

Glacé fruit

Glacé cherries, per 28g (1oz)	2½

Honey, syrup and treacle

Honey, syrup and treacle, per 28g (1oz)	3
Honey, syrup and treacle, per 15ml (level tablespoon)	2½
Honey, syrup and treacle, per 5ml (level teaspoon)	1

Sugar

Sugar, all types except fruit sugar (fructose), per 28g (1oz)	4½
Sugar, all types per 5ml (level teaspoon)	½
Quick dissolving sugar, per sachet	½
Cube sugar, per 2 small cubes	½
Fruit sugar (fructose), per 28g (1oz)	4

Sweetened fruit juices
Per 115ml (4floz) glass

Apple juice	2
Grape juice	2½
Grapefruit juice	2½
Orange juice	2½
Pineapple juice	2½

Sweetened soft drinks
Per 115ml (4floz) glass

Bitter lemon	1½
Cola	2
Ginger ale and beer	1½
Glucose drink, sparkling	3½
Lemonade	1½
Orangeade	2
Tonic water	1½

Alcoholic drinks
Port

Per 28ml (1floz)	2

Spirits
Per 28ml (1floz)

Bourbon	3½
Brandy	2½
Gin	2½
Rum	2½
Vodka	2½
Whisky	2½

Wines
Per 113ml (4floz) glass

Dry red or white	3
Rose	3
Sparkling	3½
Sweet red	3½
Sweet white	4

Other drinks
Per 248ml (½pint)

Beer, mild, pale, light	3
Beer, brown ale	3½
Beer, draught bitter	4
Cider	4
Lager	3½

Little - and - often diet
(1,500 calories)

If you are a nibbler and find it almost impossible to keep to three meals a day, this diet will suit you. Here, your daily slimming calorie allowance is divided into small meals, each of 200 calories.

The little-and-often method is the one that has proved most consistently effective for women who thought they 'did not have the willpower to diet'; the main reason is that this is a diet that caters for appetite. Many diets are designed to cope with hunger — hunger being the physical discomforts that arise from an empty stomach. However, they neglect another reason for those eating urges — appetite. Appetite is what makes you want to eat, irrespective of whether you are physically hungry or not, because you see food, smell food, think of food, feel bored, happy or sad. Many slimmers who are dominated more by appetite than hunger have difficulty in keeping to three meals a day and blame it on lack of willpower.

On this little-and-often diet you can eat virtually at any time your appetite urges you to, and the comforting thought that the next meal is never far away cancels out the temptation to eat illicit extras. If you follow this little-and-often pattern of eating you also achieve a useful advantage — your metabolic rate, the rate at which your body burns up fat, increases a little after a meal, so if you eat five small meals a day instead of three larger ones, your body is in a state of high 'burn-up' more often, thus helping to speed up your weight loss.

If you have more than 12kg (2st) to lose,

you can begin on a daily allowance of 1,500 calories, which allows you seven small meals each day plus 100 calories' worth of milk for drinks. Knowing that you *can* eat often has the surprising effect of making you decide that you do not really want to eat each snack meal and therefore you consume less than your allowance. There is no need to have your full 1,500 calorie allowance each day — if you have between 6kg (1st) and 12kg (2st) to lose, start with six meals a day and when you have less than 6kg (1st) to go, reduce the number of meals to five. If you experience a day when it is impossible to follow your diet, you can cut yourself down to three or four meals the following day to undo any damage. All these meals are simple and quick to prepare and have been divided into the following groups: Bread, crispbread and breakfast-type meals; Savoury meals without meat and fish; Meat and fish meals; Salad meals; and Fruit and dessert meals.

Bread, crispbread and breakfast meals (200 calories)

Grapefruit, Toast and Marmalade
½ grapefruit
Non-sugar sweetener (optional)
2 small slices wholemeal bread (25g/1oz)each
7g (¼oz) low-fat spread
10ml (2 level teaspoons) marmalade or jam

Sweeten the grapefruit with non-sugar sweetener, if liked. Toast the bread and spread with low-fat spread and jam or marmalade.

Beans on Toast
150g (5oz) canned baked beans in tomato sauce
1 large, thin slice white or wholemeal bread (40g/1½oz)

Heat the beans and toast the bread. Serve the beans on the toast.

Orange Juice and Cereal
125ml (4floz) unsweetened orange juice
2 wheat cereal biscuits
125ml (4floz) skimmed milk

Drink the orange juice and serve the cereal with the skimmed milk.

Ham and Pineapple Open Sandwich; Snack Pizza; Peach Melba; Florentine Egg; Prawn and Egg Salad (Opposite)

Diet rules
1 Choose up to seven of any of these 200 calorie meals each day. Ideally, vary the meals each day and include one meal from each section, so that you have a good supply of nutrients.
2 In addition, you are allowed 142ml (¼ pint) pasteurized milk or 187ml (⅓ pint) semi-skimmed milk or 284ml (½ pint) skimmed milk for use in drinks of tea and coffee. You can drink unlimited tea and coffee without milk and sugar (artificial sweeteners may be used), 'low-calorie' labelled drinks and water.
3 Keep to the stated portions of ingredients for each meal. Use your kitchen scales and measuring jug to ensure accuracy. Six or seven small calorie errors each day can add up to one large mistake and slow down or even stop your weight loss.
4 Plan and shop ahead to make sure your next low-calorie meal is readily available.

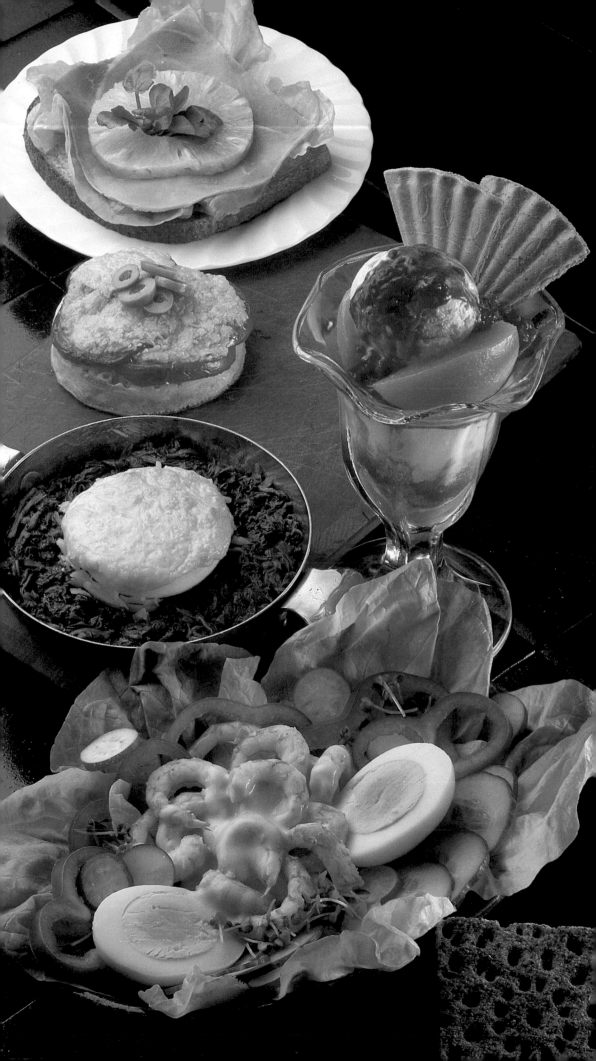

Orange Juice, Muesli and Yogurt

125ml (4floz) unsweetened orange juice
25g (1oz) muesli
1 small carton low-fat natural yogurt

Drink the orange juice. Mix the muesli with the yogurt and serve.

Crusty Roll with Cottage Cheese

1 crusty bread roll (49g/1¾oz)
50g (2oz) cottage·cheese, any flavour except
*   with added Cheddar cheese*
Mustard and cress

Split the roll and fill with cottage cheese and mustard and cress.

Creamy Mushrooms on Toast and Fruit Juice

125g (4oz) button mushrooms
125ml (4floz) chicken stock
10ml (2 level teaspoons) cornflour
5ml (1 level teaspoon) low-fat milk powder
Salt and pepper
1 slice brown or white bread
*   (40g/1½oz)*
125ml (4floz) unsweetened orange juice

Poach the mushrooms in the stock for 5 minutes. Blend the cornflour and milk powder with a little cold water and stir into the mushrooms. Continue to cook until thickened. Season to taste with salt and pepper. Toast the bread·and serve the mushrooms on toast with the orange juice.

Cheese and Pickle on Toast

1 small, thin slice wholemeal bread
*   (40g/1½oz)*
25g (1oz) Edam cheese, grated
15ml (1 tablespoon) sweet pickle or chutney

Toast the bread and top with the grated cheese. Grill until the cheese melts. Serve with the pickle or chutney.

Banana and Cottage Cheese Open Sandwich

25g (1oz) slice light rye or granary bread
50g (2oz) natural cottage cheese
1 small banana (150g/5oz), sliced
5ml (1 level teaspoon) sultanas

Spread the bread with the cottage cheese and top with the sliced banana and sultanas.

Salmon Sandwich with Tomato and Celery

50g (2oz) canned salmon, flaked
15ml (1 level tablespoon) low-calorie
*   seafood sauce*
2 small slices slimmers' bread or 1 slice
*   wholemeal bread (25g/1oz)*
Few sprigs watercress or slices of cucumber
1 tomato
2 sticks celery

Mix together the salmon and seafood sauce. Spread on one slice of bread and cover with watercress or sliced cucumber. If you use slimmers' bread, top with the second slice. Serve with the tomato and celery.

Ham and Pineapple Open Sandwich (Fresh Fruit)

25g (1oz) slice wholemeal bread
3.5g (⅛ oz) low-fat spread
Lettuce
25g (1oz) slice lean ham
1 slice pineapple canned in natural juice
Sprig watercress
1 medium orange or pear

Toast the bread if liked and lightly spread with the low-fat spread. Top with the lettuce, ham and the pineapple ring and watercress. Follow with the orange or pear.

Crispbreads with Liver Sausage (Fruit)

25g (1oz) liver sausage
3 crispbreads
1 tomato, sliced
Mustard and cress
1 medium eating apple

Spread the liver sausage on the crispbreads and top with the sliced tomato and mustard and cress. Follow with the apple.

Cottage Cheese and Crispbreads

113g (4oz) carton cottage cheese, any flavour
*   except with Cheddar cheese*
3 crispbreads
1 pickled onion or 3 spring onions
125ml (4floz) tomato juice

Serve the cottage cheese with the crispbreads and pickled onion or spring onions and a glass of tomato juice.

Breakfast Cereal and Banana

25g (1oz) cornflakes or wheat flakes
75ml (3floz) skimmed milk
1 small banana (150g/5oz), sliced

Serve the cornflakes or wheat flakes with the skimmed milk and sliced banana.

Savoury meals without meat or fish (200 calories)

Scrambled Egg and Cottage Cheese with Tomato

1 large (size 2) egg
50g (2oz) cottage cheese flavoured with chives
*   or onions and peppers*
1 tomato, sliced
2 crispbreads (unbuttered)

Beat the egg and cottage cheese together and season to taste. Pour into a small non-stick pan and heat, stirring, until the egg is just set. Turn out and serve with the sliced tomato and crispbreads.

Poached Egg and Mushrooms with Tomato Juice

1 large egg (size 2)
75g (3oz) flat mushrooms
25g (1oz) slice wholemeal bread
3.5g (1/8 oz) low-fat spread
Salt and pepper
125ml (4floz) tomato juice
Dash Worcestershire sauce (optional)

Poach the egg in some water and poach the mushrooms in stock or water. Toast the bread and spread lightly with the low-fat spread. Arrange the mushrooms on the toast. Season to taste with salt and pepper and top with the poached egg. Serve with the tomato juice seasoned with Worcestershire sauce, if liked.

Spanish Omelet

7g (1/4oz) low-fat spread
2 tomatoes, skinned and chopped
1/2 small green, pepper (capsicum), deseeded and chopped
2 medium eggs (size 4)
30ml (2 tablespoons) water
Pinch dried marjoram or basil
Salt and pepper
Chopped parsley

Melt the low-fat spread in a non-stick frying or omelet pan. Add the tomatoes and green pepper (capsicum) and fry gently until soft. Beat the eggs with the water, herbs and salt and pepper to taste. Pour over the vegetables in the pan and cook over a moderate heat until the egg is just set. Turn out and serve sprinkled with chopped parsley.

Snack Pizza

1 crumpet (40g/1½oz)
1 tomato, sliced
Salt and pepper
Pinch mixed herbs
25g (1oz) Cheshire cheese, grated
1 stuffed olive, sliced

Toast the crumpet. Cover the top with sliced tomato. Season with the salt and pepper, sprinkle with herbs, then cover with the grated cheese. Place under a hot grill until the cheese melts. Garnish with the olive.

Cheesy Tomato Treat

1 large tomato
30ml (2 tablespoons) sweetcorn
Pinch mixed herbs
25g (1oz) Cheddar cheese, grated
1 small slice slimmers' bread, or 1/2 small slice wholemeal bread
Few sprigs watercress
Few slices cucumber

Cut the tomato in half, scoop out the pips and discard them. Put 15ml (1 tablespoon) sweetcorn in each tomato half and sprinkle with mixed herbs. Cover with grated cheese and place under a hot grill until the cheese melts and is lightly browned. Toast the bread and serve the tomato halves on the toast garnished with sprigs of watercress and slices of cucumber.

Cottage Cheese, Apple and Sultanas

1 medium eating apple, cored and chopped
113g (4oz) natural cottage cheese
15ml (1 level tablespoon) sultanas
1 crispbread (unbuttered)

Mix the chopped apple, cottage cheese and sultanas. Serve with the crispbread.

Spaghetti au Gratin (Fresh Fruit)

213g (7½oz) canned spaghetti in tomato sauce
15ml (1 level tablespoon) grated Parmesan cheese
1 medium orange, apple or pear

Heat the spaghetti in a pan. Turn into an ovenproof dish. Sprinkle with the Parmesan cheese and place under a hot grill until the cheese melts. Follow with the fruit.

Vegetable Soup with Cheese and Crispbreads

1 beef or chicken stock cube
275ml (½pint) water
50g (2oz) carrot, grated
50g (2oz) onion, grated
25g (1oz) fresh or frozen peas
Pinch dried mixed herbs
Salt and pepper
25g (1oz) Edam cheese
2 crispbreads

Put the stock cube in water in a pan and bring to the boil, stirring to dissolve the stock cube. Add the vegetables and herbs, return to the boil, cover and simmer for 10 minutes. Season to taste with salt and pepper. Serve with the cheese and crispbreads.

Grapefruit and Boiled Egg

1/2 grapefruit
Non-sugar sweetener (optional)
1 large egg (size 2), boiled
2 small slices slimmers' bread, or 1 small slice wholemeal bread (25g/1oz)
7g (1/4oz) low-fat spread

Sweeten the grapefruit with the non-sugar sweetener, if liked. Serve the boiled egg with the bread spread with low-fat spread.

Cheese Topped Jacket Potato

150g (6oz) potato
50g (2oz) cottage cheese with chives
Small bunch watercress

Scrub the potato, then bake in a hot oven, 200°C, 400°F, gas mark 6, for 40 minutes, or until soft when squeezed. Cut the potato in half and top with the cottage cheese. Serve with the watercress.

Vegetable Chowder

75g (3oz) carrot, finely grated
50g (2oz) onion, finely chopped
2 sticks celery, finely chopped
1 leek, trimmed and finely sliced
125g (4oz) fresh or canned tomatoes, chopped
5ml (1 level teaspoon) tomato purée
275ml (½pint) beef or chicken stock made
* from 1 stock cube*
Salt and pepper
1 bay leaf
1 slice wholemeal bread (40g/1½oz),
* unbuttered*

Place all the prepared vegetables in a pan with the tomato purée, stock, seasoning to taste and a bay leaf. Bring to the boil and simmer for 10 minutes, stirring occasionally. Serve hot with the bread.

Florentine Egg

125g (4oz) frozen or canned chopped spinach
Salt and pepper
Pinch grated nutmeg
1 medium egg (size 4)
25g (1oz) Edam cheese, grated

Heat and drain the spinach. Season to taste with salt and pepper and stir in the nutmeg. Turn into a small ovenproof dish. Poach the egg in water and place on top of the spinach. Cover the egg with the grated cheese and place under a hot grill until the cheese melts.

Vegetables Provençale

225g (8oz) canned tomatoes with juice,
* chopped*
1 small onion sliced
1 clove garlic, crushed
175g (6oz) courgettes, sliced
Salt and pepper
10ml (2 level teaspoons) chopped parsley
25g (1oz) Cheshire cheese, grated
45ml (3 level tablespoons) fresh breadcrumbs

Put the tomatoes, onion, garlic and the courgettes in a pan. Season with salt and pepper. Cover and simmer gently for 25 minutes, stirring occasionally. Stir in the parsley and turn into an ovenproof dish. Mix the grated cheese and breadcrumbs together and sprinkle over the vegetables. Heat under a hot grill until the topping begins to brown. Serve hot.

Fish and meat meals (200 calories)

Grilled Fish and Vegetables

175g (6oz) cod, coley or haddock fillets
7g (¼oz) low-fat spread
75g (3oz) frozen mixed vegetables

Brush the fish fillets with the low-fat spread and grill until cooked. Cook the frozen mixed vegetables and serve with the fish.

Fish Steak au Gratin

1 frozen (100g/3½oz) cod, coley, haddock
* or hake steak*
125g (4oz) canned tomatoes
Salt and pepper
Pinch dried thyme
15g (½oz) Edam cheese, grated
50g (2oz) canned or frozen sweetcorn kernels
50g (2oz) broccoli

Place the fish steak in a small ovenproof casserole. Cover it with the tomatoes, season to taste and add the thyme. Sprinkle with grated cheese and bake in a moderate oven, 180°C, 350°F, gas mark 4, until the fish is cooked. Serve with the cooked vegetables.

Fish Cakes and Baked Beans

2 frozen fish cakes
125g (4oz) canned baked beans in tomato
* sauce*

Grill or bake the fish cakes without added fat. Serve with the heated baked beans.

Spicy Haddock Steaks *opposite page*

½ clove garlic, crushed
2.5ml (½ teaspoon) prepared mustard
Salt and pepper
150g (5oz) low-fat natural yogurt
7g (¼oz) butter
15ml (1 tablespoon) lemon juice
1.25ml (¼ teaspoon) paprika
1.25ml (¼ teaspoon) turmeric
2.5ml (½ teaspoon) tomato purée
1.25ml (¼ teaspoon) prepared mustard
2 haddock steaks (170g/6oz each)
Watercress to garnish

1 Make a yogurt relish to serve with the fish steaks: mix the garlic, mustard, seasoning and yogurt together in a bowl and set aside.
2 Melt the butter in a small pan and stir in the lemon juice, paprika, turmeric, tomato purée and mustard. Heat through gently but do not worry if the mixture curdles.
3 Brush the haddock steaks (you may use fresh or defrosted frozen ones) with about half of the spicy mixture.
4 Place under a hot grill and after 5 minutes, turn the steaks over and brush with the remaining spicy sauce. Continue cooking for another 5 minutes until cooked.
5 Serve the steaks very hot with the yogurt relish and garnished with watercress sprigs.
Serves 2

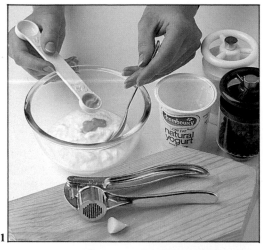

1

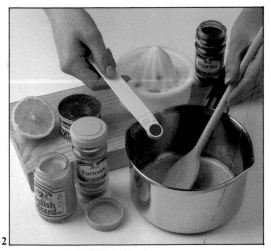

2

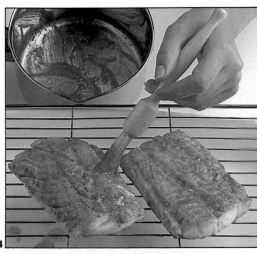

3

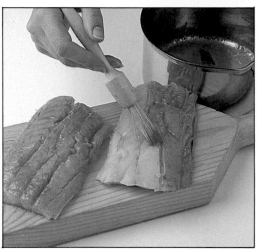

4

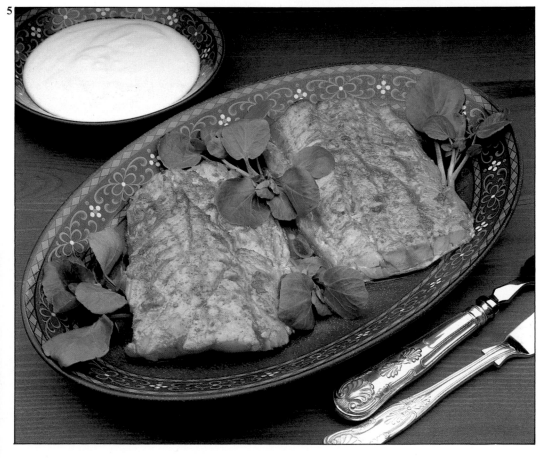

5

137

Smoked Haddock Fluff

75g (3oz) cooked smoked haddock (or other
* smoked white fish)*
5ml (1 teaspoon) tomato ketchup
1 medium egg (size 3), separated
Pepper
5ml (1 teaspoon) chopped fresh parsley
1 fresh tomato
75g (3oz) green beans, boiled

Flake the haddock and mix with the tomato
ketchup and egg yolk. Season with pepper
and add the parsley. Whisk the egg white
until stiff and fold into the fish and yolk
mixture. Turn into a small ovenproof dish
and cook it for 15-20 minutes at 190°C,
375°F, gas mark 5. Serve with the tomato
and boiled green beans.

Fish and Prawn Chowder

125g (4oz) white fish steak or fillet
225g (8oz) canned tomatoes with juice
Salt and pepper
Pinch dried basil
25g (1oz) fresh or frozen shelled prawns
30ml (2 level tablespoons) cooked or canned
* sweetcorn kernels*
1 small slice slimmers' bread or ½ slice
* wholemeal bread (unbuttered)*

Place the fish in a small pan. Roughly chop
the tomatoes and add to the fish with salt
and pepper to taste, and the basil. Cover
and simmer for 10 minutes. Remove the
fish, flake and return to the pan with the
prawns and sweetcorn. Heat through and
serve with the bread.

Seafood Salad *opposite page*

175g (6oz) white fish fillet
10ml (2 teaspoons) lemon juice
Salt and pepper
5ml (1 level teaspoon) diced gherkin
1 tomato
50g (2oz) cucumber
5ml (1 level teaspoon) chopped onion
5ml (1 level teaspoon) capers
15ml (1 tablespoon) low-calorie seafood sauce
5ml (1 teaspoon) anchovy essence
15ml (1 tablespoon) natural yogurt
50g (2oz) cucumber
15g (½oz) unpeeled prawns

Wash and skin the fish and cut it into cubes.
Poach the cubed fish in the lemon juice, a
little water and seasoning for 10-15 minutes.
Dice the gherkins and tomato; chop the
cucumber and onion. Mix with the capers in
a bowl. Blend the seafood sauce, the anchovy
essence and natural yogurt together and stir
into the chopped vegetables. Drain the fish,
allow to cool and coat with the sauce mixture.
Pile the fish mixture into a serving dish and
garnish with cucumber twists and prawns.

Fish Fingers with Mushrooms and Peas

2 frozen fish fingers
15ml (1 tablespoon) tomato ketchup
213g (7½oz) canned mushrooms in brine,
* or 125g (4oz) fresh button mushrooms*
125g (4oz) peas, boiled

Grill the fish fingers without added fat. Serve
with the tomato ketchup and heated canned
mushrooms, or fresh mushrooms poached
in stock, and the boiled peas.

Roast Beef and Vegetables

75g (3oz) roast lean beef
50ml (2floz) thin, fat-free gravy
125g (4oz) cauliflower
125g (4oz) carrots
50g (2oz) runner beans

Trim all the visible fat from the roast beef.
Serve with the gravy and boiled cauliflower,
carrots and runner beans.

Roast Chicken and Vegetables

75g (3oz) roast chicken
50ml (2floz) thin, fat-free gravy
125g (4oz) Brussels sprouts or broccoli
40g (1½oz) sweetcorn kernels

Remove all skin from the roast chicken and
serve with the gravy and boiled vegetables.

Drumstick Casserole

2 chicken drumsticks
25g (1oz) onion, sliced
25g (1oz) green pepper (capsicum), sliced
50g (2oz) button mushrooms
25g (1oz) carrot, sliced
275ml (½pint) chicken stock made from
* ½ stock cube*
Salt and pepper
Bay leaf

Skin the drumsticks and place in a small
ovenproof casserole dish with the other
ingredients. Cover and cook in a moderate
oven at 180°C, 350°F, gas mark 4, for 40
minutes, or until the chicken is tender.

Kidneys in Sherry Sauce

2 lamb's kidneys
7g (¼oz) low-fat spread
25g (1oz) onion, chopped
25g (1oz) mushrooms, chopped
50ml (2floz) beef stock
15ml (1 tablespoon) dry sherry
15ml (1 tablespoon) tomato purée
Salt and pepper
5ml (1 level teaspoon) cornflour
175g (6oz) cauliflower

Wash, skin, core and quarter the kidneys.
Heat the low-fat spread in a small pan and
gently fry the kidneys and onion for 2-3
minutes. Add the mushrooms, stock, sherry,

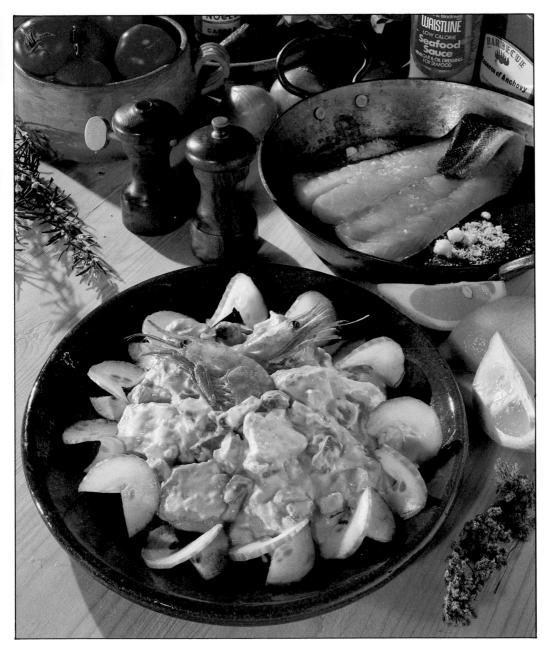

tomato purée and seasoning and stir well. Cover and simmer for 10 minutes. Blend the cornflour with a little cold water and stir into the saucepan. Continue to heat until thickened, stirring all the time. Break the cauliflower into florets and boil in salted water. Arrange the cauliflower in a border and serve the kidneys in the centre.

Baked Egg with Mushrooms and Chicken Livers

50g (2oz) mushrooms
50g (2oz) chicken livers
50ml (2floz) tomato juice
Dash Worcestershire sauce
1 medium egg (size 3)
Salt and pepper
1 crispbread (unbuttered)

Chop the mushrooms and chicken livers and place in a small saucepan with the tomato juice and Worcestershire sauce. Cover and simmer for 10 minutes. Turn into a small ovenproof dish and season to taste. Break the egg on top of the liver and mushrooms. Bake at 180°C, 350°F, gas mark 4, for about 10 minutes, or until the egg is set. Serve with the crispbread.

Grilled Chicken and Salad Vegetables

225g (8oz) chicken joint
Lettuce leaves
Watercress
1 tomato, sliced
Few spring onions or onion rings
½ small green or red pepper (capsicum)
15ml (1 level tablespoon) oil-free French dressing
1 crispbread (unbuttered)

Grill the chicken joint without added fat until cooked through. Skin the chicken joint and serve with the salad vegetables, salad dressing and crispbread.

Liver Casserole

75g (3oz) lamb's liver, sliced
25g (1oz) onion, sliced
1 medium carrot, sliced
1 stick celery, chopped
125g (4oz) canned tomatoes
50ml (2floz) water
Salt and pepper
75g (3oz) cauliflower

Place the liver, onion, carrot, celery, tomatoes, water and seasoning to taste in a small ovenproof casserole. Cover and cook in a moderate oven, 180°C, 350°F, gas mark 4, for 40 minutes. Boil the cauliflower and serve with the liver casserole.

Grilled Sausage, Bacon and Tomato

2 pork chipolata (small) sausages
1 rasher streaky bacon
1 tomato, halved
50g (2oz) button mushrooms

Grill the sausages until well done, the bacon until crisp, and the tomato halves until softened. Poach the mushrooms in salted water or stock, and serve with the sausages, bacon and tomato.

Bacon Steak with Apple Slices

1 bacon steak, 99g (3½oz) raw weight
1 small (75g/3oz) eating apple
75g (3oz) Brussels sprouts
50g (2oz) broad beans

Grill the bacon steak on both sides until cooked. Core and slice the apple and arrange the apple slices over the top of the bacon steak. Replace it under the grill and cook until the apple is softened and beginning to brown. Serve with the cooked Brussels sprouts and broad beans.

Salad meals (200 calories)

Pasta and Prawn Salad

25g (1oz) pasta rings or shells
50g (2oz) fresh or thawed frozen prawns
50g (2oz) button mushrooms, sliced
½ small red pepper (capsicum), diced
1 stick celery, chopped
30ml (2 tablespoons) natural yogurt
Pinch curry powder
Salt and pepper
Lettuce leaves

Boil the pasta until just tender, then drain and rinse under cold water and drain again. Mix the pasta with the prawns, mushrooms, pepper and celery. Mix the yogurt with the curry powder, salt and pepper. Mix with the pasta and prawns until well blended. Serve on a bed of lettuce.

Prawn and Egg Salad

50g (2oz) fresh or thawed frozen prawns
1 medium egg (size 4), hard-boiled and halved
15ml (1 tablespoon) low-calorie salad cream
    or seafood sauce
Lettuce leaves
Mustard and cress
½ small green pepper (capsicum), sliced
Cucumber, sliced
Few radishes
1 crispbread (unbuttered)

Arrange the prawns and halved egg on a bed of lettuce. Spoon over the low-calorie salad cream or seafood sauce. Arrange the remaining salad vegetables around the plate. Serve with the crispbread.

Corned Beef Salad

50g (2oz) corned beef, sliced
50g (2oz) grated carrot
50g (2oz) pickled beetroot
Lettuce leaves
Few spring onions or onion rings
Watercress
2 sticks celery, chopped
1 crispbread (unbuttered)

Arrange the corned beef with the salad vegetables on a plate and serve with the unbuttered crispbread.

Cheese, Tomato and Mushroom Salad

40g (1½oz) Edam cheese, diced
2 tomatoes, cut in wedges
1 stick celery, chopped
25g (1oz) button mushrooms, quartered
25g (1oz) small gherkins
30ml (2 tablespoons) oil-free French dressing
Watercress
1 crispbread (unbuttered)

Put the cheese, tomatoes, celery, mushrooms, gherkins and oil-free French dressing in a bowl and toss well together. Serve with a small bunch of watercress and the crispbread.

Beef Salad

50g (2oz) cold roast lean beef
2.5cm (1in) piece cucumber, diced
1 tomato, cut in wedges
4 radishes, sliced
25g (1oz) pickled beetroot, chopped
15ml (1 tablespoon) cocktail onions
30ml (2 tablespoons) tomato juice
5ml (1 teaspoon) vinegar
Salt and pepper
1 small, thin slice wholemeal bread (25g/1oz)
3½g (⅛ oz) low-fat spread

Remove any visible fat from the beef and cut into bite-sized pieces. Mix with the prepared cucumber, tomato, radishes, beetroot and onions. Mix the tomato juice and vinegar together and stir into the beef salad with seasoning to taste. Serve with the bread scraped with the low-fat spread.

Ham Rolls with Salad

2 slices lean boiled ham (25g/1oz each)
50g (2oz) cottage cheese, any flavour except with Cheddar
1 stick celery, chopped
1 head chicory
1 tomato, sliced
15ml (1 tablespoon) oil-free French dressing

Trim any visible fat off the ham. Mix the cottage cheese with the celery and spread on the slices of ham. Roll up the ham and serve with the chicory and tomato dressed with the oil-free dressing.

Cottage Cheese and Orange Salad

1 medium orange, peeled and segmented
113g (4oz) natural cottage cheese
Salt and pepper
Lettuce leaves
Mustard and cress
Cucumber slices
½ small green or red pepper (capsicum), sliced
2 crispbreads, unbuttered

Mix the orange segments with the cottage cheese and season to taste with salt and pepper. Serve with the salad and crispbread.

Pear and Curd Cheese

1 medium pear
Lemon juice
50g (2oz) curd cheese
25g (1oz) lean boiled ham, chopped
2 walnut halves, chopped
Few lettuce leaves

Peel the pear, cut in half and remove the core. Brush all over with lemon juice to prevent it from browning. Mix the curd cheese, chopped ham and walnuts together, and fill the hollows in the pear halves. Serve on a bed of lettuce.

Sardine and Coleslaw Salad

2 canned sardines in tomato sauce
125g (4oz) white cabbage, shredded
1 carrot, grated
5ml (1 teaspoon) chopped onion, or 1 chopped spring onion
15ml (1 level tablespoon) low-calorie salad cream
1 tomato, sliced
Watercress sprigs
1 crispbread (unbuttered)

Arrange the sardines on a plate. Mix the cabbage, carrot, onion and the salad cream together and place on the plate with the sardines. Garnish with the sliced tomato and watercress. Serve with the crispbread.

Salmon Salad

100g (3½oz) canned pink salmon
3 small gherkins, chopped
1 stick celery, chopped
15ml (1 level tablespoon) low-calorie salad cream or seafood sauce
Lettuce leaves
1 tomato, sliced
Cucumber, sliced
4 black olives

Flake the salmon and mix with the chopped gherkins, celery and salad cream or seafood sauce. Arrange a bed of lettuce on a plate and pile the salmon mixture in the centre. Arrange the sliced tomato and cucumber around the salmon and garnish with olives.

Oriental Chicken Salad

50g (2oz) cooked chicken, all skin removed
75g (3oz) fresh or drained canned bean sprouts
5ml (1 teaspoon) finely chopped onion
1 ring canned pineapple in natural juice, chopped
30ml (2 tablespoons) low-fat natural yogurt
5ml (1 teaspoon) lemon juice
Freshly ground pepper
Head of chicory
1 small slice slimmers' bread
3½g (⅛ oz) low-fat spread

Chop the chicken into bite-sized pieces, and mix with the bean sprouts, onion, pineapple, yogurt and lemon juice. Season to taste with pepper. Serve on a plate surrounded by the chicory leaves. Serve with the slice of bread scraped with low-fat spread.

Chicken and Grape Salad

75g (3oz) cooked chicken
50g (2oz) grapes
2 sticks celery, chopped
45ml (3 tablespoons) low-fat natural yogurt
Salt and pepper
Lettuce leaves
Chopped fresh parsley

Remove any skin from the chicken and chop into bite-sized pieces. Halve and deseed the grapes. Mix the chicken, grapes, celery and yogurt together, and season to taste with salt and pepper. Serve on a bed of lettuce and garnish with the chopped parsley.

Sweet meals (200 calories)

Drinking Chocolate and Biscuits

20ml (2 rounded teaspoons) drinking chocolate
225ml (8floz) skimmed milk (extra to drinks allowance)
2 ginger or 2 malted milk biscuits

Make a cup of chocolate with the drinking chocolate and milk. Serve with the biscuits.

Apple and Chocolate

25g (1oz) piece chocolate
150g (5oz) eating apple

Eat the chocolate with the apple.

Fresh Fruits

1 medium (175g/6oz) banana
1 medium orange
150g (5oz) grapes
Low-calorie lemonade or ginger ale

Eat the fresh fruits in any order liked. Alternatively peel and slice the banana, peel and segment the orange, halve and deseed the grapes and mix together with low-calorie lemonade or ginger ale to make a fruit salad.

Peach Melba

50g (2oz) vanilla ice-cream
1 large fresh peach, halved and stoned, or
*   2 canned peach halves*
50g (2oz) fresh or frozen raspberries
5ml (1 level teaspoon) caster sugar
2 ice-cream wafers

Place the ice-cream in a serving dish and top with the peach halves. Using a fork, crush the raspberries with the sugar and spoon over the peach. Serve with the 2 wafers.

Banana Split

50g (2oz) vanilla ice-cream
1 small banana (150g/5oz)
10ml (2 level teaspoons) raspberry or
*   strawberry jam*

Place the ice-cream in a dish long enough to take the banana lengthwise. Peel and halve the banana lengthwise and arrange one half on each side of the ice-cream. Spoon the jam on top of the ice-cream and serve.

Rice Pudding

15g (½oz) short-grain rice
15ml (1 level tablespoon) sugar
200ml (7floz) skimmed milk
Pinch grated nutmeg
10ml (1 rounded teaspoon) jam

Rinse the rice in water and place in a small ovenproof dish. Add the sugar, milk and grated nutmeg and stir well. Bake in the bottom of a warm oven, 170°C, 325°F, gas mark 3, for 2 hours, stirring twice during cooking time, or, alternatively, cook in the top of a double boiler for 2 hours. Serve topped with the jam.

Stewed Prunes and Custard

25g (1oz) dried prunes
10ml (2 level teaspoons) custard powder
150ml (¼ pint) skimmed milk
10ml (2 level teaspoons) sugar
2 plain finger biscuits

Soak the dried prunes overnight in cold water or for 2 hours in hot water, then cook in water until tender. Blend the custard powder with a little of the milk. Bring the remainder of the milk and the sugar to the boil in a saucepan. Pour onto the blended custard powder, stirring. Return to the pan and boil for 1 minute, or until thickened, stirring all the time. Serve the prunes with the custard and biscuits.

Banana and Yogurt

1 small carton low-fat fruit yogurt, any flavour
*   except banana or black cherry*
1 small (5oz/150g) banana

Peel and slice the banana and serve with the fruit flavoured yogurt.

Orange and Honey Yogurt

1 medium orange
1 small carton low-fat natural yogurt
10ml (2 level teaspoons) clear honey
2 sponge fingers

Peel and segment the orange. Stir the orange segments into the yogurt with the honey. Serve with the sponge fingers

Strawberry Fare

50g (2oz) vanilla or strawberry ice-cream
50g (2oz) strawberries
50g (2oz) seedless grapes
2 plain finger biscuits

Cut the ice-cream into cubes and mix with the fruit. Serve with the biscuits.

Gooseberry Fool

125g (4oz) gooseberries
30ml (2 tablespoons) water
15ml (1 level tablespoon) sugar
1 small carton low-fat natural yogurt
Artificial sweetener (optional)
2 sponge fingers

Top and tail the gooseberries and place in a small pan with the water. Cover and cook gently until the gooseberries are tender. Sieve the gooseberries to make a puree. Stir in the sugar and yogurt until blended. Check the flavour and add artificial sweetener, if liked. Serve with sponge fingers.

Stuffed Baked Apple

15g (½oz) sultanas or raisins
5ml (1 level teaspoon) clear honey
70ml (2½floz) unsweetened orange juice
175g (6oz) cooking apple

Put the dried fruit, honey and orange juice in a basin and stand for at least 10 minutes to soak. Peel and core the apple and stand it in a small ovenproof dish. Spoon the sultanas or raisins into the hole in the centre of the apple and pour the remaining orange juice over the top of the apple. Cover the dish with a lid or foil and bake at 170°C, 325°F, gas mark 3, for 45 minutes, or until the apple is tender. Serve the apple in its juices.

Do as you're told diet

This diet guarantees success because it tells you precisely what to eat. Firm discipline can drive you to your goal when more subtle coaxing fails. If you do as you are told and follow this diet to the letter, you will be rewarded with a speedy weight loss.

You must be prepared to co-operate and follow it precisely. It does not allow you to substitute any foods so you cannot cheat, however innocently. Because it is so precise, it means you must plan and shop before you start so that you have every food you need at hand. It is best to get in a whole week's supply of foods in one go if you can but, if for any reason you need to shop more frequently, take the greatest care to buy only those foods (in the right quantities) that you are allowed. Once you have all the foods you require, the diet is simplicity itself. Do as you are told, eat only what the diet offers and you *will* lose weight.

Diet rules

1 Each day's menus must be followed precisely. Don't substitute one food for another or change anything.

2 You may choose the times you eat your meals. The breakfast or snack meal may be eaten later in the day if you wish; and the main and light meals may be taken either in the middle of the day or in the evening, whichever suits you best.

3 As well as three meals a day, you are allowed one medium-sized orange, an apple or pear and 142ml (¼pint) whole milk or 284ml (½pint) skimmed milk for use in tea and coffee. You can also drink unlimited water, black coffee, tea without milk and sugar (artificial sweeteners may be used) and soft drinks labelled 'low-calorie'.

4 Shop ahead and weigh and measure *all* foods accurately.

Day 1

Breakfast or Snack Meal
Grapefruit, Boiled Egg and Toast

½ grapefruit, sprinkled with
5ml (1 level teaspoon) sugar
1 medium egg (size 3), boiled, served with
1 slice of bread (40g/1½oz), toasted and
spread with
7g (¼oz) low-fat spread

Light Meal
Cottage Cheese and Tomato Sandwich

2 slices bread (40g/1½oz each), spread with

15g (½oz) low-fat spread, filled with
50g (2oz) cottage cheese, any flavour, and
1 tomato, sliced, and
5ml (1 level teaspoon) yeast extract

Main Meal
Chicken, Sweetcorn and Baked Potato

225g (8oz) chicken joint, grilled
125g (4oz) canned or frozen sweetcorn,
cooked
175g (6oz) jacket-baked potato

Day 2

Breakfast or Snack Meal
Grapefruit, Toast and Marmalade

½ grapefruit, sprinkled with
5ml (1 level teaspoon) sugar
2 slices bread (40g/1½oz each), spread with
15g (½oz) low-fat spread and
15ml (1 level tablespoon) marmalade

Light Meal
Cottage Cheese and Egg Salad

113g (4oz) cottage cheese, any flavour
except with Cheddar, mixed with
1 medium egg (size 3), hard-boiled and sliced,
served with
Mixed salad of tomato, lettuce, cucumber
and celery, dressed with
15ml (1 tablespoon) low-calorie salad cream

Main Meal
Liver Casserole with Potatoes

125g (4oz) lamb's liver
225g (8oz) canned tomatoes
50g (2oz) mushrooms
25g (1oz) chopped onion
Dash Worcestershire sauce
Salt and pepper
Pinch of herbs
200g (7oz) potatoes, boiled

Place all the ingredients except the potatoes in an ovenproof dish and cook at 180°C, 350°F, gas mark 4, for 45 minutes. Serve with boiled potatoes.

Day 3

Breakfast or Snack Meal
Bacon and Baked Beans

2 rashers back bacon, well grilled
142g (5oz) canned baked beans in tomato
sauce

Light Meal
Salmon Salad

100g (3½oz) canned salmon, served with
Mixed salad of tomato, lettuce, cucumber and celery, dressed with
15ml (1 tablespoon) low-calorie salad cream
1 slice of bread (40g/1½oz), spread with
7g (¼oz) low-fat spread

Main Meal
Pork Casserole and Mashed Potato

175g (6oz) pork fillet, all visible fat removed
50g (2oz) mushrooms, sliced
¼ red or green pepper (capsicum), chopped
¼ stock cube
50g (2oz) carrots, sliced
150g (5oz) boiled potatoes
30ml (2 tablespoons) skimmed milk

Place the pork fillet, mushrooms, pepper, stock cube, carrots and 75ml (3floz) water in an ovenproof casserole. Bake at 180°C, 350°F, gas mark 4, for 1 hour. Serve with the potatoes mashed with skimmed milk.

Day 4

Breakfast or Snack Meal
Grapefruit, and Poached Eggs on Toast

½ grapefruit, sprinkled with
5ml (1 level teaspoon) sugar
2 medium eggs (size 3), poached and served on
1 slice bread (40g/1½oz) spread with
7g (¼oz) low-fat spread

Light Meal
Kidney and Spaghetti Savoury
See step-by-step recipe opposite

Main Meal
Grilled Fish, Beans and Chips

175g (6oz) cod or haddock fillets, spread with
15g (½oz) low-fat spread and grilled or baked
125g (4oz) cooked runner beans
75g (3oz) frozen oven chips, baked in the oven

Day 5

Breakfast or Snack Meal
Breakfast Cereal

40g (1½oz) bran breakfast cereal, served with

150ml (¼ pint) skimmed milk (additional to allowance) and
5ml (1 level teaspoon) sugar

Light Meal
Cheese, Crispbreads and Fruit

50g (2oz) Edam cheese, served with
2 crispbreads and
30ml (1 rounded tablespoon) pickle and
2 sticks celery, followed by
1 medium orange or apple or pear

Main Meal
Grilled Sausages and Kidneys

2 pork chipolatas, well grilled and
2 lamb's kidneys, grilled, served with
15ml (1 tablespoon) tomato ketchup and
2 tomatoes, grilled and
125g (4oz) cooked peas and
175g (6oz) potato, baked in its jacket, served with
7g (¼oz) low-fat spread

Day 6

Breakfast or Snack Meal
Orange Juice and Scrambled Egg on Toast

150ml (¼ pint) unsweetened orange juice
1 slice bread (40g/1½oz), toasted and topped with
1 medium egg (size 3), scrambled with
45ml (3 tablespoons) skimmed milk, and
7g (¼oz) low-fat spread

Light Meal
Sausages and Coleslaw

2 pork chipolatas, well grilled and cooled
Coleslaw of 125g (4oz) white cabbage, shredded; 1 medium carrot, grated; 1 stick celery, finely chopped; mixed with
15ml (1 tablespoon) low-calorie salad cream
1 slice bread (40g/1½oz), spread with
7g (¼oz) low-fat spread

Main Meal
Beef Casserole and Mashed Potato

125g (4oz) lean stewing steak
5ml (1 level teaspoon) plain flour
25g (1oz) onion, chopped
1 stick celery, chopped
1 medium carrot, chopped
Salt and pepper and pinch of herbs
¼ beef stock cube
200ml (7floz) boiling water
175g (6oz) potatoes, boiled
30ml (2 tablespoons) skimmed milk

Place the steak, flour, vegetables, seasoning,

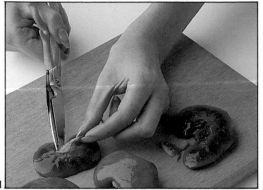
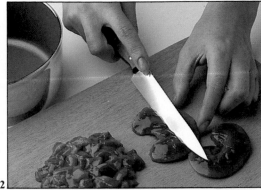

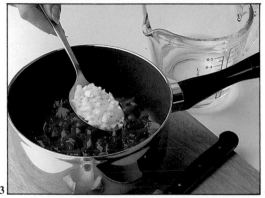
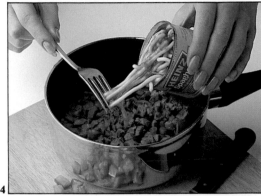

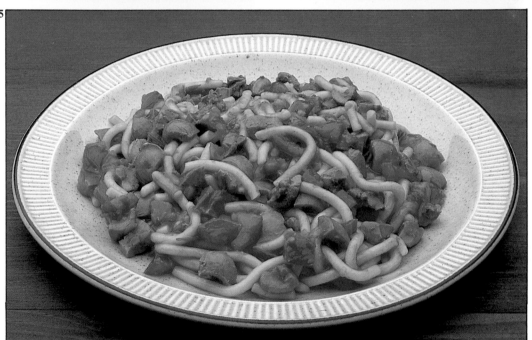

Kidney and Spaghetti Savoury

3 lamb's kidneys
15ml (1 tablespoon) chopped onion
150ml (¼ pint) water
1 tomato
142g (5oz) canned spaghetti in tomato sauce
Salt and pepper

1 Cut the lamb's kidneys in half lengthways. Carefully peel off the skin and membranes and, using kitchen scissors, remove the hard inner core of each kidney.

2 Chop the kidneys into small pieces and place them in a small saucepan.

3 Add the finely chopped onion to the chopped kidney in the pan and cover with the water. Cover the pan with a lid and simmer gently for about 15 minutes until the kidney is cooked.

4 Drain off the water from the kidney mixture. Peel and chop the tomato roughly and add to the kidney mixture in the pan together with the canned spaghetti. Heat through gently, stirring all the time. Season.

5 Serve the Kidney and Spaghetti Savoury on a serving dish piping-hot.

Serves 1

145

stock cube and the water in an ovenproof casserole. Bake at 170°C, 325°F, gas mark 3, for two hours. Serve with the potatoes mashed with the skimmed milk.

Day 7

Breakfast or Snack Meal
Grapefruit, Egg and Crispbread

½ grapefruit
1 medium egg (size 3), boiled or poached
2 crispbreads, spread with
7g (¼oz) low-fat spread

Light Meal
Beans on Toast (Apple)

1 slice bread (40g/1½oz), toasted and topped with
225g (8oz) canned baked beans in tomato sauce
1 medium eating apple

Main Meal
Pork Chop and Vegetables

213g (7½oz) pork chop, well grilled, and served with
125g (4oz) button mushrooms, poached in stock, and
125g (4oz) boiled cabbage and
175g (6oz) boiled or canned new potatoes

Day 8

Breakfast or Snack Meal
Grapefruit, Toast and Marmalade

½ grapefruit, sprinkled with
5ml (1 level teaspoon) sugar
1 slice bread (40g/1½oz), spread with
7g (¼oz) low-fat spread, and
10ml (1 rounded teaspoon) marmalade

Light Meal
Bacon Sandwich

2 slices bread (40g/1½oz each), filled with
2 rashers back bacon, well grilled, and
15ml (1 tablespoon) tomato ketchup

Main Meal
Fish Fingers, Peas and Oven Chips
4 fish fingers, grilled without added fat, served with
15ml (1 tablespoon) tomato ketchup, and
125g (4oz) cooked peas, and
1 tomato, grilled, and
75g (3oz) frozen oven chips, baked in oven

Day 9

Breakfast or Snack Meal
Orange Juice, Egg and Bread

150ml (¼ pint) unsweetened orange juice
1 medium egg (size 3), boiled or poached
1 slice bread (40g/1½oz), spread with
7g (¼oz) low-fat spread

Light Meal
Cheese and Tomato Toast (Fresh Fruit)

1 slice bread (40g/1½oz), toasted and topped with
1 sliced tomato and
40g (1½oz) grated Edam cheese, and grilled
1 medium pear

Main Meal
Bacon Steaks with Pineapple (Fruit and Ice-cream)

2 bacon or ham steaks (100g/3½oz each raw weight), well grilled, served with
2 rings canned pineapple in natural juice heated under grill, and
Small bunch watercress, and
50g (2oz) button mushrooms, poached in stock or water, and
50g (2oz) cooked peas
125g (4oz) fresh or frozen raspberries or strawberries, served with
50g (2oz) vanilla ice-cream

Day 10

Breakfast or Snack Meal
Grapefruit, Boiled Egg and Toast

½ grapefruit, sprinkled with
5ml (1 level teaspoon) sugar
1 medium egg (size 3), boiled
1 slice bread (40g/1½oz), toasted and spread with
7g (¼oz) low-fat spread

Light Meal
Sardine and Olive Sandwich

2 slices bread (40g/1½oz each), filled with
2 mashed sardines in tomato sauce, and
2 stuffed olives, chopped, and
5ml (1 level teaspoon) finely chopped onion, and
1 tomato, sliced

Main Meal
Grilled Liver and Bacon

125g (4oz) lamb's liver, brushed with
15g (½oz) low-fat spread, and grilled

2 rashers back bacon, well grilled
1 tomato, grilled without fat
75g (3oz) green beans

Day 11

Breakfast or Snack Meal
Breakfast Cereal

40g (1½oz) bran breakfast cereal, served with
150ml (¼ pint) skimmed milk, and
5ml (1 level teaspoon) sugar

Light Meal
Orange Juice and Cottage Cheese Salad

150ml (¼ pint) unsweetened orange juice
113g (4oz) cottage cheese, any flavour except with Cheddar
Mixed salad of lettuce, cucumber, watercress, few radishes and spring onions, dressed with
15ml (1 tablespoon) oil-free French dressing
1 slice bread (40g/1½oz), spread with
7g (¼oz) low-fat spread

Main Meal
Grilled Fish with Vegetables (Pineapple and Ice-cream)

175g (6oz) cod, coley or haddock fillets spread with
15g (½oz) low-fat spread, and grilled or baked
50g (2oz) cooked peas
50g (2oz) canned or frozen sweetcorn, cooked
2 canned pineapple rings in natural juice and
50g (2oz) vanilla ice-cream

Day 12

Breakfast or Snack Meal
Tomatoes on Toast

1 slice bread (40g/1½oz), toasted and spread with
7g (¼oz) low-fat spread, and topped with
225g (8oz) canned tomatoes

Light Meal
Egg and Prawn Salad

1 medium egg (size 3), hard-boiled, sliced and mixed with
50g (2oz) fresh or frozen (thawed) prawns, and
Lettuce, cucumber, spring onions, grated carrot, sliced tomato, few radishes and mustard and cress, dressed with
15ml (1 tablespoon) low-calorie salad cream
1 slice bread (40g/1½oz), spread with
7g (¼oz) low-fat spread

Main Meal
Grilled Lamb Chop with Vegetables

150g (5oz) lamb chump chop, grilled, served with
10ml (2 teaspoons) mint sauce, and
175g (6oz) boiled or canned new potatoes,
125g (4oz) boiled broccoli, and
75g (3oz) boiled carrots
1 small banana (150g/5oz)

Day 13

Breakfast or Snack Meal
Breakfast Cereal

40g (1½oz) bran breakfast cereal, with
150ml (¼ pint) skimmed milk (in addition to allowance) and
5ml (1 level teaspoon) sugar

Light Meal
Beefburgers and Beans

2 frozen beefburgers, well grilled
225g (8oz) canned baked beans in tomato sauce

Main Meal
Chicken Salad with Jacket-baked Potato

225g (8oz) chicken joint, baked
Mixed salad of lettuce, tomato, cucumber, onion rings and green or red pepper (capsicum), dressed with
15ml (1 tablespoon) oil-free French dressing
175g (6oz) jacket-baked potato, topped with
15g (½oz) low-fat spread
1 medium eating apple to follow

Day 14

Breakfast or Snack Meal
Breakfast Cereal

40g (1½oz) bran breakfast cereal, with
150ml (¼ pint) skimmed milk (additional to allowance) and
5ml (1 level teaspoon) sugar

Light Meal
Hot Mushroom Roll (Orange and Yogurt)
See step-by-step recipe overleaf

Main Meal
Chicken Drumsticks with Vegetable Rice

3 chicken drumsticks, grilled and skin removed
25g (1oz) long-grain rice, cooked in
75ml (3floz) water with
¼ chicken stock cube. Mix with
50g (2oz) cooked peas and
50g (2oz) frozen or canned sweetcorn, cooked

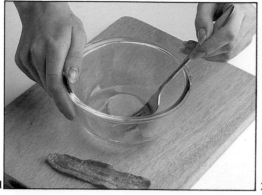

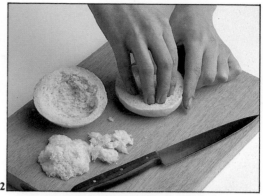

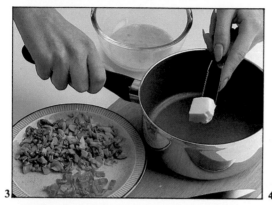

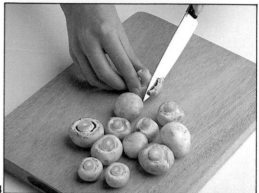

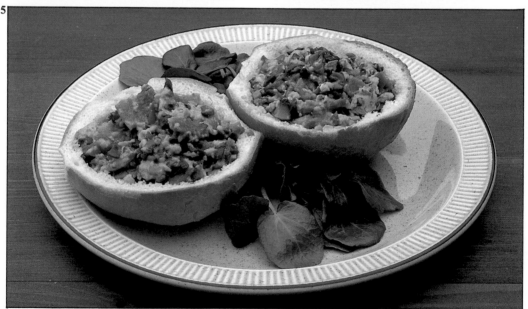

Hot Mushroom Roll

1 crusty bread roll
1 rasher streaky bacon
1 medium egg (size 3)
75g (3oz) button mushrooms
60ml (4 tablespoons) water
7g (¼oz) low-fat spread
Salt and pepper
Watercress for garnish
1 medium orange
1 small carton low-fat yogurt

1 Place the bread roll on a baking sheet and heat in a moderate oven. Grill the bacon rasher until crisp, and then crumble it. Lightly beat the egg.

2 Chop the mushrooms and place in a small saucepan with the water. Simmer gently for 5 minutes and strain off the water.
3 Melt the low-fat spread in another pan over a gentle heat. Add the mushrooms, bacon, beaten egg and seasoning to taste. Cook over a low heat, stirring occasionally, for about 5 minutes until the mixture sets.
4 Halve the hot bread roll and remove the soft centre and discard. Fill the roll with the cooked mushroom mixture.
5 Serve the Hot Mushroom Roll garnished with sprigs of watercress. Complete the meal with a segmented orange and the yogurt.

Serves 1

Super-healthy diet
(1000 calories)

Pork and Bean Medley (Fruit); Nutty Fruit Sandwich; Smoked Haddock and Wholemeal Macaroni Bake (Fresh Fruit)

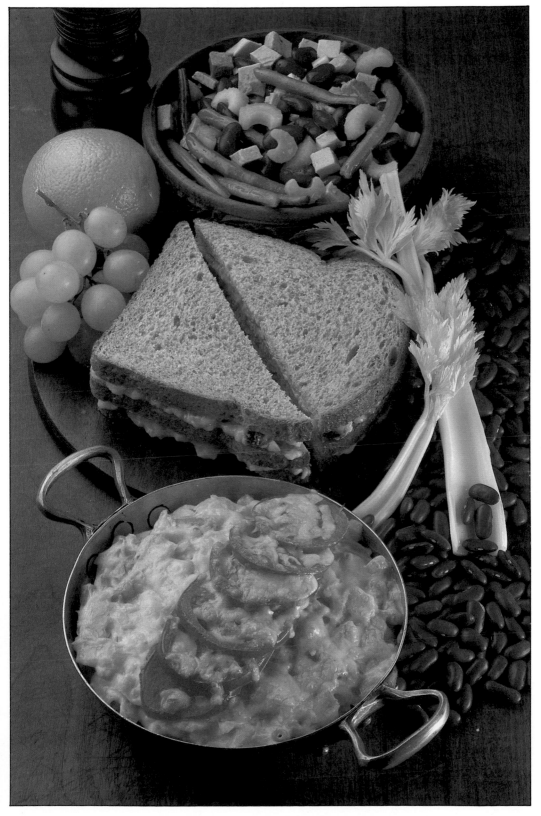

Super-healthy diet

If you want to be slim and build up new habits which will keep you sparkling with health and vitality, then here is the diet to match that resolve. Included in this diet are all the foods to which top nutritionists and medical experts attach major priority: wholemeal bread and cereals, fruit and vegetables, beans and pulses, all of which are low in fat and rich in fibre.

This is a very palatable diet with many interesting dishes and menus. Indeed, you will probably find the meals and menus so attractive that it will encourage you to change your eating habits permanently — with consequent benefit to your health and figure. If you set your sights high and aim for a health-improving slimming diet that provides a permanent source of maximum vitality, your best guide is scientific fact — that is what this diet is based on. No slimming diet can do more than the *Super Healthy Diet* to put you, and keep you, in sparkling good health as it peels off excess weight. Following the guidelines recommended by leading world health authorities, all the meals which have been devised here are:

1 Low in fat and low in cholesterol, because excess fat in Western diets is one of the major causes of health and weight problems.
2 High in fibre, because it is essential for the healthy functioning of the body and prevents constipation and many digestive disorders.
3 High in fresh fruit and vegetables, because these are excellent sources of both health-giving vitamins and fibre.

4 High in wholefood cereals, because modern research has upgraded these foods as an important factor in healthy eating, due to their high fibre content.
5 High in all the essential vitamins to make certain that you have your full requirement.
6 Low in sugar, because it is universally agreed that too much sugar is bad for health.

Diet rules
1 Choose one breakfast and two meals from the lunches and dinners listed on the following pages. If you do not want to eat breakfast, save that meal for a late-night snack or whenever you feel particularly hungry.
2 It is important that you vary your meals as much as possible to ensure that you have all the nutrients you need.
3 In addition to the three meals, which add up to 1,000 calories per day, you are allowed 284ml (½ pint) skimmed milk for use in tea and coffee, which adds 100 calories. Water, tea and coffee, taken either black or with milk from your allowance, are unlimited. Please do not put sugar in *any* drink. Use an artificial sweetener if you must.
4 Weigh and measure all foods carefully. The only exceptions to this important rule are some salad vegetables — for example, lettuce, cress and cucumber — which are so low in calories that you may eat as much as you need.
5 Do not overcook the vegetables or some of their natural goodness will be lost in the cooking process. Eat them while they are still firm and just tender.

Breakfasts (150 calories)

Cereal

2 wheat cereal biscuits or
40g (1½oz) bran cereal
125ml (4floz) skimmed milk (additional to allowance)

Serve the milk over the cereal.

Yogurt Muesli

10ml (2 level teaspoons) raisins
1 small carton low-fat natural yogurt
30ml (2 level tablespoons) muesli

Mix all the ingredients together and serve.

Honey Toast

1 slice wholemeal bread (40g/1½oz)
7g (¼oz) low-fat spread
10ml (2 level teaspoons) honey, jam or marmalade

Top the toasted bread with the spread and honey, jam or marmalade.

Cheesy Toast

1 slice wholemeal bread (40g/1½oz)
50g (2oz) cottage cheese, plain or flavoured

Toast the bread and cover the top with the cottage cheese.

Savoury Toast

1 slice wholemeal bread (40g/1½oz)
5ml (1 level teaspoon) yeast extract
25g (1oz) curd cheese

Toast the bread and spread with yeast extract and curd cheese.

Lunches and dinners (425 calories)

Nutty Fruit Sandwich

1 large banana
15ml (1 level tablespoon) raisins or sultanas
15ml (1 level tablespoon) chopped walnuts
3 slices wholemeal bread (40g/1½oz)

Mash the banana and mix with the raisins and walnuts. Make into a double-decker sandwich with the bread.

Chicken Liver Pâté with Toast

125g (4oz) chicken livers
15g (½oz) onion
30ml (2 tablespoons) chicken stock made
 from 1 stock cube
Pinch mixed herbs
50g (2oz) curd cheese
Salt and pepper
2 slices wholemeal bread (40g/1½oz each)
1 tomato

Roughly chop the chicken livers and finely chop the onion. Place in a saucepan with the stock and herbs. Cover the pan and simmer gently for 5 minutes. Cool, drain off any excess liquid and then mash the livers with the curd cheese. Season with the salt and pepper. Toast the bread and serve with the pâté and the tomato.

Peanut Butter Sandwich (Fresh Fruit)

2 slices wholemeal bread (40g/1½oz each)
25g (1oz) peanut butter
Lettuce
125g (4oz) grapes or 1 large eating apple

Make a sandwich with the peanut butter and lettuce. Follow with the grapes or apple.

Carroty meat salad

75g (3oz) lean, cold cooked meat (roast beef,
 pork, lamb or corned beef)
75g (3oz) carrots
25g (1oz) raisins
15g (½oz) hazelnuts
15ml (1 tablespoon) oil-free French dressing
Salt and pepper
2 bran crispbreads
7g (¼oz) low-fat spread
5ml (1 level teaspoon) yeast extract

Remove all the visible fat from the meat, grate the carrots and mix with the raisins, hazelnuts and dressing. Season. Spread the crispbreads with low-fat spread and yeast extract and serve with the meat salad.

Pork and Bean Medley (Fruit)

75g (3oz) cold cooked meat (lean roast pork
 or ham)
50g (2oz) French beans
1 stick celery
5ml (1 teaspoon) finely chopped onion
213g (7½oz) canned red kidney beans
45ml (3 tablespoons) oil-free French
 dressing
Salt and pepper
125g (4oz) grapes or 1 large eating apple

Remove all visible fat from the meat. Cook the French beans in salted water until just tender, drain and rinse. Roughly chop the celery. Drain the kidney beans and rinse under cold water. Mix all the vegetables together with the dressing and season. Serve with the meat. Follow with the fruit.

Cheesy Crispbreads (Fruity Yogurt)

113g (4oz) cottage cheese, any flavour except
 with Cheddar
4 bran crispbreads
1 small carton low-fat natural yogurt
25g (1oz) dried apricots
1 large orange

Spread the cottage cheese on the crispbreads. Make the fruity yogurt for dessert: chop the dried apricots, peel and roughly chop the orange. Stir the fruit into the yogurt.

Macaroni and Celery Bake

40g (1½oz) macaroni
Half 142g (5oz) can condensed celery soup
15ml (1 tablespoon) skimmed milk
50g (2oz) cooked green beans
50g (2oz) steamed white fish
Salt and pepper
1 tomato
5ml (1 level teaspoon) dried breadcrumbs
7g (¼oz) grated Edam cheese
125ml (4floz) dry wine

Cook the macaroni in boiling salted water until it is tender. Drain and return to the pan. add the soup, milk and beans. Flake the fish and add to the pan. Mix well and season with salt and pepper. Heat the mixture through gently, then turn it into an ovenproof dish and top with the sliced tomato. Sprinkle over the breadcrumbs and grated cheese and bake for 15 minutes at 190°C, 375°F, gas mark 5. Serve with a glass of dry red wine.

Macaroni and Celery Bake

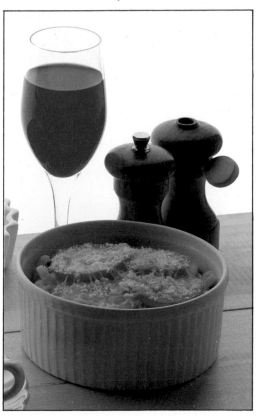

Corned Beef and Cheese Grill (Baked Apple)

1 slice wholemeal bread (40g/1½oz)
1 tomato
50g (2oz) corned beef
25g (1oz) Cheddar cheese, grated
1 medium cooking apple
15ml (1 level tablespoon) sultanas or raisins

Toast the bread on one side. Slice the tomato and place on the untoasted side with the corned beef. Grill until hot. Grate the cheese, sprinkle on top of the meat and grill until melted. Follow with the baked apple, prepared in advance. Core the apple and cut the skin around the middle. Stand the apple in an ovenproof dish and fill the cavity with dried fruit. Place 30ml (2 tablespoons) water in the dish and bake at 180°C, 350°F, gas mark 4, for 30 minutes.

Ham Sandwich (Banana)

2 slices wholemeal bread (40g/1½oz each)
15g (½oz) low-fat spread
50g (2oz) cooked ham
1 tomato
1 small banana

Spread the bread with low-fat spread. Remove all visible fat from the ham and make into a sandwich with the tomato. Follow with the banana.

Grilled Fish and Vegetables

175g (6oz) potato for baking
175g (6oz) cod or haddock fillet (or any firm-fleshed white fish)
15g (½oz) low-fat spread
125g (4oz) frozen peas
125g (4oz) carrots

Bake the potato in its jacket until soft when pinched. Dot the fish with half the low-fat spread and grill until it flakes easily (about 10 minutes). Cook the peas and carrots. Top the potato with the remaining spread, and serve with the fish and vegetables.

Smoked Haddock and Wholewheat Macaroni Bake (Fresh Fruit)

25g (1oz) wholewheat macaroni
175g (6oz) packet frozen buttered smoked haddock (or any smoked fish)
15ml (1 level tablespoon) cornflour
30ml (2 level tablespoons) powdered skimmed milk
Salt and pepper
1 tomato
15g (½oz) Edam cheese, grated
1 medium orange or apple or pear

Cook the macaroni in boiling salted water. Drain. Cook the smoked haddock. Discard the skin and flake the fish. Make the liquid from the fish up to 150ml (¼ pint) with water. Blend the cornflour and skimmed milk powder with a little liquid to make a smooth paste and then add to the remaining liquid. Bring to the boil, stirring all the time, and then cook for 2 minutes. Add the fish and macaroni, season and heat through. Turn into an ovenproof dish and arrange the sliced tomato on top. Sprinkle with the cheese and grill until melted.

Bacon and Bean Toastie (Fruit Yogurt)

220g (7¾oz) canned baked beans in tomato sauce
1 rasher streaky bacon
1 slice wholemeal bread (40g/1½oz)
1 small carton fruit yogurt

Heat the baked beans and crisply grill the bacon. Toast the bread and serve the beans and bacon on top. Follow with the yogurt.

Wholewheat Pasta and Tuna Salad (Raspberry Yogurt)

99g (3½oz) canned tuna in brine
40g (1½oz) wholewheat pasta rings or macaroni
50g (2oz) frozen peas
¼ red or green pepper (capsicum)
30ml (2 tablespoons) low-calorie salad cream
Salt and pepper
125g (4oz) frozen raspberries, thawed
1 small carton low-fat natural yogurt
Granulated non-sugar sweetener, to taste

Drain the tuna and flake roughly. Cook the pasta in boiling water until just tender. Drain, rinse under cold water and drain again. Cook the peas and drain. Remove the white pith and seeds from the pepper (capsicum) and chop into small squares. Mix together the tuna, pasta, peas, pepper (capsicum), low-calorie salad cream and a little chopped parsley. Season. To follow, mix together the raspberries and yogurt and sweeten with artificial sweetener if liked.

Fish and Tomato Wholemeal Pie

150g (5oz) potato
175g (6oz) cod or haddock fillet (or any firm-fleshed white fish)
125g (4oz) drained canned, tomatoes
Pinch mixed herbs, salt and pepper
25g (1oz) mushrooms
25g (1oz) wholemeal breadcrumbs
25g (1oz) Edam cheese

Bake the potato at 180°C, 350°F, gas mark 4, until soft when pinched. Place the fish in an ovenproof dish, then roughly chop the drained tomatoes and mushrooms. Season with herbs, salt and pepper and spread over the fish. Cover the dish with foil and bake with the potato for 15 minutes. Cover with the breadcrumbs and grated cheese. Return to the oven for 10-15 minutes.

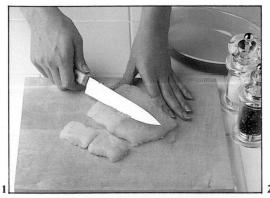

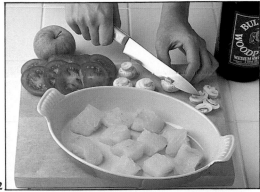

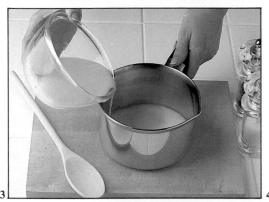

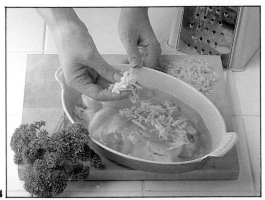

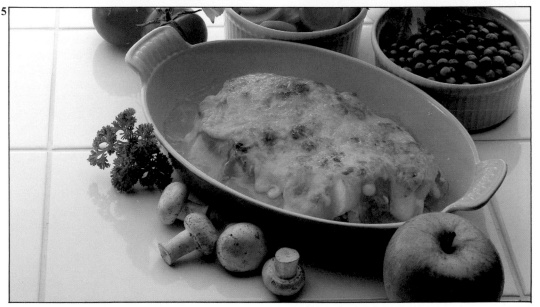

Cider Saucy Fish

225g (8oz) cod or haddock fillet
Salt and pepper
2 tomatoes
25g (1oz) button mushrooms
1 medium eating apple
175ml (6floz) dry cider
15g (½oz) low-fat spread
15g (½oz) cornflour
25g (1oz) grated Edam cheese
2 large (198g/7oz) bananas

1 Remove the skin and bones from the fish and cut into 2.5cm (1in) pieces. Place in an ovenproof dish and season with salt and pepper.
2 Slice the tomatoes and mushrooms thinly, and peel, core and slice the apple. Place the sliced vegetables and fruit on top of the fish and add the cider. Dot the top with the low-fat spread and cover the dish. Bake at 190°C, 375°F, gas mark 5, for 25-30 minutes.
3 Strain a little of the cooking liquor into a bowl containing the cornflour and blend until smooth. Gradually stir in the remaining liquor and pour into a pan. Bring to the boil, stirring until thick. Cook for 2 minutes and pour over the fish.
4 Sprinkle over the cheese and place under a hot grill until brown and bubbling.
5 Garnish with parsley and serve with boiled peas and carrots. Follow with the banana.

Serves 2

153

Chicken, Sweetcorn and Potato

225g (8oz) chicken joint
175g (6oz) potato
7g (¼oz) low-fat spread
125g (4oz) sweetcorn

Bake the chicken at 190°C, 375°F, gas mark 5, without added fat for 30 minutes. Bake the potato and top with low-fat spread. Cook the sweetcorn and serve.

Herby Liver with Brown Rice (Fresh Fruit)

125g (4oz) lamb's liver
10ml (2 level teaspoons) flour
50g (2oz) mushrooms
15g (½oz) onion
1 large tomato
½ beef stock cube
75ml (3floz) water
Salt, pepper and pinch mixed herbs
25g (1oz) brown rice
125g (4oz) French beans
1 medium orange or pear

Slice the liver and toss in flour. Place in a casserole dish. Slice the mushrooms and chop the onion and tomato. Add to the liver. Dissolve the stock cube in water and pour over the vegetables. Season with salt, pepper and herbs. Cover and cook in the oven at 180°C, 350°F, gas mark 4, for 45 minutes. Cook the rice and beans separately and serve with the casserole. Follow with fruit.

Bacon Steaks and Pineapple

2 bacon steaks (100g/3½oz each)
2 pineapple rings, canned in natural juice
125g (4oz) sweetcorn
125g (4oz) fresh or frozen broad beans

Grill the bacon steaks until well done. Drain the pineapple rings and grill for a minute until hot. Cook the sweetcorn and broad beans and serve.

Chicken and Fruity Coleslaw

225g (8oz) chicken joint
2 rings pineapple, canned in natural juice
75g (3oz) cabbage
25g (1oz) carrot
50g (2oz) celery
15ml (1 tablespoon) raisins
30ml (2 tablespoons) low-calorie salad cream
15ml (1 tablespoon) low-fat natural yogurt
Salt and pepper
1 slice wholemeal bread (40g/1½oz)
7g (¼oz) low-fat spread

Bake the chicken joint without fat, discard the skin. Cool. Drain the pineapple and cut into small pieces. Shred the cabbage, grate the carrot and chop the celery. Mix all the vegetables with the raisins, salad cream and yogurt. Season. Serve with the chicken joint and the slice of bread.

Minced Beef and Bean Casserole

125g (4oz) minced beef
25g (1oz) mushrooms
206g (7¼oz) canned baked beans in tomato sauce
Pinch chilli powder
125g (4oz) cooked potato

Brown the minced beef in a non-stick pan and drain off the fat. Chop the mushrooms and mix with the mince and beans. Add a pinch of chilli powder and turn into a small ovenproof dish. Slice the potato and arrange on top to cover the beans and mince. Cook at 190°C, 375°F, gas mark 5, for 20 minutes.

Chinese Chicken Salad (Biscuits and Fruit)

125g (4oz) cooked chicken
50g (2oz) cucumber
1 stick celery
50g (2oz) bean sprouts
30ml (2 tablespoons) oil-free French dressing
1.25ml (¼ teaspoon) soya sauce
3 wholemeal bran biscuits
1 medium pear or orange

Discard the chicken skin and cut the chicken into small pieces. Dice the cucumber and celery and mix it with the chicken, bean sprouts, dressing and soya sauce. Follow with biscuits and fruit.

Stuffed Ham Rolls with Coleslaw *opposite*

1 stick celery
3 small gherkins
50g (2oz) cottage cheese
2 slices cooked ham (25g/1oz each)
75g (3oz) white cabbage
25g (1oz) carrot
15ml (1 tablespoon) natural yogurt
Salt and pepper
1 slice wholemeal bread (40g/1½oz)
7g (¼oz) low-fat spread
1 large eating apple

1 Chop the celery and gherkins and mix with the cottage cheese.
2 Remove all the visible fat from the cooked ham slices and spread them thickly with the cheese mixture. Roll them up lengthways.
3 Make the coleslaw: shred the white cabbage finely and grate the carrot, then mix them together in a bowl.
4 Mix in the low-calorie salad cream and the low-fat yogurt and season to taste with salt and pepper.
5 Serve the ham rolls on a plate with the coleslaw, and accompany with the wholemeal bread spread with low-fat spread. Complete the meal with an eating apple.

Serves 1

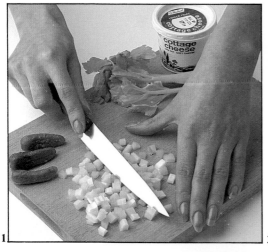

1

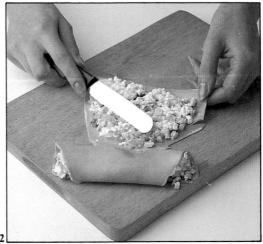

2

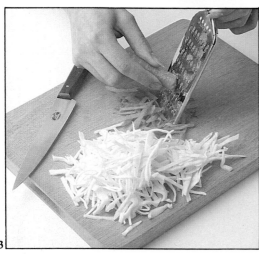

3

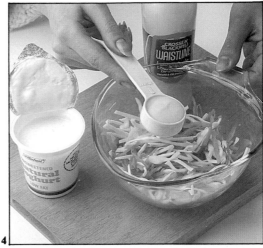

4

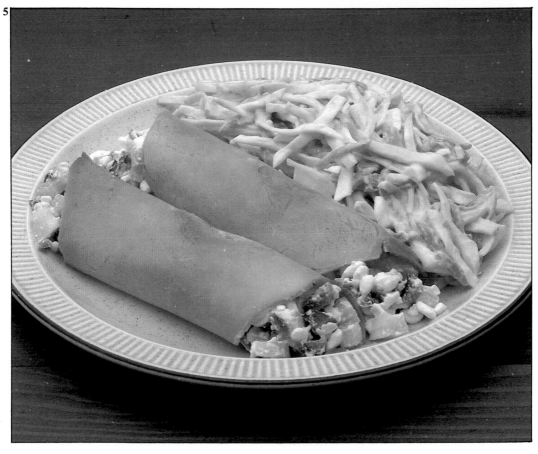

5

1000 calories diet

This is the ideal diet if you have 6kg (1st) of surplus weight or less to lose, or if you have already shed a great deal of weight and are now finding that it is coming off slowly.

On a 1,000 calorie diet everyone should achieve a reasonably speedy weight loss, but do not set your target any higher than 1kg (2lb) per week. As you get slimmer you need fewer calories to move your body around, so the last little bit of weight tends to be the toughest to shift. If you manage to lose more than the goal you set yourself you will feel very pleased, but if this is all that comes off you will not feel a failure. Accuracy is needed to keep to 1,000 calories a day. All foods have to be weighed and measured, for generous over-estimation can quickly add hundreds of extra calories to your daily intake. It is the many unintentional calorie mistakes that lead some dieters to swear that they cannot lose weight on any diet.

What is the best way in which to eat your 1,000 calories a day? There is only one answer to that question: the way that is easiest for you. Some people will find a conventional eating pattern of breakfast, lunch and evening meal the easiest. Others may prefer to have their first meal mid-way through the morning or at lunchtime and keep a small meal until late evening or bedtime when they feel most hungry.

Whatever your eating pattern, you can adapt our 1,000 calorie diet to it. Each day your 1,000 calories are divided into three meals, a breakfast/supper meal, a light meal and a main meal plus a milk allowance. You can eat these meals at any time of the day.

Just follow the simple rules, stick to your allowance, and you are sure to reach your target weight.

Diet rules

1 You are allowed three meals a day. Choose *one* meal only from each of the following sections each day: one breakfast/supper meal; one light meal; and one main meal. These meals can be eaten in any order and at any time of day to suit your lifestyle.

2 Add 284ml (½ pint) skimmed milk for use in tea and coffee. Coffee and tea may be drunk freely, provided that your milk allowance is not exceeded and that saccharin sweeteners are used instead of sugar. Drinks labelled 'low-calorie' and water (including the bottled kind) are also unrestricted.

3 Keep to the stated portions for each meal. Weigh and measure all foods (except very low-calorie salad vegetables, such as lettuce and cucumber) which do not come ready-packed in individual portions. Take special care when measuring fats for cooking or spreading. If you do not have scales that accurately measure very small quantities, for example, 3½g (⅛ oz) or 7g (¼ oz), then weigh out a 25g (1oz) portion and divide equally into 8 or 4 smaller portions to give you the correct portion size. (This is easiest done when the fat is taken from the refrigerator.)

4 Vary your choice of meals each day to ensure that you have a balanced diet, but remember to choose only one meal from each section.

5 Plan and shop ahead so that you always have the right foods available — in this way you will be less tempted to break your diet.

Breakfast/supper meals (200 calories)

Note: Milk given in any of these meals is in addition to your drinks' allowance.

Orange Juice and Wheat Cereal Biscuits
125ml (4floz) unsweetened orange juice
2 wheat cereal biscuits, served with
125ml (4floz) skimmed milk

Breakfast Cereal and Banana
25g (1oz) cornflakes, served with
75ml (3floz) skimmed milk
1 small banana (150g/5oz)

Grapefruit, Bread and Marmalade
½ grapefruit, with non-sugar sweetener
  (optional)
2 small slices wholemeal bread
  (25g/1oz each), lightly spread with
7g (¼oz) low-fat spread, and
10ml (2 level teaspoons) marmalade or jam

Yogurt with Banana, Nuts and Raisins
1 small carton natural yogurt, mixed with
1 small (150g/5oz) banana, peeled and sliced,
15ml (1 level tablespoon) raisins and
15ml (1 level tablespoon) roughly chopped
  nuts

Boiled or Poached Egg on Toast
1 medium egg (size 3), boiled or poached
1 large thin slice white or wholemeal bread
  (40g/1½oz) toasted and spread with
3½g (⅛oz) low-fat spread

Fruit Juice, Muesli and Yogurt
125ml (4floz) unsweetened orange juice
25g (1oz) muesli, served with
1 small carton low-fat natural yogurt

Yogurt with Banana, Nuts and Raisins; Egg Benedict; Turkey Breast with Mushroom Sauce, Ice-cream (Opposite)

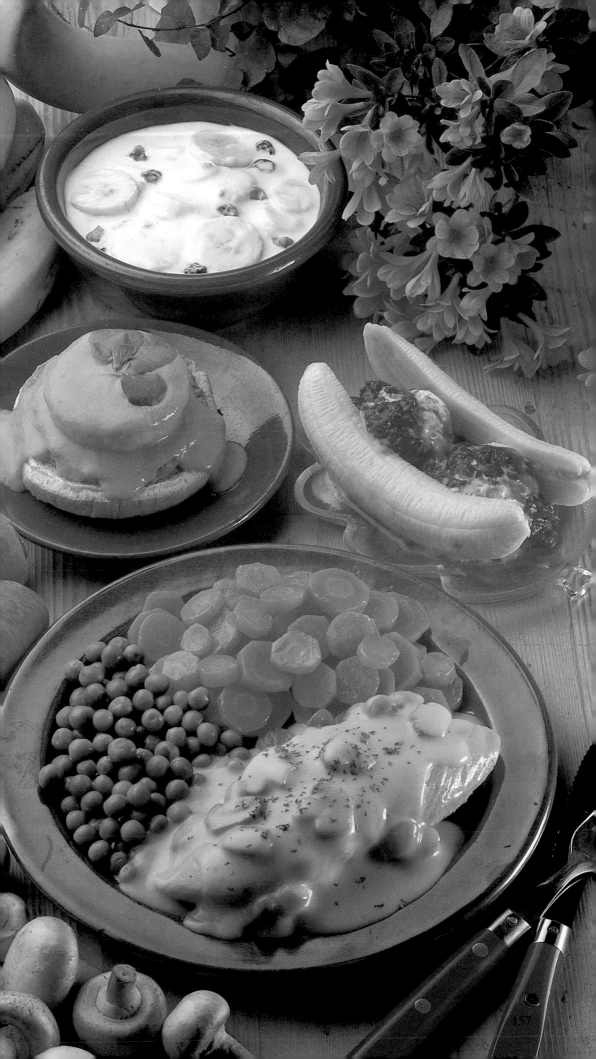

Beans on Toast
150g (5oz) canned baked beans in tomato sauce
1 large thin slice white or wholemeal bread (40g/1½oz), toasted (unbuttered)

Creamy Mushrooms on Toast (Grapes)
125g (4oz) button mushrooms, simmered in
125ml (4floz) chicken stock for 5 minutes
10ml (2 level teaspoons) cornflour and
5ml (1 level teaspoon) low-fat milk powder, blended with a little cold water. Stir into the mushrooms. Boil for 1 minute, stirring continuously
1 large thin slice brown or white bread (40g/1½oz), toasted (unbuttered)
75g (3oz) grapes

Mushroom Omelet
2 medium eggs (size 3), beaten with
15ml (1 tablespoon) water and
Salt and pepper, cooked in
1.25ml (¼ teaspoon) oil to brush omelet or frying pan, and served with
50g (2oz) button mushrooms, poached in stock
1 crispbread (unbuttered)

Cheese on Toast
1 small thin slice wholemeal bread (40g/1½oz), toasted and topped with
25g (1oz) Edam cheese, grated, then grilled until the cheese is melted
15ml (1 tablespoon) sweet pickle or chutney

Crusty Roll and Cottage Cheese
1 crusty bread roll (49g/1¾oz), split and filled with
50g (2oz) cottage cheese, any flavour except with Cheddar

Smoked Haddock and Tomato
150g (5oz) smoked haddock (or any smoked fish) poached in water
2 tomatoes, halved
1 small slice slimmers' bread or ½ slice wholemeal bread (unbuttered)

Fish Cakes and Vegetables
2 frozen fish cakes, grilled or baked in the oven without added fat
125g (4oz) canned tomatoes and
15ml (1 tablespoon) boiled peas

Fruit Juice and Scrambled Egg
125ml (4floz) unsweetened orange juice
1 medium egg (size 3), scrambled in a non-stick pan with
45ml (3 tablespoons) skimmed milk and
Seasoning to taste, served on
1 small slice wholemeal bread (25g/1oz), toasted (unbuttered)

Grapefruit and Bacon Sandwich
½ grapefruit, sweetened with non-sugar sweetener (optional)
2 rashers streaky bacon, grilled until crisp
2 small slices slimmers' bread or 1 slice wholemeal bread (unbuttered), filled with the bacon and
15ml (1 level tablespoon) tomato sauce

Light meals (250 calories)

Herring Roes on Toast
125g (4oz) herring roes, gently fried in
7g (¼oz) butter, or 15g (½oz) low-fat spread, served on
1 large, thin slice white or brown bread (40g/1½oz), toasted (unbuttered)
Few sprigs of watercress

Crusty Roll with Egg and Cress
1 crusty bread roll (49g/1¾oz), split and filled with
1 chopped medium hard-boiled egg (size 4), mixed with
15ml (1 tablespoon) low-calorie salad cream and
Mustard and cress

Scrambled Egg and Tomato on Toast
2 medium eggs (size 4), scrambled with
30ml (2 tablespoons) skimmed milk and
Salt and pepper to taste in a non-stick pan, then stir in
1 skinned and chopped tomato, and serve on
1 large, thin slice wholemeal bread (40g/1½oz), toasted (unbuttered)

Cheese and Pickle Toasty with Salad
1 small, thin slice wholemeal bread (25g/1oz), toasted and spread with
30ml (1 rounded tablespoon) mixed pickle covered with
25g (1oz) Cheddar cheese, grated, and grilled
Mixed salad prepared from lettuce, watercress, 2 tomatoes and 1 grated carrot

Double-decker Ham and Cheese Sandwich
3 small slices slimmers' bread, or 1½ slices wholemeal bread with a filling of
3½g (⅛oz) low-fat spread
25g (1oz) lean boiled ham and
1 sliced tomato, and a second layer filling of
3½g (⅛oz) low-fat spread, and
15g (½oz) Edam cheese, grated, and
Mustard and cress

Cottage Cheese, Crispbreads and Fruit
113g (4oz) carton cottage cheese, any flavour except with Cheddar, served with
4 crispbreads, and
1 medium apple, orange or pear

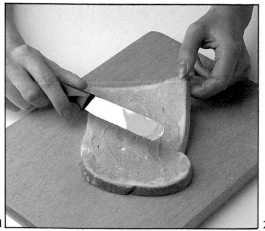

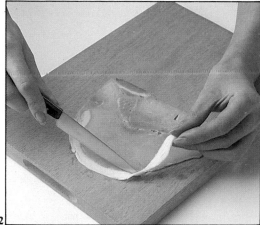

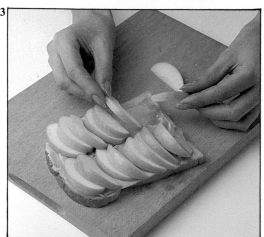

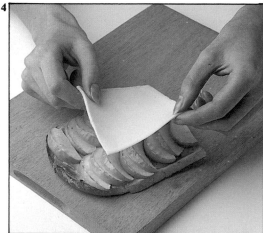

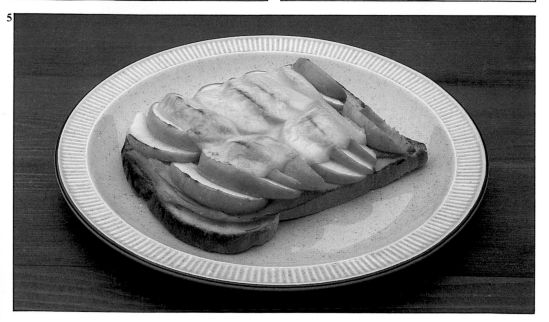

Cheese, Apple and Ham on Toast

1 small slice white bread (25g/1oz)
1.25ml (¼ teaspoon) prepared mustard
25g (1oz) slice lean boiled ham
1 medium eating apple, cored and sliced
1 slice processed cheese
Sprigs of watercress

1 Toast the bread on one side only and spread the untoasted side with a little prepared mustard.

2 Trim fat from ham and throw it away.

3 Place the slice of ham on top of the bread and arrange the apple slices on top. Place under a hot grill for about 2 minutes until the apple starts to soften.

4 Cover with the slice of processed cheese and return to the grill until the cheese has melted and starts to brown.

5 Serve garnished with sprigs of watercress.

Serves 1

159

Salmon and Tomato Salad

*100g (3½oz) canned pink salmon, drained
   and flaked and mixed with
2 tomatoes, sliced or roughly chopped, and
15ml (1 level tablespoon) low-calorie
   seafood sauce or salad cream, and a
Generous squeeze lemon juice and a
Little chopped parsley. Arrange on a bed of
Lettuce, and garnish with
4 black olives and
1 crispbread, spread with
3½g (⅛oz) low-fat spread*

Cheese Salad

*50g (2oz) Edam cheese served with a
Mixed salad prepared from lettuce, or
   chicory, watercress, a few radishes, onion
   rings, sliced tomato, and dressed with
15ml (1 tablespoon) low-calorie salad cream
1 crispbread (unbuttered)*

Chicken Salad

*125g (4oz) sliced cold roast chicken, all skin
   removed, served with
50g (2oz) button mushrooms, sliced and
   tossed in
30ml (2 tablespoons) oil-free French dressing
Green salad prepared from lettuce, spring
   onions, sliced cucumber, served with
1 small slice slimmers' bread or ½ slice
   wholemeal bread, spread with
3½g (⅛ oz) low-fat spread*

Corned Beef Salad

*75g (3oz) corned beef, sliced, served with
Chinese leaves, shredded, or lettuce and
50g (2oz) pickled beetroot and
50g (2oz) grated carrot
1 crispbread spread with
3½g (⅛ oz) low-fat spread*

Ham Salad

*50g (2oz) boiled ham, served with
125g (4oz) shredded white cabbage and
50g (2oz) grated carrot mixed with
15ml (1 tablespoon) low-calorie salad cream
2 crispbreads, spread with
7g (¼oz) low-fat spread*

Fish Fingers and Vegetables

*4 fish fingers, grilled without added fat and
   served with
15ml (1 level tablespoon) low-calorie tartare
   sauce or tomato ketchup, and with
125g (4oz) boiled runner beans or 50g (2oz)
   boiled peas*

Pork Chipolatas and Baked Beans

*2 pork chipolata sausages, well grilled and
   served with
150g (5oz) baked beans in tomato sauce and
1 crispbread (unbuttered)*

Bacon and Eggs

*1 medium egg (size 3), poached, served with
2 rashers streaky bacon, well grilled and
1 tomato, grilled without fat
1 small slice wholemeal bread (25g/1oz),
   unbuttered*

Cheesy Baked Potato

*200g (7oz) jacket-baked potato, split in half
   and topped with
50g (2oz) cottage cheese with chives or with
   onions and peppers (capsicums)
Mixed salad of lettuce, or Chinese leaves,
   watercress, cucumber, 1 stick celery, ½
   small green pepper (capsicum), sliced, and
1 tomato, sliced*

Beefburger Sandwich (Fruit)

*50g (2oz) beefburger, well grilled and
   served in/on
2 small slices slimmers' bread or 1 slice
   wholemeal bread with
30ml (1 rounded tablespoon) hamburger
   relish or mixed pickle
1 small (150g/5oz) banana*

Egg Benedict

*40g (1½oz) dressed crab, spread on
Half a toasted bap, topped with
1 medium egg (size 4), poached, then covered
   with sauce made from
15ml (1 tablespoon) tomato ketchup mixed
   with
15ml (1 tablespoon) low-fat natural yogurt
Sprigs of watercress*

Prawn Sandwich and Fresh Fruit

*2 small, thin slices white or brown bread
   (25g/1oz each), filled with
50g (2oz) peeled prawns, mixed with
15ml (1 level tablespoon) low-calorie
   seafood sauce or salad cream and
Lettuce or mustard and cress
150g (5oz) eating apple*

Main meals (450 calories)

Grilled or Baked Chicken and Chips (Fresh Fruit)

*225g (8oz) chicken joint
125g (4oz) frozen oven chips
75g (3oz) Brussels sprouts
1 fresh peach, apple or pear*

Grill or bake the chicken joint without added fat until it is cooked through. Bake the oven chips as directed. Boil the Brussels sprouts. Remove the skin from the chicken and serve with the chips and the Brussels sprouts. Complete the meal with the fresh fruit.

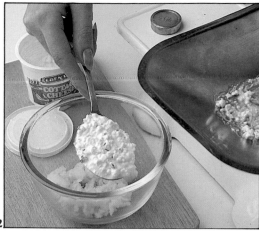

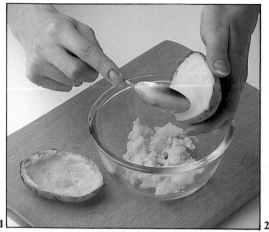

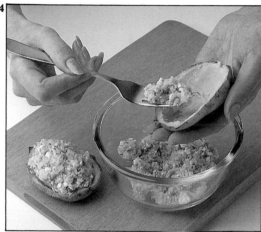

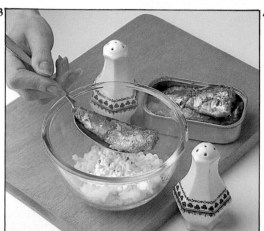

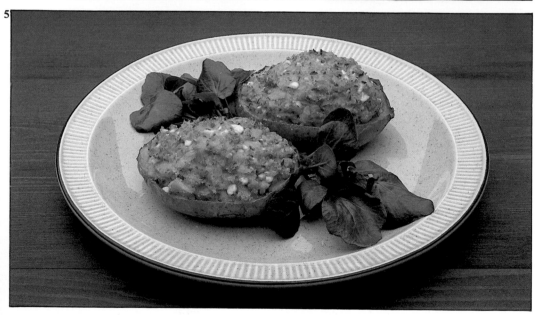

Sardine Stuffed Potato

One 170g (6oz) jacket-baked potato
50g (2oz) cottage cheese with chives
1 canned sardine in tomato sauce
Salt and pepper
Sprigs of watercress

1 Cut the baked potato in half lengthways and scoop out the soft centre. Place in a dish and retain the potato skins.
2 Mix the cottage cheese with the potato.

3 Add the canned sardine and mash together with a fork. Season to taste with salt and pepper.
4 Pile the mixture back into the potato cases and place in a medium oven at 190°C, 375°F, gas mark 5, for about 15 minutes until heated through thoroughly.
5 Serve the Sardine Stuffed Potato garnished with sprigs of watercress.

Serves 1

Turkey Breast with Mushroom Sauce (Ice-Cream Dessert)

175g (6oz) raw turkey breast, skinned and
  boned
150ml (¼ pint) chicken stock made from
  ¼ chicken stock cube
25g (1oz) onion, chopped
50g (2oz) mushrooms, sliced
7g (¼ oz) low-fat spread
10ml (2 level teaspoons) flour
30ml (2 level tablespoons) skimmed milk
  powder
Salt and pepper
50g (2oz) peas, boiled
125g (4oz) carrots, boiled
50g (2oz) vanilla ice-cream
1 small banana (150g/5oz)
50g (2oz) fresh or frozen raspberries
5ml (1 level teaspoon) sugar

Place the turkey breast in a small saucepan with the stock, onion and mushrooms. Bring to the boil, cover and simmer gently for 30 minutes. Remove the turkey and mushrooms and keep warm. Drain the stock into a measuring jug and make up to 150ml (¼ pint) with water. Pour into a saucepan and add the low-fat spread, flour and milk powder. Bring to the boil, whisking all the time and cook for 2-3 minutes. Season to taste and stir in the mushrooms. Pour over the turkey breast and serve with the peas and carrots. Complete the meal with the ice-cream dessert: place the ice-cream on a serving dish, peel and cut the banana in half lengthwise and arrange one half on each side of the ice-cream. Crush the raspberries with a fork, stir in the sugar and spoon over the ice-cream.

Oven-baked Chicken (Fruit and Cream)

225g (8oz) chicken joint
200g (7oz) potato
30ml (2 level tablespoons) low-fat natural
  yogurt
Chopped chives
Lettuce
Cucumber
Watercress
½ small green pepper (capsicum)
2-3 spring onions
15ml (1 tablespoon) oil-free French dressing
125g (4oz) fresh or frozen (thawed)
  raspberries or strawberries
15ml (1 tablespoon) single cream or top of the
  milk or 45ml (3 level tablespoons) low-fat
  natural yogurt

Wrap the chicken joint in foil. Scrub the potato. Bake the chicken joint and potato in a moderately hot oven at 200°C, 400°F, gas mark 6, for 45 minutes or until the chicken and potato are cooked. Split the potato in half and top each half with 15ml (1 tablespoon) yogurt and a pinch of chopped chives. Prepare a green salad from the salad vegetables and dress with the oil-free French dressing. Serve the baked chicken with the potato and green salad. Complete the meal with the fruit served with single cream, milk or yogurt.

Parsnip-topped Cottage Pie (Canned Fruit)

125g (4oz) raw minced beef
1 small onion, peeled and finely chopped
25g (1oz) mushrooms, sliced
5ml (1 level teaspoon) flour
Salt and pepper
70ml (2½ floz) beef stock made from ¼ beef
  stock cube
15ml (1 tablespoon) tomato ketchup
175g (6oz) parsnips, peeled
7g (¼ oz) low-fat spread
15ml (1 tablespoon) milk
125g (4oz) cauliflower
75g (3oz) carrots
220g (7¾ oz) canned fruit cocktail in low-
  calorie syrup

Fry the minced beef in a non-stick pan until well browned, then drain and discard the fat. Add the onion, mushrooms, flour and seasoning to taste to the beef in the pan. Blend the stock with the tomato ketchup and add to the pan. Heat to boiling point, stirring continuously, then cook for five minutes until the mixture thickens. Turn into an individual ovenproof dish. Cook the parsnips in boiling salted water until tender. Drain and mash them with the low-fat spread and milk. Season to taste. Spoon over the top of the meat and fork the top. Bake in a moderately hot oven, at 200°C, 400°F, gas mark 6, for 20-30 minutes or until the top is browned. Meanwhile, boil the cauliflower and carrots in lightly salted water until tender. Serve the cottage pie with the vegetables. Serve the canned fruit as a dessert.

Smoked Haddock with Spaghetti (Banana)

175g (6oz) smoked haddock (or any smoked
  fish)
213g (7½ oz) canned spaghetti in tomato sauce
15g (½ oz) Edam cheese, grated
125g (4oz) runner beans
1 small banana (150g/5oz)

Poach the smoked haddock in a little water until cooked, about 12 minutes. Drain the haddock and place in a small heatproof dish. Heat the spaghetti in a pan and spoon on top of the smoked haddock. Sprinkle the grated cheese over the spaghetti, place under a moderate grill and cook until the cheese has melted. Boil the runner beans. Serve the smoked haddock and spaghetti with the beans. Complete the meal with the banana.

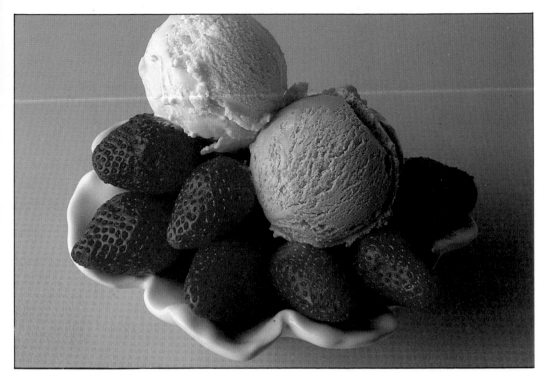

Strawberries and Ice-cream

Beef Casserole (Fresh Fruit)

125g (4oz) lean braising steak
5ml (1 level teaspoon) flour
Salt and pepper
125g (4oz) frozen casserole vegetables
10ml (2 level teaspoons) tomato purée
150ml (¼pint) stock
130g (4½oz) potatoes, peeled
125g (4oz) cabbage
1 medium orange or pear

Trim any visible fat from the meat and cut the flesh into cubes. Season the flour with salt and pepper and toss the meat in it. Place the meat in a small ovenproof casserole with the casserole vegetables. Stir the tomato purée into the stock and pour over the meat and vegetables. Cook in a slow oven at 160°C, 325°F, gas mark 3, for 1½-2 hours until the meat is tender. Boil the potatoes in lightly salted water until tender, then mash. Boil the cabbage until just tender and drain. Serve the beef casserole with the mashed potato and boiled cabbage. Follow with an orange or pear

Liver, Leek and Tomato Casserole (Grapefruit)

200g (7oz) potato, unpeeled
125g (4oz) lamb's liver
1 leek
225g (8oz) canned tomatoes with juice
Salt and pepper
Pinch mixed herbs
½ grapefruit

Scrub the potato well and bake in a moderately hot oven at 200°C, 400°F, gas mark 6, for about 1 hour, or until soft when pinched. Wash and slice the liver. Trim most of the green part off the leek, and wash thoroughly and slice. Put the liver, leek and canned tomatoes in a small ovenproof casserole. Season well and sprinkle in the mixed herbs. Cover and cook in the oven with the potato for 40 minutes. Serve the baked potato (no butter) with the liver casserole. Start or complete the meal with the grapefruit, sweetened if liked, with the non-sugar sweetener.

Stuffed Chicken Parcel (Strawberries and Ice-Cream)

2.5ml (½ level teaspoon) low-fat spread
125g (4oz) chicken breast fillet
15g (½oz) onion
15g (½oz) red or green pepper (capsicums)
25g (1oz) fresh breadcrumbs
3.75ml (¾ level teaspoon) mixed dried herbs
15ml (1 tablespoon) chicken stock
5ml (1 level teaspoon) grated lemon rind
Salt and pepper
125g (4oz) frozen mixed vegetables
75g (3oz) ice-cream
75g (3oz) strawberries, fresh or frozen

Lightly grease a square of foil with the low-fat spread and place the chicken in the middle. Chop the onion and pepper (capsicums) and mix with the breadcrumbs, herbs, stock and lemon rind. Season with salt and pepper and pile onto the chicken. Wrap up to form a loose parcel. Place on a baking tray and cook in the oven at 190°C, 375°F, gas mark 5, for 25-30 minutes. Cook the vegetables as instructed on the packet and serve with the chicken. Follow with the strawberries and ice-cream.

Cauliflower with Beef Sauce (Orange with Yogurt)

175g (6oz) raw minced beef
½ beef stock cube
90ml (6 tablespoons) boiling water
2 spring onions, chopped
1 carrot, grated
Salt and pepper
25g (1oz) mushrooms, chopped
225g (8oz) cauliflower
1 medium orange
1 small carton low-fat natural yogurt

Fry the minced beef in a pan until well browned, then drain off any fat. Dissolve the stock cube in the boiling water and pour onto the beef. Stir in the spring onions and carrot. Bring to the boil, season to taste, cover and simmer gently for 20 minutes. Add the mushrooms and simmer for a further 5 minutes. Meanwhile, cook the cauliflower in lightly salted water until just tender then drain. Serve topped with the meat sauce. Complete the meal with the peeled and segmented orange mixed with the yogurt and sweetened to taste, if necessary, with non-sugar sweetener.

Ham and Pineapple au Gratin (Fresh Fruit)

2 bacon or ham steaks (100g/3½oz raw weight each)
2 rings canned pineapple in natural juice, drained
25g (1oz) Edam cheese, grated
1 tomato, halved
Watercress
1 orange or pear

Grill the bacon or ham steaks until well done. Top each bacon steak with a ring of pineapple and half the quantity of grated cheese. Heat under the grill until the cheese melts. Grill the tomato halves without added fat. Serve the Ham and Pineapple au Gratin with the tomato and a small bunch of watercress. Complete the meal with the fresh fruit.

Cauliflower Cheese with Mushrooms

225g (8oz) cauliflower
15g (½oz) low-fat spread
15g (½oz) plain flour
150ml (¼ pint) skimmed milk
50g (2oz) Cheddar cheese, grated
Salt and pepper
1.25ml (¼ level teaspoon) prepared mustard
30ml (1 rounded tablespoon) fresh breadcrumbs
50g (2oz) button mushrooms

Break the cauliflower into florets and cook in boiling salted water until just tender, about 10 minutes. Drain and place in an ovenproof dish and keep warm. Place the low-fat spread, flour and skimmed milk in a saucepan and bring to the boil, stirring continuously. Cook for 2 minutes. Reserve 30ml (1 rounded tablespoon) grated cheese and add the remainder to the sauce in the pan. Season with salt and pepper and the mustard and stir well. Pour over the cauliflower. Mix the reserved cheese with the breadcrumbs and sprinkle on top. Brown under a moderate grill. Poach the mushrooms in a little lightly salted water or stock, drain and serve with the cauliflower.

Fish Casserole (Fruit Yogurt)

175g (6oz) coley fillet (or any firm-fleshed white fish)
125g (4oz) leek, well washed and sliced
25g (1oz) green pepper (capsicum), diced
1 stick celery, chopped
Pinch garlic salt
Pinch dried thyme
Freshly ground pepper
2.5ml (½ teaspoon) salt
175g (6oz) potatoes, peeled and thinly sliced
90ml (6 tablespoons) dry cider
1 small carton low-fat fruit yogurt (any flavour except banana or black cherry)

Skin the fish and cut into 7.5cm (3in) pieces. Lightly grease a small ovenproof casserole. Put the sliced leeks in the bottom and then the fish. Sprinkle the green pepper (capsicum), celery, tomato, herbs and seasoning over the fish. Top with the sliced potato and pour in the cider. Cover and bake at 180°C, 350°F, gas mark 4, for about 1 hour, uncovering the dish for the last 10 minutes. Check that the potato is tender and the fish is cooked. Serve hot. Complete the meal with the yogurt.

Lemon and Parsley Stuffed Herring (Fruit and Ice-cream)

175g (6oz) whole herring (or any oily fish)
Salt and pepper
25g (1oz) fresh breadcrumbs
1 small onion, finely chopped
Grated rind and juice of 1 lemon
15ml (1 tablespoon) chopped parsley
7g (¼oz) low-fat spread
125g (4oz) frozen mixed vegetables, thawed
50g (2oz) fresh or frozen (thawed) raspberries or strawberries
50g (2oz) vanilla ice-cream

Remove the head, tail and fins of the herring, then clean it thoroughly and remove the backbone (or ask the fishmonger to do this for you). Season inside the herring with salt and pepper. Mix together the breadcrumbs, onion, lemon rind and juice and parsley. Spoon the stuffing into the herring and fold into its original shape. Grease one side of a piece of foil with a little of the low-fat spread and lay the fish upon it. Place the mixed vegetables alongside the fish and top with the remaining low-fat spread. Wrap the foil around the fish and vegetables and seal. Bake in a moderate oven at 180°C, 350°F, gas mark 4, for 30 minutes. Unwrap, lift onto a warm serving dish and serve. Complete the meal with the raspberries or strawberries and ice-cream.

Mixed Grill (Fresh Fruit)

125g (4oz) lamb's liver, sliced
1 lamb's kidney
2.5ml (½ teaspoon) oil
2 rashers streaky bacon
1 tomato, halved
50g (2oz) mushrooms
125g (4oz) broccoli
1 medium apple, pear or orange

Wash and dry the liver, and halve and core the kidney. Brush the liver and kidney halves lightly with the oil and place on a grill rack with the bacon. Grill until cooked on one side, then turn over and add the tomato halves. Continue to grill until the liver and kidney are cooked, the bacon is crisp and the tomatoes are soft. Poach the mushrooms in a little stock or water and boil the broccoli. Serve the mixed grill with the vegetables. Complete the meal with the fresh fruit.

Grilled Lamb Chop with Vegetables (Crispbreads and Cheese)

150g (5oz) lamb chump chop (raw weight)
1 tomato, halved
50g (2oz) mushrooms
125g (4oz) frozen mixed vegetables
2 crispbreads
15g (½oz) Edam cheese
1 stick celery

Trim off any fat from the lamb chop and grill the chop, turning once, until cooked. Add the tomato halves to the grill pan for the last 3 minutes of grilling time. Poach the mushrooms in a little stock or water and cook the mixed vegetables as directed. Serve the lamb chop with the tomato and vegetables. Complete the meal with the crispbreads, cheese and the celery.

Cheese Medley Salad

25g (1oz) long-grain rice (raw weight)
2 sticks celery, chopped
2 carrots, grated
2 canned pineapple rings, drained and
    chopped
50g (2oz) green grapes, halved and deseeded
30ml (2 tablespoons) oil-free French dressing
Few lettuce leaves
50g (2oz) Edam cheese, cut into triangles
2 tomatoes, cut in wedges

Cook the rice in boiling salted water until just tender (about 12 minutes for white rice, 30 minutes for brown rice), then drain. Rinse under cold water and drain again. Mix together the rice, celery, carrot, pineapple, grapes and dressing in a large bowl. Turn out onto a bed of lettuce and surround with the triangles of cheese and tomato wedges.

Smoky Fish Pie

175g (6oz) smoked haddock
    (or any smoked white fish)
150ml (¼ pint) skimmed milk
15g (½oz) low-fat spread
15g (½oz) plain flour
10ml (2 teaspoons) chopped fresh parsley
Freshly ground black pepper
150g (5oz) potatoes, peeled
15ml (1 tablespoon) low-calorie tomato
    ketchup
Salt

Put the smoked haddock fillets and milk in a small pan. Bring to the boil, cover and simmer gently for 15 minutes. Drain off the milk, reserve and allow to cool slightly. Meanwhile, boil the potatoes in lightly salted water until tender. Place the low-fat spread, flour and milk in which the fish was cooked in a small pan and bring them to the boil, whisking continuously. Cook for 2 minutes, then stir in the chopped parsley and pepper to taste. Flake the haddock, removing skin and bones, and stir into the sauce. Pour into a small ovenproof dish. Drain and mash the potatoes, then beat in the tomato ketchup and seasoning to taste. Spoon on top of the fish and fork level. Brown the top of the potato under a hot grill, then serve.

Fish Hawaiian-style (Melon)

125g (4oz) canned pineapple in natural juice
Water
50g (2oz) long-grain rice (raw weight)
1 tomato, skinned and chopped
50g (2oz) green pepper (capsicum), chopped
175g (6oz) coley or cod fillet (or any
    firm-fleshed white fish)
5ml (1 teaspoon) lemon juice
Salt and pepper
Green salad: lettuce, watercress, cucumber,
    spring onions or onion rings
15ml (1 tablespoon) oil-free French dressing
200g (7oz) slice melon

Drain and chop the pineapple and reserve the juice. Make the juice up to 150ml (¼ pint) with water and put in a small pan with the rice. Cook the rice for 10 minutes, then add the pineapple, tomato, green pepper (capsicum) and a little more water if necessary. Continue to cook for a further 5 minutes or until the rice is just tender. Meanwhile, cook the fish in a shallow pan with the lemon juice and sufficient water to cover for 10 to 15 minutes. Drain and flake the fish and stir into the rice mixture and season to taste. Serve hot with the green salad. Complete the meal with the melon.

Sue's fishing for compliments

Sue Dunn's life changed completely when she shed over 38kg (6st). Now her husband, Charlie, and her daughter, Clare, have a 'fun person' to accompany them on fishing trips — before, she was always a stick-in-the-mud-Mum who would not go anywhere. Sue came from a family of sailing enthusiasts and one of her earliest memories is of being given a boat of her own as a Christmas present — her size, as always, spoilt her fun. There were no Wellington boots wide enough to pull over her heavy calves and so she had to slop around in soggy gym shoes. On chillier days her feet were perpetually half frozen. At nine-years-old, she weighed 66.7kg (10½st), which did not help when she started learning to sail. It is essential to be able to react quickly in an open boat and it takes great agility, particularly in a heavy life-jacket, to be in the right place at the right time to avoid the boat keeling over. She later trained to be a nurse and met Charlie when she was 20 years old and hovering around 79.4kg (12½st). The following year they were married and then pregnancy gave her weight another upwards push. She had always had a weakness for chocolate eggs, and pregnancy gave her an excuse for over-indulgence — she munched her way through half-a-dozen or more chocolate eggs a day. A few days after Clare was born, Sue had to steel herself to the horrifying fact that she weighed nearly 101.6kg (16st). She decided to join forces with her mother who had a 12.7kg (2st) surplus and they joined a slimming club together. It was a gradual process but Sue's diet cleverly catered for her main weakness — chocolates. She saved her small chocolate treat to eat during the evening and found that she enjoyed it far more than the mounds of chocolates she used to demolish so fast that she hardly tasted them. Sue found that when she reached her 62.6kg (9st 12lb) target, which was just right for her 1.73m (5ft8in) medium frame, she could join in with Charlie and Clare without worrying all the time about her weight slowing them down. She is not above fishing for compliments now that she knows Charlie is proud of her achievement.

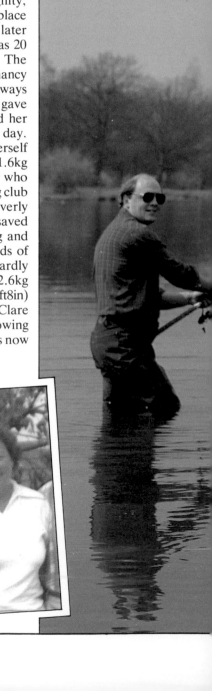

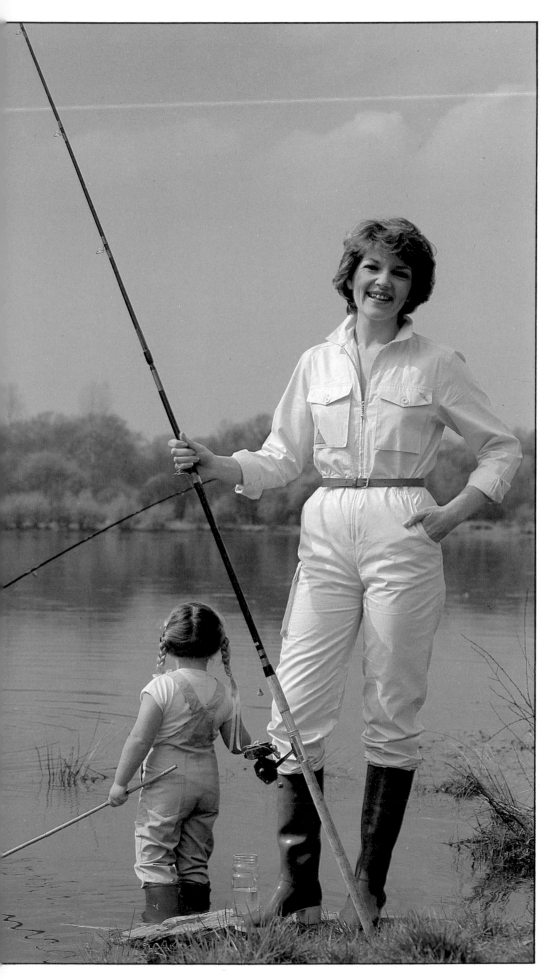

Joyce was the farm's prize pig

Life really began at 40 for farmer's wife Joyce Fletcher, when she slimmed from a middle-aged and matronly shape down to the trim and youthful figure on the right. Joyce came from a farming family and, as a child, she loved tucking into her mother's home-baked cakes.

By the time she was 15 years old she weighed 66.5kg (10½st). Joyce met her husband, John, through a friend, and although her size did not make her feel self-conscious and speechless, she could not quite believe it when John asked her to marry him. Her sister was also engaged and so they agreed on a double wedding. At 73kg (11½st), Joyce could not help envying her sister's beautifully slim figure. However, she wore her tightest corselet beneath her wedding dress, held her breath throughout the long ceremony and moved very carefully! During her two pregnancies Joyce's weight rose to over 82.5kg (13st). Working on a sixty-acre farm with her husband did not keep Joyce automatically slim, either. The energy she burned in planting celery, picking potatoes and running behind the seed driller was amply compensated for by hearty meals and hastily grabbed snacks. Ignoring all those people who warned her that if she slimmed she would 'lose all her strength', Joyce eventually decided that she had had enough of carrying her excess weight round the farm. At l.68m (5ft6in) she had never weighed below 66kg (10½st) since she was a child and it was a great revelation to find that she was not naturally 'big boned' after all. In three months, she lost nearly 19kg (3st) and immediately felt healthier and more energetic.

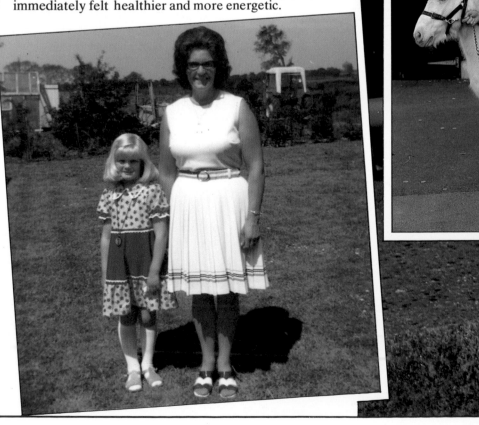

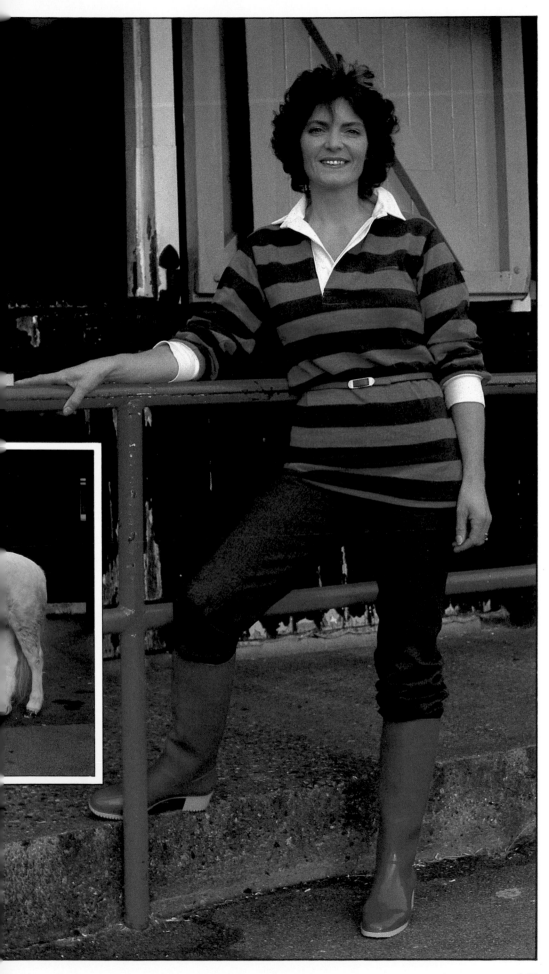

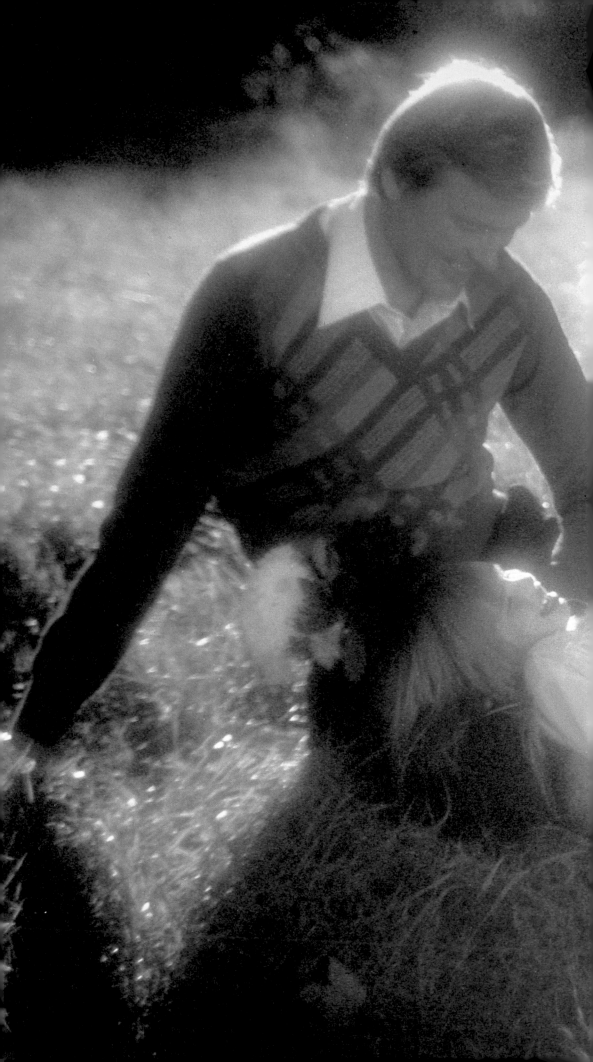

CHAPTER 8

Slimming and your health

Is it necessary to consult your doctor before you embark on a slimming campaign? If you do so, what help can he give? Is it healthier to eat foods raw wherever possible? What causes water retention? Will your stomach shrink? Here are the answers to many questions that slimmers ask about how dieting will affect their health.

For the normal overweight person to ask her doctor for permission to shed surplus fat makes just about as much sense as asking permission to give up smoking. However, if you do decide to ask your doctor for help in your slimming, what can you expect?

It is unrealistic to imagine that every doctor will actively help and encourage you to slim. Some may hand you a typed standard diet and whisk you out of their surgery before you have time to sit down. The amount of slimming support that doctors give is variable but most are helpful if you are heavily overweight, or if you have an associated illness like heart trouble or high blood pressure, in which case they take the problem seriously. However, few doctors can afford the time to see you each week to give psychological support to your slimming efforts, and this is why many doctors recommend that you join a slimming club for advice and moral support. All experts agree that some effective psychological support has to be given on a weekly basis. Monthly visits give you time to cheat on your diet with the optimistic idea that you will make up for it in the remaining weeks. A few years ago, doctors and dieticians tended to regard slimming clubs as cranky and commercial, but nowadays these clubs are widely accepted in medical circles and have acquired a good reputation. In fact, scientific investigations have shown that clubs are more effective and supportive to slimmers in their fight against calories than are most doctors.

Slimming clubs usually meet once a week and take the form of a weigh-in session followed by a talk on slimming by the person in charge of the group. What they offer is expert advice from someone who has had a weight problem herself, proven diets and the comradeship and competitiveness of other people who are also trying to lose weight. The diets offered vary with the different organizations that run clubs. Whereas some clubs have a set dieting programme, others offer a wide variety of diets tailored to meet members' special requirements. Doctors' diets rarely take into account personal whims, and you cannot expect your doctor to know the number of calories in a fish fillet or a chocolate éclair. Thus although doctors' diets are generally sound, they are usually dull.

So what can a doctor do that no one else can do for you? Obviously he can check whether excess weight is causing health complications, and he can prescribe pills, although many doctors now refuse to do this for slimming, and for good reasons. There is nothing new about the idea of slimming drugs. As far back as the 1890's medicinal miracles, such as Dr. Grey's Electric Fat Reducing Pills, 'capable of rapidly and quite safely dissolving superfluous fat and permanently curing corpulence', were advertised. If only that were possible! Nowadays, the law insists that claims are a good deal more realistic.

Appetite suppressants come in many varieties but can be obtained only on a doctor's prescription and may cause a number of nasty side-effects, such as nausea. Remember, if you are still contemplating using these drugs, that they do not effect any cures. If you are able to lose weight only because your appetite is artificially suppressed, then it is likely that you will regain the weight when the pills are eventually withdrawn and your appetite returns to its normal level.

Derek Miller, Research Fellow of London University's Department of Nutrition, foresees the eventual availability of safe, non-addictive drugs for use in certain cases to boost metabolic rate. They could help a slimmer, for instance, over the so-called 'plateau problem' when, despite much conscientious calorie limitation, weight loss progress tends to slow up or stand still. However, whatever drugs are developed as slimming aids, they will never be an adequate substitute for good eating habits.

Some private clinic doctors may even treat overweight patients with diuretics, but these cannot remove fat although they lower the fluid content of the body temporarily and, therefore, the body's weight. As soon as you stop taking the pills, usually after your course of treatment has finished, the fluid weight will return.

Most women retain extra water before their monthly period but, apart from the depressing psychological effect of this, a temporary weight gain need not present a real problem (the psychological aspects of this are dealt with in the section on *Your mind*). Research has shown that by severely limiting one's salt intake during the week preceding menstruation, the symptoms of fluid retention can be alleviated significantly. Salt (sodium chloride) should, in any event, be cut down for your health's sake, and most of us consume 10 times more than we need. If you find food very unpalatable without salt, look out for potassium chloride, which is sold as a salt substitute and does not have its fluid-retaining properties. Also restrict your intake of salted foods at this time, including salted butter, salted meats and fish, and ready-prepared meals.

If you experienced a swift weight gain after starting to take a contraceptive pill,

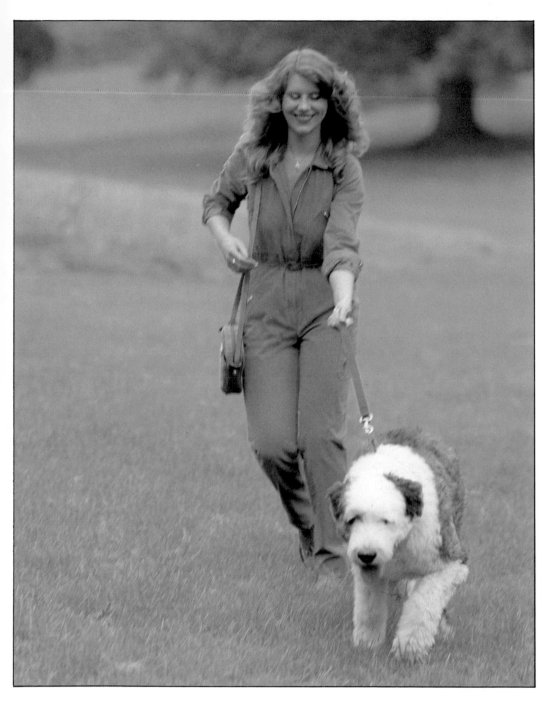

this could also be due to fluid retention. Trying another type of contraceptive pill is the only sensible solution. Some medically prescribed drugs, like cortisone, can cause fluid retention as can such medical conditions as anaemia, kidney or heart disorders.

There are so many types of laxatives readily available at a chemist that most people do not bother to consult their doctor if they feel constipated when dieting. However, many people who take laxatives regularly may become dependent on them and may even reach a stage where their bowels will not function without them. This is not conducive to good health and laxatives should be used only occasionally. It is better to increase the fibre in your diet — try the *Super healthy diet* in the dieting section.

Fat people often blame their figure on a mild thyroid deficiency and this is a question that Professor Yudkin deals with on page 179. However, any person with sufficient deficiency to cause fatness will also notice such symptoms as feeling cold, sleepy and generally unwell. There are other glandular disturbances that can cause fatness, the most important of which is when the pituitary gland fails to function correctly. The effects of such a deficiency are more obvious and serious than being simply overweight.

Doctors cannot work miracles — only in extreme cases can they admit people to hospital to slim, and only then if they are excessively overweight. In the final analysis, it is you who has to learn to cope with slimming and staying slim in the outside world.

Professor John Yudkin is famous world-wide as an authority on dieting and nutrition and for giving a straight answer to a straight question and never dodging an issue. The vast postbag of mail he receives on health and slimming reveals that many people share the same source of worry about their body. So we have selected 30 of the most frequently asked questions in the belief that the answers will be a universal source of help and reassurance.

Please tell me Professor...

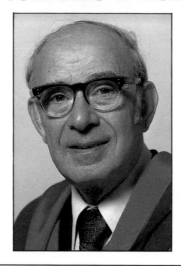

Dear Professor...should I try to slim?

Up to three years ago, I always weighed about 61.7kg (9st 10lb). When I started to gain, I went to see my doctor; but he says the fact that I'm now 76.2kg (12st) is 'just my age' — I'm 48. I'm reluctant to accept this but must admit that although I've been on a daily 1,000 calories for the past six weeks, I haven't lost any weight at all. I'm a very active person too. Can you advise me?

You don't tell me a vital fact: your height. So I'm assuming that you are not 1.90m (6ft4in) and that your former weight was about right. If this is so, I'm forced into doing something I dislike: disagreeing with a doctor. I hate doing this because he (or she) is the one with the full facts of the case; I have to judge on incomplete second-hand evidence from, usually, a non-medical person. This is the reason for my hesitation. But if you are healthy, I really don't believe that becoming 48 years old should make your weight 76.2kg (12st). Reaching any particular age is no reason, no

excuse, to become at all heavier than you ought to be. Ideally, we should weigh the same at 48 as at 20 or so. And at 68... Now I'm going to disagree with you! If you are at least 12.7kg (2st) overweight, as you imply, and have kept faithfully to 1,000 calories a day for the past six weeks, I simply don't believe that you 'haven't lost an ounce'. It's not at all easy to be sure that you are indeed taking 1,000 calories a day unless you really weigh or otherwise measure everything you eat and drink. It's no good just guessing: you can so easily deceive yourself about your intake, which is what I am pretty well certain you have done.
Never let 'it's your age' lead you to dismiss some symptom. The amount of preventable, curable misery that many people put up with quite unnecessarily these days is appalling. If a strictly counted 1,000 calories a day doesn't reduce you, and you honestly can't think of any change in lifestyle to account for your weight gain, then I suggest you go back to your doctor and ask him to reconsider.

Could you suggest, please, the main ingredients of a high-energy diet which will let me lose weight? I lead a very active life and don't want to risk feeling lethargic while slimming. What foods should I eat?

If you remember that a 'calorie' is, in fact, really another name for 'energy' — calories are units of energy — you will see that what you are seeking is a diet that is both high and low in its calorie content. I'm stumped! But there is no reason why you should feel lethargic on a reducing diet if you choose one that has been sensibly devised to provide all the protein and other nutrients you need.
On a sound reducing diet you should feel extra energetic and fit as the surplus pounds begin to disappear.
If you are in normal good health apart from surplus weight and still feel a bit 'down' after a week or two's efforts to slim by a method we suggest, then it's worth realizing that 'feeling lethargic' is for some people an unconscious protest at going on a diet — any diet. If you bring

your feelings out into the open, honestly balancing the effort slimming usually involves against the undoubted rewards of a body in good shape, then you may emerge with a more positive mental attitude — and no more of that lethargy you fear.

Q **How should I deal with my husband? He says women are stupid to bother about being a stone or two overweight — they are much more attractive very well covered! He hates my dieting, though I feel much better and livelier at the proper weight for my height; I'm now within 2.3kg (5lb) of it again, thank goodness. But it is tough going when you are fighting a weight problem and your husband. Have you any suggestions?**

I don't think there is any simple answer; the reaction of husbands to their wives' shape is such a complicated question. Without knowing a great deal more about you, I can't be very specific. But here are some suggestions you may find useful.
First, it seems clear that you are aiming at a sensible weight; your husband can't claim that you are dieting towards an unhealthily low level. But is it, I wonder, a level much below your weight when you were married? If so, your slimmer shape — plus the increased confidence and vivacity your 'livelier' feelings imply — may strike him as a threat. Is the new you going to love and need the old him as much as before? While many husbands much prefer a slim wife, others are not nearly as sure of themselves as they may appear; they may well feel 'safer' with an overweight wife. If she becomes slim and better-looking, they start biting their nails and wondering if she'll run off with another man! I'm not exaggerating; it's a genuine problem. Some husbands express their insecurity by getting very angry. I think that a wife faced with this sort of problem — well, this sort of husband — must work out what is worthwhile to her. A fiercely anti-slimming husband could be a very insecure husband. If she cannot reassure him to accept that her slimness is not a threat, then perhaps she will be wise to accept the real inconvenience and health

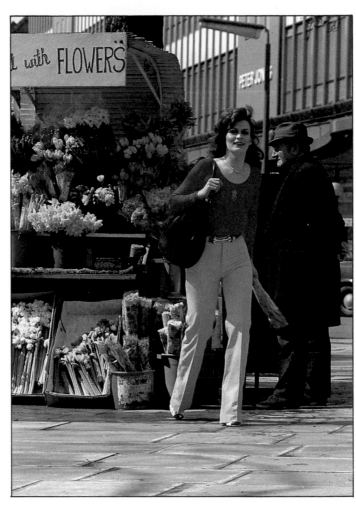

disadvantages that go with overweight. This is not, I must stress for any husband reading this, a desirable answer in the strictly medical sense. Sometimes, though, one must make a choice of evils. A very great pity, isn't it?

Q **Don't you think there's too much emphasis these days on encouraging people to slim, and isn't it dangerous?**

By 'dangerous', I take it you mean anorexia nervosa, which, I am sorry to see, is often called 'slimmer's disease'. However, I am sure that the number of lives saved by people deciding not to be fat enormously outweighs the minute number of cases that may come to grief. If you are overweight, then the risk of developing this condition is not a sensible reason for deciding against slimming. You are certainly not playing safe by deciding to stay as you are. In fact, unless you happen to come within a very well-defined and tiny section of the population,

you are really not at risk from this condition at all.
The majority of anorectics are between about 15 and 20 years old. They tend to be of well above average intelligence. They come from 'good' homes in the sense that their background is well-educated and fairly comfortably off. And they tend to have led what you could call sheltered lives. Usually, their parents have sent them to fee-charging schools. You could say that much has been given them. But it's been made clear that much is expected of them. Either directly or indirectly, their parents have usually put a lot of pressure on them to excel academically. It is highly significant, I think, that one survey of anorectic girls has revealed that the bizarre eating habits in about three-quarters of them dated from the year in which they were working very hard for a major examination. Examinations, however, may be only part of the pressure pattern. In the likeliest candidate for anorexia nervosa, the years of hard study coincide with other, more personal stress areas.

175

Besides competing academically, she is pressured by many sources nowadays to compete in another very real sense — as a young adult, as an attractive young woman. Her developing sexuality, the strains of moving into the increasingly competitive grown-up league and having to face new kinds of relationships with the opposite sex, may make an unconfident girl feel she has 'too much on her plate'. But remember that we are talking of an odd girl out. Though occasional storms and upsets are to be expected, the vast majority of girls do cope with growing up more or less competently. Less 'sheltering' earlier on has made them reasonably self-reliant and less tense about life in general. They probably have the big advantage of a mother who is fairly settled and relaxed in her role: she is not always pushing, not trying to re-live her own life or to realize earlier frustrated ambitions of her own through her children.

Probably what makes an anorectic girl most hard to treat is that her condition is usually part of a family disturbance. Something has gone wrong right at the heart of her closest relationships. If a family is disturbed in some way, the member most affected is often the one who happens to be most vulnerable at that particular time. An adolescent girl is very vulnerable. Most anorexia nervosa specialists accept that they really have to treat a family rather than just one thin, pathetic and often exasperating girl. It is significant that one specialist found a survey of his patients' mothers revealed three out of four to be suffering from clinical depression; these mothers needed psychological help just as much as their more obviously ill daughters.

It is pointless to look for scapegoats or to talk in terms of 'the girl's fault' or 'the parents' fault' in cases of anorexia nervosa, as uninformed outsiders often do; blame is a meaningless word in such situations. Taking the long view, it is often eventually helpful that a family need has been brought out into the open by the daughter's symptoms. I would like to emphasize here that soonest helped is soonest cured. And it is professional help that should be quickly sought — in the first instance, from the family doctor. There is no set treatment. Each case must be dealt with, and urgently, as its own particular needs dictate. Treatment is inevitably a long dose of psychotherapy, helping the girl to come to terms with the pressure she faces. When the physical symptoms are severe, hospital treatment may be necessary. There is then the patient's retraining in normal eating habits; and, as every slimmer knows, altering eating behaviour is often not easy. There are no plain and simple answers to this condition, but I can honestly make one simple final statement. If you are overweight, then for your health's sake — let alone your vanity's — do try to shift the surplus. The only way to do this and to stay healthily slim is to make a permanent change in the eating habits that have made you fat, There must have been something wrong with them or you would be in shape. Yes, there is a risk in any course of positive action. But don't let the bogey of anorexia nervosa ever prevent you slimming.

Dear Professor… what should I eat when dieting?

 Is it healthier to eat foods raw whenever possible?

The 'raw is best' brigade have got a bit out of hand lately, I think! I can tell you straight away that some foods are far less healthy if eaten raw or underdone. Pork and some sorts of fish, especially if you eat them in Japan or Scandinavia, may contain some parasites that proper cooking kills. It's most unlikely these days, thank goodness, that you will get TB from drinking raw milk, since our cattle in the United Kingdom are now very well cared for. But untreated milk can carry other harmful germs; pasteurization is a most important safeguard.

As far as vegetables are concerned, it's true that cooking reduces their Vitamin C and other nutrients, though not as much as most people imagine. If cooked fast in minimum water and if served immediately, vegetables don't lose much in the way of nutrients. Another factor is that one tends to eat more of cooked vegetables than of raw. For example, a reasonable helping of nicely cooked cabbage is 175g (6oz) but you'd be likely to find 50g (2oz) of the raw stuff — in coleslaw, perhaps — quite enough. So even if the cabbage were carelessly cooked, you would probably end up getting more nutrients than by eating an average raw portion. I'm not saying you shouldn't eat raw vegetables. I'm just stressing that raw isn't automatically right. There's a special reason for laying off raw eggs. They contain 'avidin', a substance that greedily grabs hold of a B vitamin called 'biotin' and stops the body absorbing it. If you ate a lot of raw eggs, you could suffer from the very rare condition called biotin deficiency. As cooking destroys the avidin in eggs and most people aren't mad about raw eggs, this isn't a major health hazard, however.

Luckily most people's taste buds stop them fancying starchy food, such as potatoes and cereals, uncooked. Human beings aren't good at digesting these raw.

 Surely I'm right in believing that a good hot meal is better and more warming for you than a cold one?

Certainly, you do feel warmed when you eat a hot meal. So I go along with those advertisements which show people sipping hot soup, etc. as the snowflakes lash against the window pane. But, in fact, the extra warmth contributed to the body by eating something hot instead of eating it cold is minimal. It's not difficult to calculate, for instance, that a largeish portion of thick soup — my own favourite is lentil — could give you about 250 calories when it's been metabolized by the body. But if you drank it down piping-hot rather than at room temperature, you might possibly get 255 calories from it. If hot food makes you feel good, fine: I'm all for that. Nutritionally speaking, through, a good hot meal isn't superior to a good cold one.

If you eat a very high-fibre diet, is the whole digestive process then 'speeded up'? If so, would this faster flow of food and waste material through the body usually hasten the slimming process?

There tends to be a certain contradiction in what people are told about the speed of passage of food with a lot of fibre along the alimentary canal.

It's true that it is likely to stay a little longer than usual in the stomach, so that it gets rather more slowly into the small intestine (next part of its journey). Because of this, some people believe that such high-fibre food is more 'satisfying', thus helping to reduce your appetite and therefore aid slimming. There is no good evidence for this; I, for one, don't believe it.

Later on, the presence of lots of fibre in the diet speeds the passage of food through the intestine; the stools therefore appear sooner, and also emerge rather bulkier. The result is indeed a greater amount of unabsorbed food. But this, in terms of calories, is a fairly minor factor; meanwhile, you

will have taken in quite a few extra calories if your dietary fibre is eaten in the form of added bran, since one-third or more of this could well be starch or other digestible material. Besides supplying some calories, dietary fibre is likely to combine with certain mineral elements of the diet — such as calcium, zinc and iron — and reduce the amounts of these essential nutrients you will absorb from food.

The only time you get a significant reduction in the amount of calories the body absorbs when food is 'speeded up' along the gut is if you take so much of a laxative that diarrhoea results. A daft thing to do for any reason and, as a slimming aid, potentially very dangerous. Never consider it, please.

I'm told that you should be sure to drink at least two pints of water a day when you are slimming in order to assist the elimination of the toxins which are released when you start using stored body fat. Is this true?

It's amazing how many people advocate 'flushing the system' as if it were some dirty old drain… Still, there is no reason at all why you should not drink lots of water. But there is also no reason to suppose that it will do anything like you have been told. The fat in the body and all its other components are constantly being broken down and built up again; this is what

happens in the process called metabolism. On a sensible reducing diet, the rate of burning is faster than the rate of building up. But, in any case, the burning does not produce toxins. So you don't have to worry about 'washing them away' with lots of water.

Are fats in the diet essential for health? And, if this is so, in what kind of quantity?

Human diets are rarely very low in fats, except in some exceedingly poor lands. Even there, no obvious signs suggest that people suffer in any way from this. On the other hand, animal experiments show that diets containing no fat lead to illness and, ultimately, death. It does look as if we need some fat in our diet, particularly a small amount of so-called polyunsaturated fat. But let me repeat that, in the western industrialized societies, it would be practically impossible to eat a diet so low in fat that a deficiency would result. This is because fat occurs in many un-obvious foods, not just in butter, cheese, milk, etc. For practical purposes, unless you are eating in a totally weird way, this is a food fear you can entirely dismiss.

Does skimmed milk have fewer vitamins/nutrients in it than creamy milk?

Vitamins A and D are dissolved in the fatty part of the milk and almost all the fat is missing from skimmed milk. There are, of course, other foods containing these vitamins, so there is no need for you to become deficient in them if you decide to economize on calories by a switch to skimmed milk. All the other components of milk — its calcium, for instance — stay there when it is skimmed.

Though my husband eats lots of very fattening foods — sweets, cakes, sugar — he never puts on any weight. I say too much sweet stuff is harmful, but he says he burns it up and therefore it can't hurt him. Who is right, please?

Tell him tactfully that you are the one who has got it right. There are three important things to bear in mind about sugary foods and drinks. One is that,

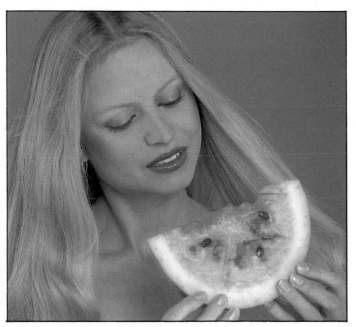

for most of us, they are the most tempting items. So they're the ones most likely to lead people to take more calories than they need. Some people don't put on surplus weight even if they eat lots of these foods — partly because, as your husband states, they can burn up at least some of the sugar. But it's also because they tend to eat less of other foods. And since sugary foods and drinks don't have much in the way of nutrients, merely a load of calories, a sugary diet is likely to be poor in proteins and vitamins and minerals. Thirdly, and I think most importantly, sugar in itself is harmful except in quite small amounts. It increases cholesterol in the blood, also the uric acid level, and makes the blood clot more easily. So even if he isn't fat, your husband would be much better off if he avoided so many sweets and cakes.

Dear Professor…is my health stopping me slimming?

Q I suffer badly from migraine , and my attacks don't seem to be triggered off by any particular food. But the moment that I try to slim, a migraine begins. Yet why should this be? I'm 26, with two children; I take the contraceptive pill and have 12.7kg (2st) to lose. I have been dieting on and off for years and fail because of the migraine pain rather than from any lack of willpower. How can I slim down to my ideal weight?

Migraine is a most tricky condition to treat; we still don't understand all the causes. If any people with bad migraine can be called lucky, they're the ones who can identify their particular 'trigger' and thus avoid eating garlic, avocado or whatever gets their pain going. But a lot of sufferers can't, despite many medical tests, pinpoint the causes so easily.
I doubt if a reducing diet, which doesn't involve eating new stuff but, rather, just cuts your intake of familiar foods, could of itself produce migraine. So, if you always diet sensibly and don't shock your system by silly regimes, I am inclined to suspect that — without your being aware of it — dieting and/or its consequences worries you in some way. In many sufferers, hidden stress of this type could be enough to trigger an attack. Your years of on-off dieting suggests you may have a somewhat ambivalent attitude to losing weight. Perhaps, though your conscious self wants to be slim, the inner you finds your present state useful in some way? For instance, a woman may find being over-weight is something of a protection against sexual advances which she doesn't much welcome. Or it could be that, just by unlucky chance,

an early dieting attempt happened to coincide with a migraine and that you have subconsciously expected the two to go together ever since.
I have no idea whether any of this applies in your case. All I suggest is that it's often a big help to try to see what lies behind a problem. A chat with your doctor could help, but I think you may find you can manage on your own. It isn't easy to bring out hidden worries honestly into the clear light of day, but it's worth the effort. A worry honestly faced is very often a worry halved.

Q I am a 20-year-old girl with a nine to five job, so three meals a day suit me. My only problem is that I have high cholesterol (I have no other medical condition) and need to devise a low-cholesterol diet for myself. As yet, I've not seen you give one. Can you please help?

When you say 'diet', do you also imply a reducing diet? In other words, are you seeking to cope with surplus weight as well as a cholesterol problem? And, as measuring cholesterol in the body is a complicated process, I must assume that this isn't a condition you have 'diagnosed' for yourself — which would not be sensible of you — but that it is your doctor who has decreed a low- cholesterol regime. In which case, I'm a bit surprised that you haven't been given any dietary advice already.
Anyway, in general terms, a person on a low-cholesterol regime can eat a fairly ordinary diet with some modifications. Firstly, there are certain things you needn't change at all. For instance, like everyone else, include in your diet all sorts of fish, fruit, bread and vegetables. You can also eat lean meat,

especially chicken and turkey. The changes you must make are to eat no fatty meat and not more than two or three eggs a week. And you should substitute certain soft margarines — those labelled 'high in polyunsaturates' — for butter. And use a vegetable oil for cooking instead of butter or cooking fat.

Q The hospital told me I was much too overweight to have a hysterectomy that I need and so I went on a diet and lost 22.2kg (3½st). I'm so pleased with the 'new me', but I keep hearing that I'm bound to put on a lot of weight after this particular 'op'. Is this true?

I'm glad to say there is no medical reason why you should not keep your nice shape, though you may have to be slightly extra strict with your food intake. If the hysterectomy involves the removal of just your womb, then you should have no extra-weight worries as a result of the surgery. But this operation very often involves the removal of the ovaries too; as their function includes the secretion of hormones, surgical removal produces the effect of an 'instant menopause'. The resulting change in hormone balance can mean that some patients tend to put on weight and others tend to lose it.
It's probable that your doctor may give you replacement hormones, gradually tapering off the dosage to mimic the effects of a natural menopause. It's difficult to do this in a precisely balanced way and your metabolism may be temporarily altered to some extent. If you find yourself gaining weight, you may not be burning up your food quite as efficiently as before, so you may need to cut your intake a little. Or you may be retaining

178

a bit more water than previously, in which case the doctor can prescribe pills. If you carry on with your new eating habits, you won't in any case put on a large amount. What's more, any gain is correctable. Please don't think me unsympathetic when I mention that some ladies do tend to seize on this 'op' as an excuse for middle-aged spread. If you want to, you can stay in trim.

Q Surely many women are overweight due to a glandular or fluid retention problem?

The straight answer is no, they're not. No normal person in good health, insofar as one can be considered healthy if overweight, can legitimately blame a weight problem on 'fluid retention' or on 'glands' (except salivary glands!). Glands are the body organs which produce hormones; and some disturbance or disease affecting, say, the pituitary gland could indeed cause a gain in body fat. But, in such a case, being fat would be among the least of one's worries. In other words, a glandular disorder that can be properly blamed for weight gain will have already sent you to your doctor with much more urgently serious

symptoms. If your only symptom is surplus weight, then I can confidently predict that you are kidding yourself if you are blaming it on your 'glands'. Because the contraceptive pill is a hormone treatment that induces a continuing state of mock pregnancy, a few women using this birth-control method may experience an unacceptable weight gain. They should see their doctor; a switch to another sort of pill should solve the problem.
As an excuse for fatness, 'fluid retention' ranks even higher than 'glands'. If your body keeps retaining enough excess water to account for more than a very few pounds of surplus weight, you have serious medical problems — and fatness is likely to be the least worrying of your physical symptoms.
Other constantly recurring excuses for fatness that I'm always hearing include: 'Two weeks ago, I went to this party' (trotted out to account for a whole 3.2kg (½st) gain); 'I have to eat with the children' (someone stands there with a gun, I gather); and 'I'm sure dieting would make be bony and haggard' (implying that great lumps are lovely). And when a woman at least 25.4kg (4st)

overweight confides, 'My husband likes me a little plump', it is hard to remain a properly polite professor.
You are extremely unlikely to achieve slimness if you don't face up to the fact that you're fat.

Q Years ago, I shed weight well but now it doesn't seem to work. Could the menopause be the reason? After two years of 'hot flushes', I feel my personal thermostat has got stuck, putting my metabolism out of balance. And I need to practically starve to lose any weight. Well, I can't do that — but at 1.64m (5ft4½in) and 69.9kg (11st) I must do something. What do you suggest?

You're right in thinking that the menopause can make your hormone balance go somewhat haywire for a while. To this extent, weight control may be a bit more difficult temporarily. But because weight is more difficult to control, this doesn't mean impossible. Nor does it mean that you need 'to starve'. You may find you do better if you try a different diet for a while. The good news is that, however trying your difficulties, your hormones and metabolism will eventually settle down.

Dear Professor...what will happen when I diet?

Q What causes water rentention and how can I prevent it?

Retention of small quantities of water - say, not more than two or three extra pints — occurs chiefly because of hormonal changes during a woman's menstrual cycle. This could mean a weight gain (temporary, of course) of up to about 2kg (4lb), usually in the two or three days before a menstrual period. This is an entirely natural phenomenon. Any longer-lasting retention may be due to having had to take a hormone such as cortisone for some inflammatory condition or an allergy perhaps. Water retention can occur, too, from the low-dose hormones in the contraceptive pill. If hormone preparations aren't being taken, then a sizable degree of water retention indicates some serious disease of kidney or heart — in

which case, other symptoms will have put you under medical care. Healthy kidneys do a remarkably good job of keeping the body's water level exactly right. Normally, you should let them get on with it without worrying.

Q We are often warned against eating out of habit rather than hunger, suggesting that it's OK for a slimmer to miss any meal she is not actually eager for. But I've been told that regular meals are important, otherwise the gastric juices become lazy and don't function properly. Is this correct?

Healthy people vary enormously in the number and the regularity of the meals they eat or want to eat. I go along with the idea that if you really feel hungry, then you should eat. I am also strongly for not eating if you're not really hungry. I

don't think one should either leave out or include a meal just because the clock happens to be pointing to a certain time. But when I say 'hungry', I do mean hungry. I'm not referring to a craving for a bar of chocolate or a piece of rich cake that's lurking in the kitchen. If you fancy some such goody, that's not true hunger. Your point about gastric juices implies that the stomach won't produce much digestive juice unless stimulated by a meal. This is quite true, but it's amazing how rapidly your stomach rolls up its sleeves and gets on with the job when it's asked to. There are a lot of things in life to worry about these days, but concern over whether one's tum could get too lazy in the digestive-juice production department is honestly not worth the tiniest furrowing of the brow. Your stomach and I are delighted to pass on such good news.

Q My problem is the so-called 'plateau problem'. I always get stuck at 57.2kg (9st). I've been there for four weeks on my latest diet and haven't lost an ounce, despite keeping to 1,000 calories a day. I'm getting very depressed. What can I do?

I think it's true that many slimmers do hit a 'plateau', but there is no good reason why you should 'get stuck' except at your body's ideal weight. So please stop thinking that you are the helpless victim of some primeval force of Nature! If you're stuck, there is a reason for it — and one you can discover.
There are two vital bits of information you don't give me. The first is how tall you are: from your letter, I've no idea of what you should weigh. The second (and more important) omission is how do you make sure you're eating 1,000 calories daily and not 1,200 or 1,500? Do you weigh or measure out each item you eat? Many people

fondly imagine they can guess 1,000 calories accurately. I'd say 99 per cent eat far more.
It might help you to change your diet method; you can go a bit 'stale'. But, as you'll have gathered, I'm rather sceptical of 'plateau' talk till I know for sure that a slimmer has some surplus weight to lose and is truly averaging no more than 1,000 calories a day.

Q When will my stomach shrink? Or, rather, how long do you have to eat less before your stomach wants less food?

I'm not sure how the Great Shrinking Stomach Myth ever got going, but it has no scientific basis. In fact, you may have noticed that 'shrinking stomachs' are no longer prominent in advertisements for so-called slimming aids. The law, prodded by an occasional sharp kick, is gradually ensuring that people are not so misled. Because you mention the size of your

stomach, I assume that you reckon a tinier tum would help you to eat less. But stomach size governs only the maximum you can stuff at a sitting; you could indulge in umpteen fill-ups in a day, if you desired. Though the factors governing how often and how much an adult eats are still not fully understood, we do know that total food intake has normally nothing to do with stomach size unless it has been vastly decreased by an operation. You mention later in your letter that your stomach felt quite sore when, after following a fairly strict diet for some weeks, you had a birthday blow-out. Well, that wasn't a shrunken stomach grumbling at being forcibly enlarged; it was simply your same-sized stomach protesting at an unusually heavy load. It's much the same as if, after weeks of minimum physical exertion, you asked your legs to take you out on a 10 mile jog. I suspect that you would get a fairly sharp complaint from them too.

Dear Professor...suppose I get pregnant?

Q If you are on 1,000 calories a day and have only 3.2kg (7lb) to lose, do you have less chance of conceiving a baby than if you weren't dieting at all? In other words, could dieting be affecting my fertility?

What you eat can reduce your chances of conceiving in two opposite ways. If you eat too much and thus become significantly overweight, you may well be infertile. There are many women who will tell you that they produced their first baby only after getting their weight nearer normal. On the other hand, infertility also occurs in people who have not eaten enough — as in war conditions or in famine or if they suffer from the self-induced semi-starvation impulses symptomatic of the condition known as anorexia nervosa.
On a well-balanced reducing diet your fertility should not be affected. The fact that your intake is low in calories need not mean that it is low in all the

nutrients you require.
In general, getting yourself as fit and healthy as you can is obviously important to your chances of becoming pregnant: being the right weight is, of course, a major sign of health. But I think you should be sure that you are indeed half a stone or so too heavy that you are on a sensible diet and aren't aiming at a weight a bit too low for your height. In a woman, a good sign of fertility is if your menstrual periods continue normally.

Q So many weight problems seem to be aggravated by pregnancy. So could you please advise me as to the lowest number of calories it is safe to have when pregnant?

If you can raise your right hand high and assure me that you are an Exactly Average Woman — in height, 'background', weight, activity, the number of hours you sleep, pulse rate and temperature, etc. — then I can tell you how many calories you

will need when pregnant. For the average woman, 2,200 calories a day would be right for the first three months of pregnancy and 2,400 calories a day for the rest of the time. But, in practice, no one can really say how many calories *you* need — a totally average woman is so rare!

Q I'm 1.63m (5ft 4in) and 69.9kg (11st), about 15.9kg (2½st) too heavy. Yet, even so, my doctor says I must on no account attempt to diet while I am breast-feeding. My baby is two months old and I hope to feed him for another four months. Frankly, as I am carrying so much surplus weight, this advice seems daft. So I've tried to diet but feel very hungry and irritable even on 1,500 calories a day. Can you give me advice?

The trouble is that most people think of a 'diet' in terms of a general restriction of food. For this reason and not being safely able to take for granted a fair standard of nutritional know-how in those they advise, medical experts understandably worry that people with special needs — a pregnant woman, a nursing mother, a growing child — may be 'nutritionally deprived' if given an OK to diet. When you hear of the amazingly potty and harmful ways in which some people try to lose weight, you can understand this 'official' caution. But it is, of course, perfectly possible for anyone to eat fewer calories but stay well nourished.

Your baby's demands may amount to about 500 calories a day, so it looks as if you have been trying to diet on the equivalent of a super-strict 'net' of 1,000 calories. A carefully counted 2,000 calories a day should see you getting back into shape. Cut down on the sweet and sugary things — cakes, confectionery, biscuits, buns, etc. — when you choose your food and drink. This will reduce your calories but hardly at all the nutrients you and your baby need. If you calmly explain that losing this surplus weight is important to your morale and general well-being and that, of course, you are going to do it sensibly, then I think you will find your doctor much more helpful.

Dear Professor...what diet advice have you for youngsters?

What would you say to my daughter-in-law in my place? I hate to interfere but I am certain my grandson (of 18 months) is exceedingly overweight; he has great jowls and is not as active as he should be. But the other granny is proud of his 'bonniness' — which is a kind word for great wads of fat, I'm afraid. Am I right?

I think it is high time we banished the idea that a really overweight baby is a bonny baby. A very fat baby is a malnourished baby. If your daughter-in-law takes her son for regular medical check-ups (which, of course, I hope she does), this fact is likely to be firmly pointed out to her. There is increasing emphasis on avoiding overweight problems right from the start these days.

Is it possible for a 14-year-old boy to slim? My main problem is fat thighs. Please can you help?

You are sensible to be on guard against getting really heavy. As a first step, aim to get your mother on your side; she can help you a lot once she knows that you are sensibly concerned about your weight. For one thing, she can see that cakes, biscuits, crisps, sweets and chocolates are not on the meal table or allowed to tempt you. She can keep soft drinks, apart from the special low-calorie kind, out of your way too. And she can make it easier for you to fill up with extra vegetables and fresh fruit.

You can help yourself by not spending pocket-money on the sweet and sugary things I've mentioned, and by never forgetting that plain water can quench your thirst perfectly well. Also try to be as physically active as you can: walking, running, swimming, etc.

The good news is that you don't have to lose weight. Because you are at an age when you have a lot of growing still to do, just aim to hold your weight steady for the present. Then you will find that increasing height will gradually get you into the right proportions. The eating and the exercise rules I've given you will apply all your life, even when you are in good shape — they'll help you to stay that way. And you don't need to 'take anything', except my advice!

I am 15 and have gained about 9.5kg (1½st) over the past year. I'm 1.60m (5ft 3in) and now weigh 60.8kg (9st8lb). Yet I don't eat a lot, and have tried dieting for about six months without success, though. Is it puppy fat or over-eating fat?

Girls of your age and younger do change shape as they become physically grown-up; body fat is distributed differently in an adult female. But this doesn't mean that it is natural to put on surplus weight. A healthy puppy isn't fat, by the way!

For your height, you are about 6kg (1st) too heavy at present. And I don't think you should hope for this weight to go away by 'magic'. Because your body still has some developing to do, I think your best plan is to be as active as you possibly can and to cut down hard on sweets, buns, cakes — all sugary, starchy foods and drinks and snacks.

Dear Professor...should I exercise?

How can I lose about 0.9kg (2lb) of surplus fat which hangs around my abdomen and my thighs? Dieting seems to make me lose the weight only in places where I'd rather keep it. What should I do?

I have to start by saying that, once any surplus fat has been shed and what's left of your body has had enough exercise to tone its muscles, then you're down to your God-given basic shape. And if you don't like it, then that's something to take up with the Almighty rather than me. Even slim body shapes vary enormously, of course. Some figures, for instance, don't go in much at the waist; this happens to be their natural structure. Losing one's surplus weight can make legs and thighs slimmer but it will not alter their basic conformation; this will naturally be thicker in some people than in others.

Many dieters find that the last surplus half-stone clings where it's least wanted, and that getting right down to their ideal weight is worth the final effort. If you yourself are at your ideal weight, then exercises to improve local muscle tone may help, particularly in the tummy area.

But after you have done your very best with diet and exercise, then I think you must accept your natural shape — and rely on clever clothes sense to take care of remaining imperfections that bother you. Everybody has some, you know!

Q I'm nearly 44 and quite slim — maybe because, as my job keeps me sitting at a typewriter, I make a point of walking up the eight flights of stairs to my office. But a friend says this is rather drastic exercise for my age and may do me more harm than good. I'm not exhausted but I'm a bit out of breath. Is this dangerous for my health?

If you can tackle all those stairs with only a slight shortness of breath, then keep at them — and congratulations!
In fact, I'd put it almost the other way around. If you walked up eight flights and didn't feel a bit short of breath, then the daily exercise wouldn't be doing you any real good. It's suddenly taking strenuous exercise that can do damage to a person who has previously been very inactive. By the way, tell your jolly friend from me that 43 is not exactly elderly. Of course, if she herself is 19 she won't believe it, I'm afraid — anyway, not for at least another 20 years or so.

Q My husband is a sports fanatic whe is always training, and he's under the impression he sweats off fat. When I told him that he's just losing water, replaced as soon as he drinks, he said: 'Why do they make sweat-suits for training, then?' Is he right?

Like your husband, many people believe that sweating helps fat loss. They are wrong. The confusion may come about because we talk about 'overweight' when we're really concerned about 'over-fat'. The reason for this is that we can easily pop on some scales and measure weight but we can't easily measure the amount of fat in the body. While it is true that excessive weight usually means excessive fat, fat isn't the only component of your body's total weight. And the component most easily increased or decreased is water, which accounts for about 60 per cent of the weight of a normal adult man and some 50 per cent of a normal adult woman's weight. This is why you can temporarily make yourself lose weight by drinking very little for a while or encouraging sweating. But the kidneys will correct this temporary imbalance at the first chance they get.

Dear Professor...how can I look my best?

Q My problem is that since I've started to slim my skin has become very dry. The skin round my nails is particularly hard and ragged. Please don't suggest a hand cream because I'm allergic to cosmetics. Has cutting down fat caused my skin's present dryness?

This is one of the many myths about slimming: that fat in the diet helps to keep the skin smooth, supple and non-dry. Let me assure you that the body makes all the fatty and oily material it needs for the skin from any reasonable diet. It is just possible that a skin-affecting food constituent could be lacking in a 1,000 calorie-a-day diet but only if it were a very poorly designed diet. Regarding hand creams, etc., it is quite easy nowadays to find cosmetics that don't contain any so-called 'allergens'. Consult your chemist. Sometimes, when one is starting a course of self-improvement such as a diet, one does become extra aware of body conditions that were there before but went more or less unnoticed. Now you know your dry skin can't be blamed on diet, perhaps you will take a fresh look for other causes. There's another factor I'd ask you to consider honestly. It's quite common for people subconsciously to resent the fact that they've put themselves on a diet. And, without realizing that this strong 'anti' undertone is there, they report being troubled by headaches or constipation or, in your case, dry skin — all of which are, if not imagined, considerably exaggerated. I'm not criticizing you for this possibility, just making you aware of it.

Q Though I eat sensibly, take quite a lot of exercise and am not overweight, I have cellulite around my tummy and upper thighs. Even if I did diet, I'm sure that this fatty tissue would stay. I am broad in build and just over 1.60m (5ft 3in). How is this ugly cellulite caused and how can I get rid of it?

I do understand how you feel, but my reaction to your question is the same as if you had told me that there were little green men at the bottom of your garden and wanted advice on getting them to go. As I've said before, the French word 'cellulite' can best be translated into English as plain 'fat'. That rigmarole about the big difficulty of getting rid of cellulite and the fact of the skin looking like orange peel is nothing more than an observation of how ordinary surplus fat under the skin can shift less readily from some parts of the body in some people, and how — again in certain places and people — this fat tends to pucker under the skin.
All this is the common behaviour of ordinary surplus fat; you are not suffering from some special affliction. You don't tell me your precise weight but it sounds to me as if you may have several surplus pounds to lose. So why don't you change your eating habits in order to get rid of this extra weight and keep it off for ever? Lose your surplus weight and I promise that your 'cellulite' will disappear.

Q Four weeks ago I weighed 112kg (17st 9lb). I'm now 104.8kg (16st 7lb), a long way off 60.3kg (9½st). I work out on an exercise bicycle for two hours a day and walk two miles. But I'm worried by how my figure will look when I am slim. I have stretch marks all over my body, so how can my skin shrink back to normal?

Three cheers! You obviously intend to get down to your target and know that you can do it. And that is by far the most important thing. But I don't know what your skin is going to look like. This is something which varies very much from individual to individual, just as some women get stretch marks during pregnancy and many do not. But, as a rule, people's skin is remarkably accommodating to change. Frankly, unless you eventually intend to do a streak down the High Street — in which case, let me know when — I do not think you should worry too much. It's not that I dismiss your natural concern about your skin. But, compared with the benefits to health and appearance of achieving your proper weight, it seems a fairly minor factor. Don't let any considerations stand in the way of losing those surplus stones. When you are slim, that will be the time to take stock of your skin. If you are unlucky enough to be left with any area of loose skin, there is a possible remedy in simple surgery. But you may well find that this is not at all necessary.

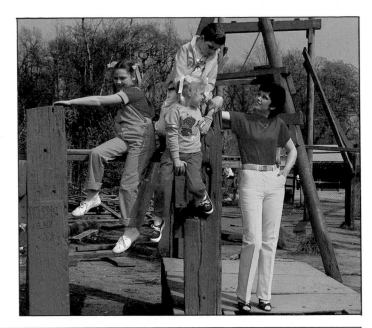

Dear Professor…what happens when I'm slim?

 I'm a very small-boned 1.45m (4ft 9in) and once weighed 60.8kg (9st 8lb). I am utterly sick of myself because I've now reached my 44.5kg (7st) target five times — and each time I then start eating till I'm at least 3.2kg (7lb) over weight. How can I stay slim?

It seems to me that you may feel a bit lost without something to aim for; you need that real sense of achievement which polishing off a surplus half-stone can bring. Are there other targets you could set, other satisfactions and interests to replace the kick you get out of conquering a weight problem? If you could build all sorts of small goals into your working life or in some hobby area, it might reduce the importance to you of reaching 44.5kg (7st) — and the subsequent letdown of being left with nothing to strive for unless you regain 3.2kg (7lb)! With this pressure off, I think that — rather paradoxically — you might find it easier to keep to your target weight. It could be helpful in your case not to think of a 'target' as such; this can seem to convey a kind of finality. For every weight-prone person, staying slim is a matter of being perpetually on-guard. Most of us need to feel that we are achieving things in various ways as we go along: try seeking your satisfactions outside slimming. I suspect this may well make staying in shape far easier. One other point needs stressing

here: your 44.5kg (7st) target is a proper one for the height and build you mention. Often, I find slimmers who moan to me that they can't stay at 'target' are, in fact, aiming at a weight way below their ideal. If you have set your sights too low, your body will battle back. Nature wants you slim, not emaciated.

I am 22 and 1.60m (5ft 3in) and always was around 50.8kg (8st) till I got married 18 months ago. Through cooking for my husband and 'picking', I went up to 57.2kg (9st) and dieted it away by sticking mainly to salads and fresh fruit. But now I find that if I eat a couple of what I'd call 'normal' meals I can put on as much as 2.3kg (5lb) in two days. What should I do?

Oh no, you haven't ruined your health. Simmer down and look at your problem calmly. First of all, the ideal weight range for your height is about 51.7kg to 58.1kg (8st 2lb to 9st 2lb) with 54.9kg (8st 9lb) as the medium-framed average. So why this talk of 'ruin'? You have never gone more than a very few pounds, at most, over your ideal size. You may have been a bit under-weight in earlier days. Secondly, for goodness' sake stop this weighing yourself every day or two. For various natural reasons, people's body weight fluctuates from day to day — even hour to hour — so such frequent checks tend to give you a false impression of your body's

fat levels. A weekly weigh-in is far more sensible.
You have changed your life-style lately and your eating habits. You need to experiment to see how much you can afford to eat to maintain an ideal weight — probably around 54kg (8½st) in your case. You may have to trim a few calories from what you've so far regarded as 'normal' meals.

How long need I stay on my diet before I can start normal eating again?

The core of this question is what do you consider 'normal'? To me, a normal eating pattern is one that provides all the nutrients necessary for your health in a balanced way that ensures you stay slim. A healthy diet is automatically a slimming diet. If you've been eating in a way that has made you overweight, it may well be your habitual eating pattern — it could even be a pattern you have followed all your life — but that doesn't make it normal. Obesity is the result of abnormal eating. That's why, when someone tells me she is trying to reduce by switching to another sort of abnormal eating (something daft like the banana and bubble-gum diet), I advise her to chuck it out and to start eating now as she ought to go on. If you want to achieve and hang on to a healthily slim shape, you can never go back to what you used to call 'normal'.

Jean's smile masked a secret despair

Jean Garrod was used to being described as a 'big girl' — at 1.73m (5ft 8in) she had weighed 76kg (12st) when she had married at 17 years old. After suffering years of thoughtless teasing and cruel remarks about her size, Jean had learned to get in first with a wisecrack about her weight and made a 'fat joke' before anyone else, although deep inside herself she was in despair. She always longed for approval and friendship from others and tried to win it in any way she could, often by being unselfish and obliging to a ridiculous extent. When she married she felt more secure, but soon her pre-married weight of 76 kg (12st) seemed quite low in comparison with her new weight gained during pregnancy, and after her daughter, Julie, was born it did not miraculously disappear. By the time Julie was trying to walk, Jean was over 95.5kg (15st). However, not wanting to bother her husband with her weight worries, Jean pretended that she did not care about being fat or, at 19 years old, not being able to wear jeans and fashionable clothes. After several years of trying unsuccessfully to diet, Jean at last discovered why her previous dieting attempts had failed — learning about counting the calories in foods was a revelation to her. After losing 25.5kg (4st) on her own, Jean joined a slimming club to get the extra support to shed her final excess weight. Soon she was down to 62.5kg (9st 12lb) (right). As her weight gradually decreased, Jean felt her self-confidence growing and began to feel like a new, elegant, slim woman as a result of her successful dieting.

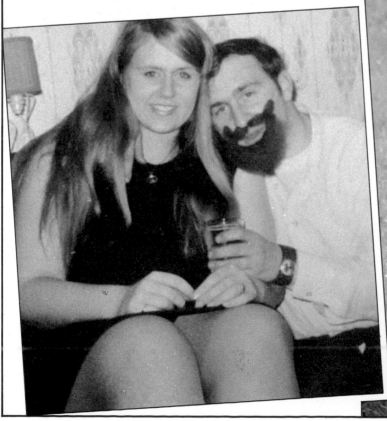

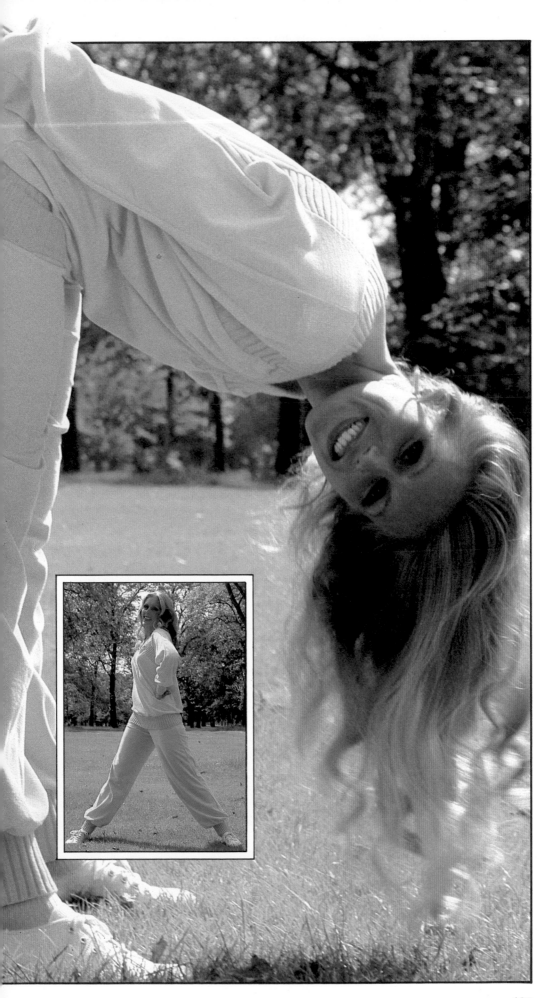

The Mason chassis trims down

Diane Mason, at 1.70m (5ft7in), had felt trapped in a mountain of fat ever since she could remember. At six years old she appeared in family photographs with a scowl on her fat face. At 12, she was a solid, plain 76.2kg (12st) lump in a short skirt which revealed great tree-trunk legs. Then there was the massive 17-year-old with tangled masses of henna'd hair and a long flowing kaftan hiding the bulges below. Diane as a bride of 19 was dressed in the biggest white cheesecloth dress an Indian boutique could provide. Later, as a young mother, she became 85.7kg (13½st) of solid misery. After binging and dieting for most of her life Diane finally discovered the new low-fat way of eating. Once down to a trim 60.3kg (9½st) she found it easy to maintain her weight, enjoyed going for long walks and exercising every day, and she still had plenty of energy left over for one of her new hobbies — stripping down the engines of old cars and motorbikes and shining them up. Her brother, Andrew, is a fellow enthusiast, yet in the old days he would not allow Diane into his garage in case she knocked something over! It is hard to feel feminine when you weigh a bulky 85.7kg (13½st) but the new Diane can wear dungarees and still feel attractive. The miracle has happened. The girl who skims out shopping for skin-tight glitter pants and is told by an envious salesgirl that they look great on a figure as slim as hers, is confident that she will not be treated like one of the lads any more.

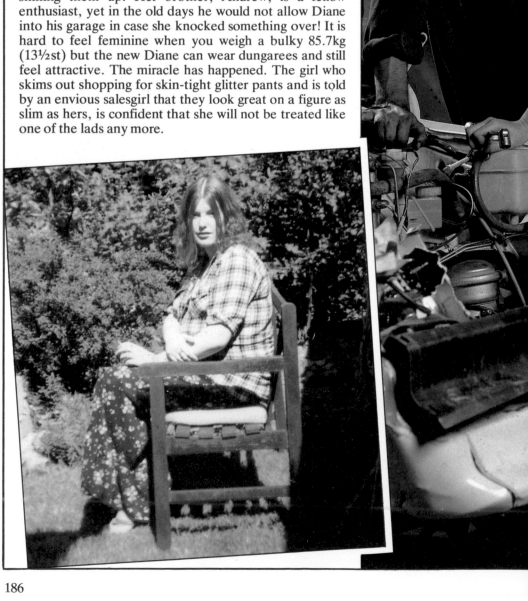

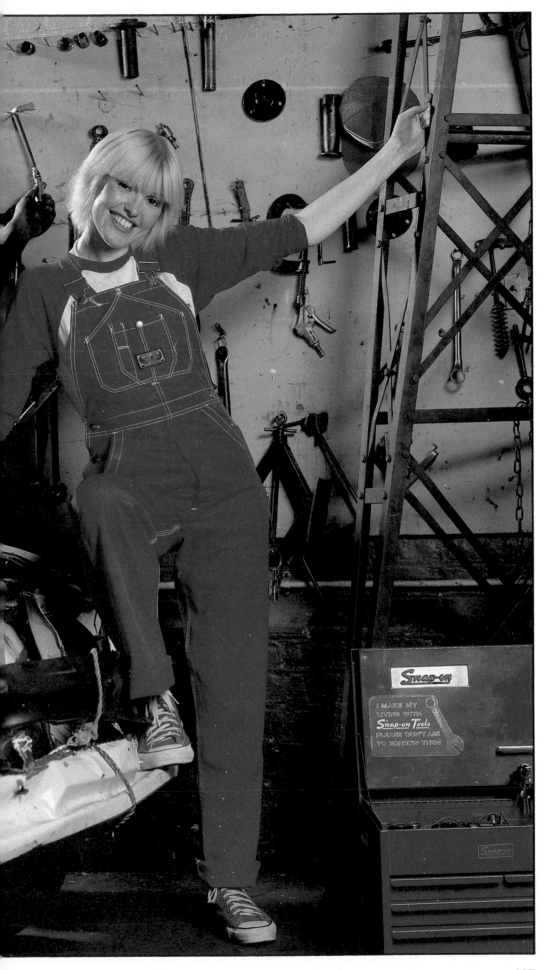

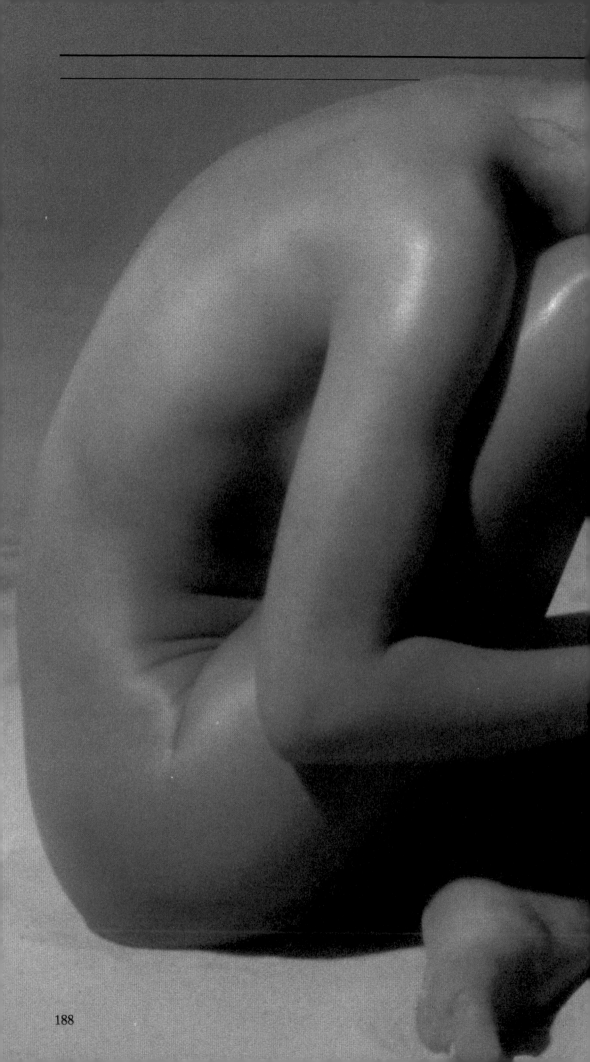

CHAPTER 9

Getting into shape

Shaping up.

Few women can say that they are totally satisfied with their body, whether they are young or old, plump or slim, or even top photographic models. It is not unusual to hear women bewailing their 'drooping pear shape', 'plump waistline' or 'flabby tummy'. As your slimming routine takes effect and the weight melts away, you may find that your shape is not as streamlined as you would wish. For as flab disappears, flabby muscles show up and these can add to your waist or hip measurements — just what you *do not* want when you have worked hard to get rid of unwanted weight.

One thing to remember is that fat seems to cling always in the places where you least want it. So if your waistline or your thighs are your biggest problem areas, you may have to get right down to your target weight before the final problem flab disappears. However, you can certainly trim your shape

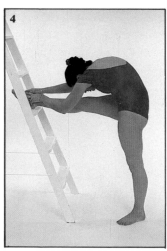

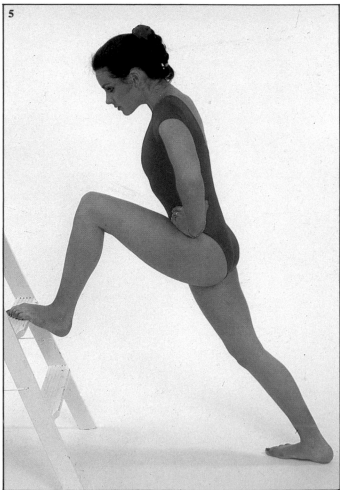

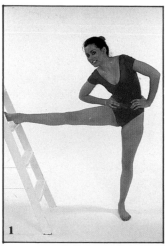

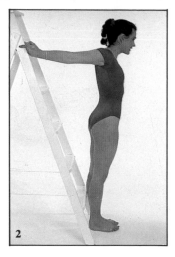

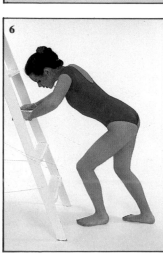

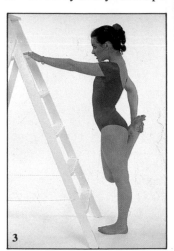

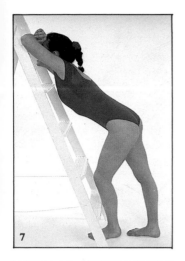

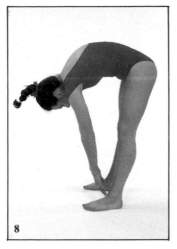

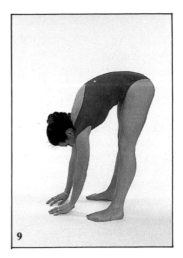

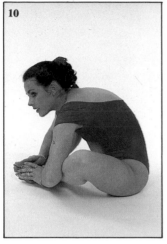

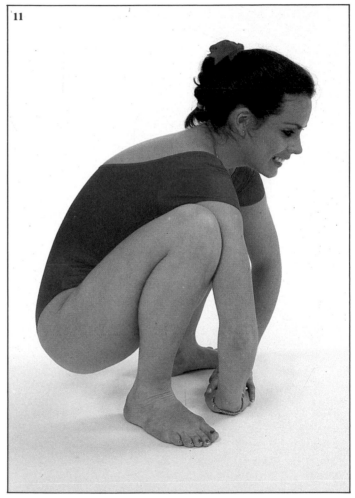

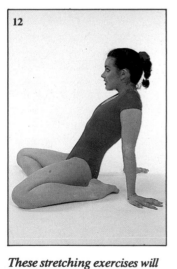

These stretching exercises will stretch your limbs and muscles before you embark on the shaping-up exercises.

1 *Stand with one foot parallel to ground, and bend at waist towards it. Each leg for 15 seconds.*
2 *Holding the support with your hands behind you at shoulder level, straighten arms as you lean forwards. Hold your chin in and your chest up for 20 seconds.*
3 *Holding your right foot in your left hand, pull your heel towards buttocks. Hold 30 seconds.*

4 *Bend forwards from the waist until you feel the pull in your raised leg. Hold for 20 seconds, relax and repeat with other leg.*
5 *Hold your raised leg straight and bend your knee as your hips move forwards. Hold 30 seconds.*
6 *Keeping your back flat and heel down, lower hips as you bend knee. Hold 15 seconds.*
7 *Stretch the right side of your hip by turning your right hip inwards. Turn your hip sideways as you lean your shoulders in the opposite direction. Hold for*

25 seconds for each hip.
8 & 9 *With feet apart, bend forwards from hips slowly. Hold and stretch for 15-25 seconds.*
10 *Feet together, hold your toes and bend forwards. Hold for 40 seconds.*
11 *From a standing position, squat down with your feet flat and toes pointed out at 15 degrees. Hold for 30 seconds.*
12 *With right leg bent and heel just outside right hip, bend left leg with left sole inside upper right leg. Hold for 30 seconds.*

191

as you lose weight with exercises designed to tone up muscles that are not as firm as they should be. Take a look in your mirror and honestly assess where muscle sag shows — tummy, thighs, bottom, upper arms? Perhaps your bust droops or you have the faintest hint of a double chin?

The no-nonsense exercises in this chapter are tailored to attack muscles where they need chivvying most. You start on them gradually, working up to full measure as your body becomes more accustomed to the effort (if you have any worries about your health, consult your doctor first). To be really successful a certain amount of effort and determination will be needed on your part. The reward will be a much trimmer shape and a new confidence that you are looking your best.

Concentrate at first on your worst problem area rather than trying to do all the exercises. As you get into the habit of exercising for a few minutes every day you will probably find that it takes very little effort to incorporate some of the other exercises if you need them.

Before you embark on any of our muscle-toning exercises, try this warm-up exercise which is an instant morale booster and also a treat for your back.

Stretch up slim

To lose several centimetres (inches) off your waist in seconds you simply need to start stretching your spine. There is nothing more instantly improving to any body.

Stand, with your feet just slightly apart, hands lightly clasped on top of your head; elbows back, shoulders down. Now try hard to push your crown up through your hands. Keeping that stretched spine upright, walk slowly about with a deliberate, high goose-stepping movement (or if you have not got room for that, just raise your knee high with each stride). Repeat this as often as possible.

Fix a motto in your mind for slim-stretch potential: *tail in, tum in, chin up!* Follow this advice and you can be sure that, whatever your weight, you are carrying it well. When you go out shopping, try to imagine that all your shopping is beautifully balanced on your head and walk tall.

Your newly stretched spine will give you an instantly slimmer look and stretching in this way gives a real mental lift.

Firming up

The following exercises are designed to tone up muscles rather than burn up lots of calories. We have suggested some high-calorie-burning exercises in the section entitled *Stepping up the calories you burn.*

You could incorporate a mixture of these exercises into your daily slimming pro-gramme. You may find that it is easiest to break your exercises into short sessions throughout the day — a muscle-toning exercise first thing in the morning before you dress, walking for half an hour at lunchtime to burn up extra calories and a second muscle-toning exercise in the evening before you go to bed. Try to establish a set routine so that exercising becomes a habit rather than a chore.

If your flab is due to the fact that you are still overweight, you must combine exercise with a diet to get satisfactory results. No form of exercise, however strenuous, will compensate for an excessive intake of food.

Firming up heavy thighs

Heavy thighs are not uncommon among many women who have otherwise good figures. They are, however, a problem that is shared by many women who have allowed themselves to become overweight. When they slim down, they may find that their thighs tend to remain big and flabby. For some women, too, the thigh is the area most vulnerable to weight gain. Whatever the cause, it is possible to trim down even the most massive thighs to a slim, firm shape by using our special thigh-reducing exercises. Continue to work at these to maintain firmness even after reducing flab in these areas. The only way to trim thighs is by using specific exercises which are designed to strengthen the weak muscles in this part of the leg. Firm flesh depends on firm muscles, and this can only come from hard work. Firming the thighs is always tough, especially at the beginning, and you must expect to experience some pain as muscles are tautened. If nothing hurts, you are being too easy with yourself.

Two warnings: if you are still very over-weight, then please diet down until you are a reasonable size before starting this exercise plan; and because the movements are very strenuous, do not overdo them at first. Do each exercise two or three times for the first few days, then gradually increase the number until you can reach the maximum target.

How much improvement may you expect? There will be a gradual but very definite improvement from the start, but if you are over 40, it will take about a year before your thighs slim down and firm up to a good shape. If you are under 40, it will take less time, perhaps about six months or so.

If you do this routine every day, you can expect to see your thighs become more shapely within a few weeks. However, at this point you are likely to reach a plateau

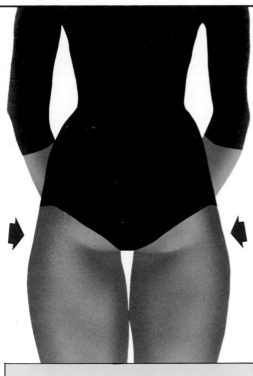

Firming up heavy thighs

1 *Stand sideways to a firm object such as a table or chair to give support at waist level. Using the right hand to steady yourself, hold your left arm at shoulder level and squat on the balls of your feet with heels together and your knees widely apart.*

2 *Keeping your back straight, bounce up and down. Start with five bounces a day and build up gradually to 40. This exercise works on the top of the thigh muscles, so persevere.*

3 *In the same squat position, raise your body until your bottom is 30cm (12in) off the floor. Hold this position and push your knees open in small movements to a count of 10. Relax, then repeat the exercise.*

4 *Stand facing the support and, with knees together, sink slowly into a squat position resting on your tiptoes.*

5 *Keeping your back straight, lift your body a little above your heels.*

6 *Now push your pelvic bone forwards and count up to 3. Relax into a squatting position and repeat five times.*

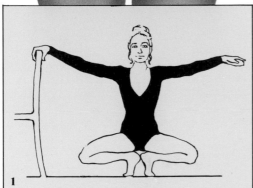

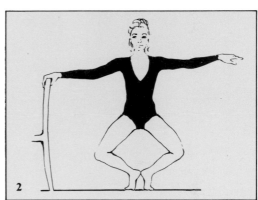

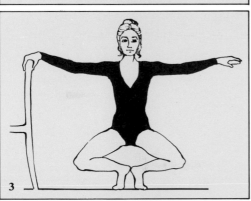

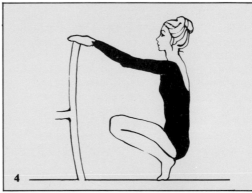

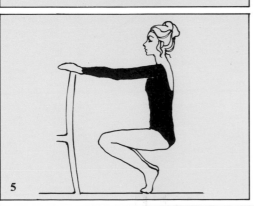

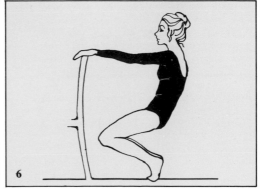

where they appear to stay the same size in spite of the exercise. If you stop, you will go right back to square one, so persevere and you will find that after a time there is suddenly a noticeable improvement again; and as weeks and months go by, your thighs will become more shapely.

Firming up the tummy and waist

Look at a slim young girl in a bikini and you will notice the almost violin-shape of the muscles at either side of the abdomen. This is the natural corset that holds the stomach beautifully in shape and, if you look after it, your corset should last as long as you do.

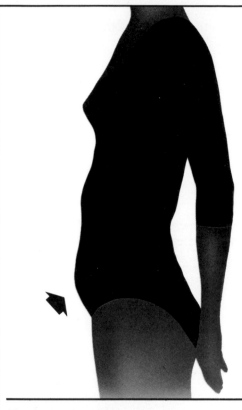

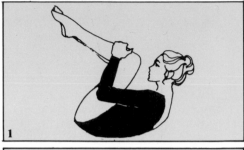

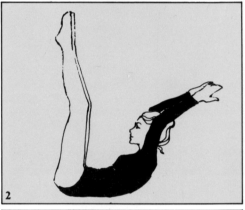

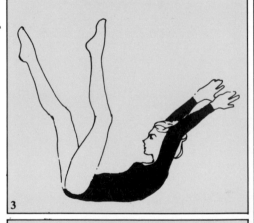

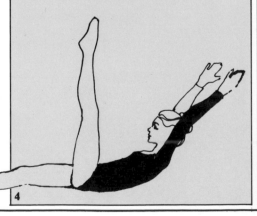

Firming up the tummy and waist

These exercises are designed to firm up slack muscles around your stomach and waist. Practise them every day if you wish to see some positive results in a short space of time.
1 Lie on a comfortable mat on your back, with your body curled up and head and knees together. If your stomach muscles are very flabby, you can do this exercise against a wall.
2 Raise your legs towards the ceiling and lift your arms above your head, while 'pushing' your spine downwards as though into the floor itself. Be sure to push down hard.
3 Now do a little 'walk' in the air with your legs, with your arms outstretched as high as possible and pulling upwards from your diaphragm all the time.
4 Move your other leg and 'walk', keeping your waist and lower leg on the floor. Begin with 20 walks and build up the number gradually until you can do 100 non-stop. If you ache across your ribs, that is a good sign. You may not feel any pull lower down at first but this exercise does firm and tighten tummy muscles eventually if you keep on persevering at it.

Most stomach muscles, however, get little natural, 'automatic' exercise, and therefore this middle area of the body is often the first to suffer from shapelessness, especially when excess fat has been allowed to accumulate. So be warned that restoring the firm shape of a neglected stomach will be hard work.

Two factors encourage the stomach to become flabby: slouching and over-eating. If you sit and stand with your spine curved over and your middle slumped downwards, the stomach muscles gradually become flaccid and relaxed. Thus whether you are overweight or not, you are likely to suffer from a spreading waistline and a noticeably flabby stomach if you slouch habitually.

The flat, youthful stomach's other main enemy, of course, is over-eating. Overweight and obesity encourage relaxed muscles all over the body, and in the midriff area, fat accumulates rapidly around the flaccid muscles. If this is your problem, you must diet to lose the excess fat, or you will never achieve a firm, flat stomach. Dieting alone is not the answer, as exercise is essential to firm and tauten the muscles and restore a youthful outline. With the simple exercise given here, you can confidently expect to lost up to 7.5cm (3inches) off your stomach relatively quickly — within two or three months if you are under 40 but maybe a little longer if you are over that age. Assuming that you have no medical problems other than a moderate degree of surplus weight — up to 12.7kg (2st) too much — you can safely tackle this exercise.

The exercise is simple, but if you do it correctly, you must expect to suffer a few minor aches and pains at first until the stomach muscles become accustomed to the increase in movement. You may groan a little when you laugh, and if there is no twinge of discomfort, then you are being too kind to yourself and are not exercising the stomach muscles properly. However, do not overstrain them to begin with — just two to three minutes at one time is enough at first. You can build up gradually to three five-minute sessions totalling 15 minutes a day. As your aim is to increase over a long period the number of times you do the exercise at one go, always do one more than you think you can, and then relax. Very soon, if you exercise every single day, you will notice that your stomach is becoming flatter and more shapely.

Nothing is achieved without constant application and self-discipline, and a firm stomach is so well worth achieving! You will feel healthier, more confident, hold your body better and walk more gracefully. Your clothes will hang better, and you will look younger and fitter too. All these benefits are worth some suffering!

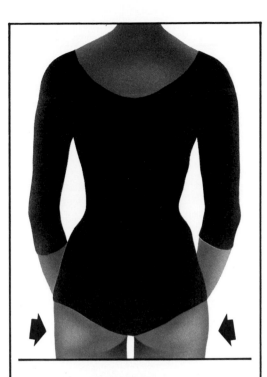

Firming up a sagging bottom
1 *Kneel on a carpet, holding onto the edge of a firm table. Now extend your left leg diagonally behind you, with the left knee slightly bent. Lean over the extended leg and, without moving your body, roll your left hip slowly forwards.*
2 *Now raise and lower the left leg a few inches above the floor. Repeat 5 times and then do it again with the other leg.*

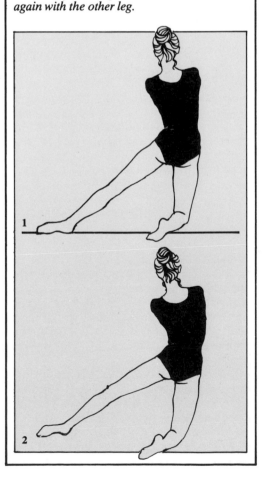

Firming up a sagging bottom

The slimmer a woman is, the quicker she will obtain results from exercise to lift a sagging bottom, caused by relaxation of the muscles due to lack of usage. Exercise can help firm those muscles up, although for everyone this is a fairly long job. Even a young girl, who has had to diet back to a sensible weight, will have to wait three or maybe four months before she sees an improvement. Most older women will have to wait up to six months. The degree of improvement depends upon the extent of sag and how long it has been sagging! Some older women may have to work at it for a year. After 55, you can do this exercise knowing that, even if it will not actively improve your sagging bottom, it will be effective in preventing the problem from getting worse.

Plan a 10-minute session of this exercise every day. That takes determination because exercising, for some women, is very boring. To be honest, only girls in their early twenties will get back a really firm bottom, but if you persevere, the results will come.

A lot of women 'bounce' their bottoms on the floor, 'walk' on their bottoms or lie full-length and roll from side to side to try to improve the shape of their bottoms. These movements will only roll the fat around and do not firm the muscles themselves.

The exercise illustrated on the previous page will hurt. In fact, if at first you do not ache from the back of the knee to the top of your leg, you are not doing the exercise properly! So start gradually and work up to 10 minutes. The foot can be raised only 7.5-10cm (3-4in) and if the leg can be raised higher, without pain, then you are not thrusting the hip forwards enough. You can practise this exercise in an easier form when you are standing about, in a queue for instance. Get into the habit of clenching your bottom, but not when sitting down as this uses the wrong muscles.

Firming up flabby upper-arms

Fat both on and around the upper arms accumulates easily and may leave unsightly, flabby flesh when it is reduced by dieting. However, neither fat nor flab are inevitable. Here, as everywhere else in the body, firm shapeliness depends on two things: correct weight and good muscle tone. This may surprise you, but before we even talk about the exercises that can make your arms shapelier, consider how you hold yourself. If you tend to slump or stoop, then whatever weight you are, you are encouraging excess fat to settle on your upper arms and your shoulders, because the muscles that keep

Firming up upper arms

1 *Stand with your feet slightly apart and your head straight. Now place your hands on your shoulders but only lightly.*
2 *Keeping your hands on your shoulders, bring the elbows down and forwards to touch each other in front of you.*
3 *Now raise the elbows, still together, up to face level in a circular movement.*
4 *Continue moving your elbows upwards and then move them outwards in a circular movement. Repeat these elbow circles between five and eight times.*

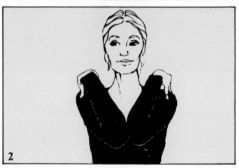

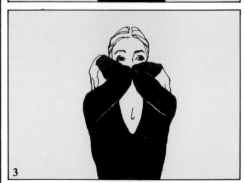

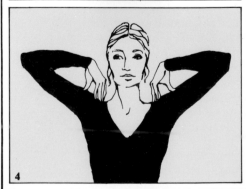

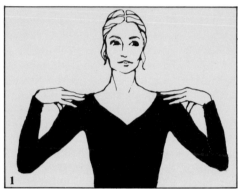

flesh firm are allowed to become slack and droopy. Only firm muscles can give firm, shapely flesh. You must retrain yourself to move 'tall' but not to stand like a soldier with head up and shoulders back — this encourages stiffness and tension.

Try to walk and move from the centre of the body. Imagine that you can feel energy flowing out from a power source in your diaphragm, and you will soon find yourself moving the way a dancer does with your head and spine in natural alignment. This form of movement makes you feel (and look) more graceful, healthier and better psychologically, but if you have got into the habit of stooping, you will have to keep reminding yourself to move like this. It is easy to slip back into bad habits!

Now for those floppy upper arms. Ask yourself whether they are really due to overweight? If so, the first thing you must do is to diet down to size. Loss of fat will not lead to flabby, loose flesh if you exercise to restore firm muscle tone while you are dieting. These exercises will encourage your upper arms to regain their beautiful shape — and when you are at your correct weight there will be no saggy flesh to remind you of how fat you were! Even if you have already lost weight and are now suffering from flabby, loose flesh, these exercises can still make your arms more shapely. However, you must be strict with yourself and do these exercises every day for three months — six months or longer if you are over 35 — if you want to see real improvement. They are not painful but you will feel a pull in the muscles of the upper arms and shoulders. Do not make them too easy — flaccid exercises without a pull on the muscles are no use and you should feel some tension.

The first exercise is very simple, and you can do it easily at any time during the day. Stand with your arms outstretched sideways at shoulder level. Now make a fist, and move the whole arm from the shoulder up and down... up and down in very fast, tiny, beating movements. You will feel the tension in the upper arm and know that it is helping muscles regain their firmness.

The second exercise, illustrated opposite, should be carried out several times a day. Remember to persevere and you will see rewarding results.

Firming up your bustline

No external appliance or exercise can affect your actual breasts because you are not dealing with the muscle tissue, which can be toned, but with twin mammary glands. You cannot alter a bust's basic siting either — some are placed high (cleavage seems to start almost at the collar-bone) and some are positioned lower. Exercise can help, however, to develop and brace the pectorals,

your bust's supporting muscles, and also to neaten your rib-cage. This helps a small bust to make the most of itself, and it stops a big bosom looking 'solid to the waist'.

Although many people believe that splashing cold water over their chest is both helpful and effective, it will not alter the size or shape of the breasts. It merely gives the pectorals a chilly surprise, makes you wince and causes an automatic reflex action. The pectorals always relax again once you stop shocking them. Both contraction and relaxation improve muscle tone, but you will achieve similar results from warming exercise sessions.

You can monitor the effect of these exercises if you perform them topless in front of a mirror. You will feel the pectorals flex and see your bosom lift if you are exercising correctly. Stand steadily, your feet slightly apart, and interlock your fingers in front with the elbows and hands at shoulder level. Now turn your knuckles inwards towards your body and clench the 'heels' of your hands together hard while, at the same time, stretching your body upwards and pulling in your stomach as if trying to fit into a very tight belt. Clench and relax them rhythmically six times.

The following exercise can benefit desk-bound women and anyone whose posture is not perfect — remember that even the most shapely bosom slumps under round shoulders. Clasp your fingertips behind your head and press your head backwards on to the palms. Then press your elbows back as far as possible, trying to make the shoulder blades overlap and pulling in turn sharply at the same time. Then repeat this action rhythmically six times as for the first exercise. Complete your routine (gradually aim to do the whole trio several times over) by interlocking your fingers with the 'heels' together just above your head and pressing upwards three times. Now release the 'heels', turn your clasped hands inside out and press up three times with your arms at full stretch to the same brisk tick-tock rhythm.

Firming up jaw-line flab

When neck and facial flab is due to excess weight, a slimmer cannot expect to see her prettiest profile until most of the surplus is shed. Exercises can help your face, though, in two worthwhile ways. First, they tone the under-chin area and elsewhere. When sag is due to slack muscles rather than to surplus flesh (often the case as you near your target weight), proper exercises can give your face, jaw-line and spirits a lovely lift. Secondly, many facial lines get embedded far too early by plain bad posture. A badly held neck and shoulders can create huge tensions, reinforce frown lines and even lead to painful head-aches. Exercises can help to alleviate this.

197

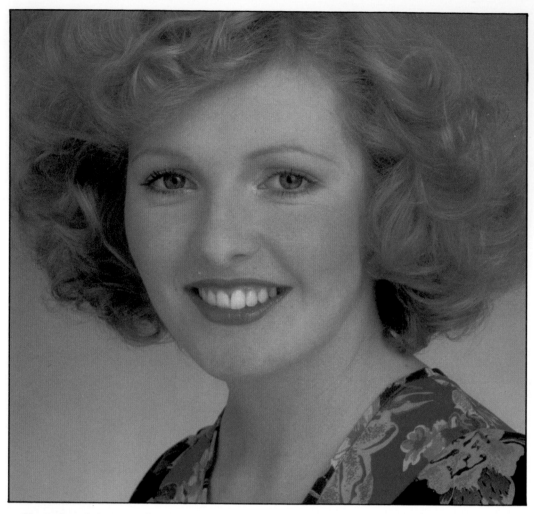

Your head is very heavy and may be compared to a concrete football resting on top of a sturdy but narrow column. If the ball is squarely balanced, then you need not lift a finger to hold it in place, but once it lurches off-centre, you will have difficulty in keeping it on the column. In the same way, balancing your head centrally above your spine by standing or sitting straight, saves the neck and shoulder muscles a great deal of unnecessary strain. Take care how you position your head until you find that an easy upright balance is second nature and you will soon notice the benefits.

Now, are your shoulders hunched? If so, un-tense them immediately — the shoulders' proper placement is back and down, giving a long slimming line between the chin and the chest. Some shoulders hunch forwards because their owners need glasses or a new lens prescription. A peering, frowning posture will spell out instant middle age in body language even if your birth certificate states that you are under 25. Work at making loose, un-tensed shoulders second nature.

● Tone away a double chin or over-chubby cheeks by practising this simple exercise. Do not be self-conscious or afraid of looking silly — just think of the beneficial end-results. Simply say, 'Oooh! Eeek!' six times, in rhythm to a clock's tick-tock sound, first pursing up your mouth to make it very round and then stretching it as wide as it will go. You should feel the muscles flexing up to your ears on the 'oooh', and tightening under your chin on the 'eeek'.

● Slowly stick your tongue straight out to its fullest extent and then bend it upwards as if to touch your nose. You will feel your under-chin area being braced. Repeat this exercise three times, building gradually up to six but do not overdo it!

● Rest your elbows on a table, then tuck both thumbs under the tip of your chinbone, with the first two fingers of each hand touching your temples. Open your mouth gently and slowly, letting your lower jaw 'fight' hard against the thumbs; you will feel the strain on many facial muscles. Relax and then repeat the exercise twice, working up gradually to six repeats.

● With your elbows still on the table, try this toner for eye-area muscles. Rest your fingertips over closed lids, then, very gently and slowly, attempt to close your eyes tightly but let your fingers stop you. Repeat this exercise only three times a day.

CHAPTER 10

Staying slim

Once you have slimmed down to the weight that suits you best, how do you keep it that way? If you have clung to the fantasy that *now* you can revert to your 'normal' pattern of carefree eating without regaining any weight, forget it. If that pattern was the cause of your putting on weight in the past, then it will have the same effect the second, third, or even the fourth time around. You have got to find a new way of eating.

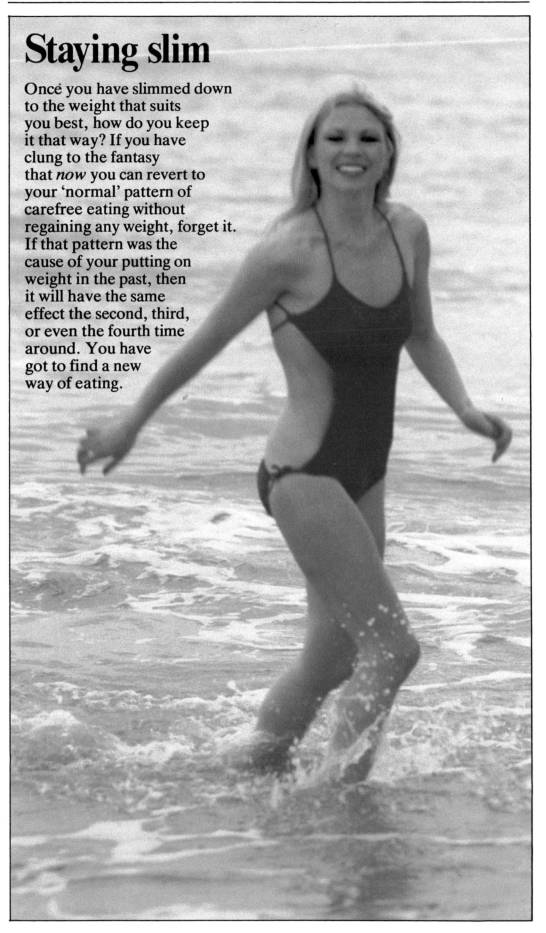

Eat either of the typical three-meal menus on these pages and you will have consumed 2,000 calories. That is the upper limit that most women can consume in a day without gaining any weight. In fact, scientists have now discovered that even this amount is more than many a modern woman can afford unless she starts burning up a few more calories. In addition, most women swallow more calories in the form of drinks and snacks. If you eat three meals each day like the ones shown, you cannot afford even the milk in your tea without putting on weight.

Although you cannot be expected to stay on a diet forever, you do need to find your own personal and successful blueprint for limiting your daily calorie intake, so that you neither gain nor lose any weight and maintain your new, trim figure.

If you have been doing some extra

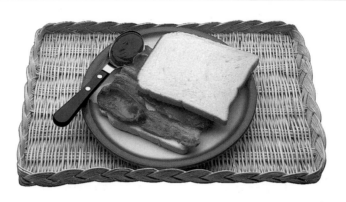

This typical three-meal daily menu contains 2000 calories — as much as most women can eat in a day without gaining weight.

Breakfast

2 slices bread	200
3 rashers grilled bacon	240
15ml tomato ketchup	15

Lunch

275ml (10floz) cream of tomato soup	225
1 small bread roll	145
7g (¼oz) butter	55

Dinner

Cheese omelet, made from 2 large eggs (size 2), 15g (½oz) butter and 75g (3oz) Cheddar cheese	645
1 large grilled tomato	15
150g (5oz) slice lemon meringue pie	460
Calorie total:	**2000**

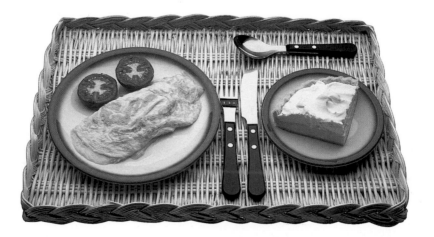

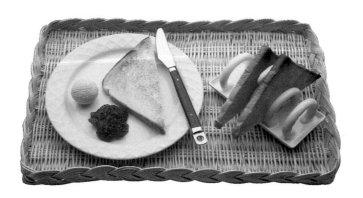

This typical three-meal menu also comes to 2000 calories.

Breakfast

1½ slices toast	150
15g (½oz) butter	105
20ml (2 rounded teaspoons marmalade	70

Lunch

75g (3oz) Cheddar cheese	360
Mixed salad	30
30ml (2 tablespoons) salad cream	90

Dinner

125g (4oz) roast beef	240
225g (8oz) roast potatoes	360
125g (4oz) sprouts	30
25g (1oz) Yorkshire pud	60
60ml (4 tablespoons) thick gravy	80
200g (7oz) canned peaches in syrup	175
50ml (2floz) double cream	250
Calorie total:	**2000**

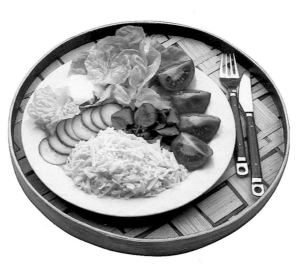

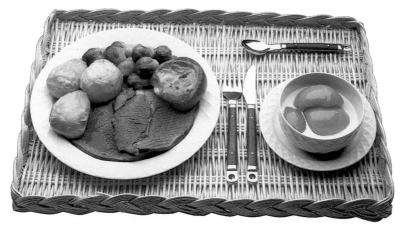

exercising while you have been slimming, please keep this up. Not only is regular exercise good for your general health and mental well-being, but the additional number of calories you burn up will enable you to eat more as you stabilize your weight.

How do they really stay trim?
The real experts on staying trim are those women who have succeeded in both their slimming and staying slim. You can learn from their example and advice.

'Quite frankly, as far as I'm concerned, eating is tied up with emotions. I find that when I am unhappy or emotionally a bit empty, I eat and eat; but when I am emotionally satisfied I just don't need stacks of food...' This comment came from a woman who was 12.7kg (2st) overweight all her life until she succeeded in solving her big weight problem. It crystallizes a major problem that many weight-prone women face by posing the question: can any normal human female eat in a restrained and weight-conscious way all the time? Many previously overweight women point to the relationship between eating and emotions.

A woman who had been overweight for 10 years, reaching more than 82.6kg (13st) at one time before getting her weight down to a slim 54.4kg (8st8lb), confessed that she has kept slim despite the fact that she still suffers from having a 'sweet tooth' and a couple of temptation days each month. She attributed these difficult days to pressures and tension rather than to a conscious craving for high-calorie foods. Another woman, who had become very slim after being moderately overweight for years, admitted to being an erratic eater, who found it relatively easy to stick to a moderate amount of food for a week or two but then dashed automatically to the biscuit tin whenever she was upset or harrassed. These are women who have succeeded nevertheless in staying slim.

On that golden day when a woman finally achieves her goal and becomes slim at last, she will feel on top of the world. She may promise herself that *nothing* will ever induce her to become fat again, but how difficult is it for the average woman to keep to her resolve? Will she find that the desire to over-eat that made her fat has disappeared automatically with her surplus weight?

A recent survey asked a sample of successful slimmers whether, during the few months immediately following their dieting, they had found that they could not eat as much food as they had consumed before slimming. Only 18 per cent said that this was the case; the remaining slimmers said that their appetites were reduced, but only to a degree. They all agreed that it would have been very easy to slip back into eating the same pre-diet quantity of food if they had not made a conscious effort to discipline themselves. However, to a certain extent, most of them did stray occasionally from their new eating pattern.

Only 15 per cent succeeded in keeping their weight steady during the first few months. For the majority, the pattern was one of gaining a little weight and then of shedding weight again by more dieting.

During the early months of staying slim, it is more realistic to accept this slight fluctuation in weight level than to become guilt-obsessed by gaining even a little weight. The key factor lies in having a set weight of maybe 3kg (½st) over your ideal weight, above which you will *never* go.

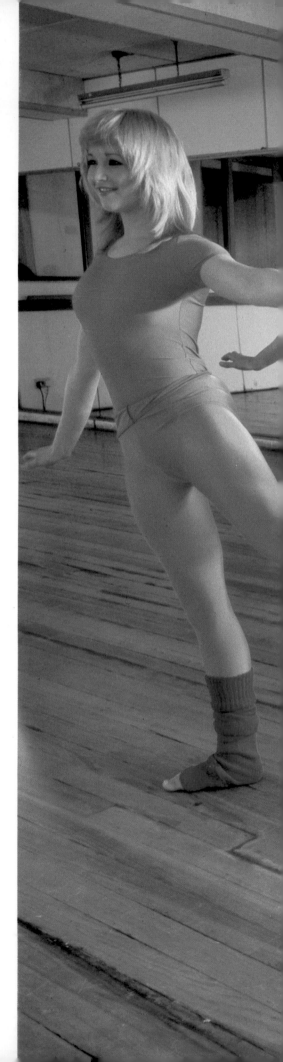

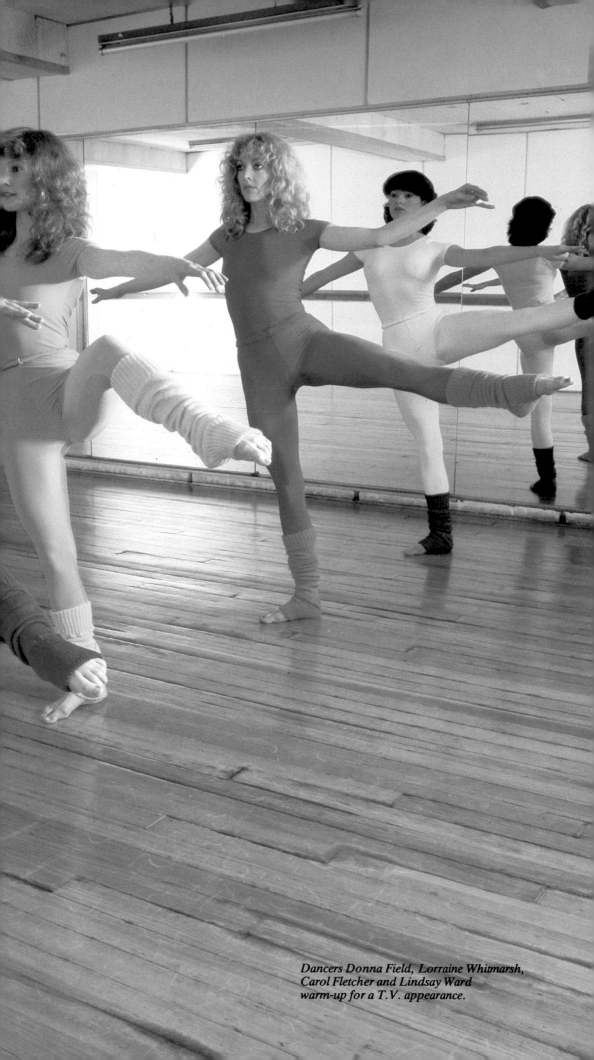

Dancers Donna Field, Lorraine Whitmarsh,
Carol Fletcher and Lindsay Ward
warm-up for a T.V. appearance.

Some women found at first that they gained 1½-2kg (3-4lb) every month, but then they would diet for a week to lose it all again. This did not prove difficult, as shedding 2kg (4lb) is simple after losing maybe 25kg (4st). Others experienced eating binges during which they would put weight on, and then diet for two weeks to take it off.

However, over the months, or even years in some cases, this habit of on-off dieting gradually merges into a more steady pattern of weight control, which rarely involves controlling food intake or choice of food on an unchanging, unerring everyday basis. Even a once-overweight woman who has succeeded in staying slim for 10 years can still admit to bad days when she finds it difficult to control her total food intake. However, these difficult days are balanced out by the good ones and as a result her weight stays fairly steady.

The majority of slimmers succeed in staying slim mainly by having learned about the calorie content of the foods they eat during dieting. This allows them to eat many of the foods they like without feeling guilty and to over-indulge a little on some days, notably at weekends, social occasions, or days when they are feeling pressurized and harrassed. They know, however, that they can make up for these dietary lapses by choosing really low-calorie foods on other easier days.

Many women are 'weekday dieters' and 'weekend-indulgers'; thus they follow their routine of eating moderately during the week but eat large amounts of food when relaxing, socializing or entertaining at the weekend. In this way, they stay slim and their weight is relatively steady.

Other slimmers, who eat a lot at weekends, diet on Mondays and Tuesdays, and then eat moderately for the rest of the week. Thus they control their weight with the minimum of effort. They may think in terms of 14,000 calories per week rather than 2,000 calories a day. In this way, if their calorie intake is high on one day, they can eat foods that are lower in calories the next day. You may find that you grudge wasting calories on foods you can do without and prefer to enjoy your social life, eating and drinking what you like, and then eat low-calorie foods on your own during the week.

Research has shown that, although many successful slimmers may slip back into a pattern of eating large quantities of food in the first few months following their dieting, those dieters who had kept slim for a longer period frequently reached a point when their appetite started to diminish and they needed less food than before.

Thirty-five per cent of the slimmers who were questioned in one survey said that they frequently left food on the plate because they felt too full to finish a large meal. These tended to be the women who had persevered in staying slim for long periods, and this evidence suggests that a form of automatic control may not set in until six months have elapsed after the end of the diet. However, some women experience immediate appetite reduction after dieting, while others are still tempted to eat over-large meals for a year or even more.

The majority of successful slimmers admit that, although they now eat less sugary and less starchy foods than when they were overweight, they still consume these foods but quite often in smaller amounts. These over-indulgences, however, make little or no difference to their weight, which remains steady. Although days of emotional distress, very often the pre-period days, are often the most dangerous for the most weight-prone women, a close runner-up is boredom. Most women discover that losing weight gives them the confidence to launch into a more active and sociable life and therefore there is less time to feel bored. Successful slimmers should be aware, however, that if they allow themselves to become inactive, uninterested or bored, they might easily resort to the eating habits that previously made them fat. Therefore, try to keep busy and active, especially by regular exercise. This will burn up your calorie output, firm up muscles and keep your figure trim while dispelling any boredom you might be feeling.

Perhaps the most important question that every slimmer will want to ask is whether the process of staying slim can ever become effortless? When this question was put to 100 women interviewed in a recent survey, 37 per cent replied that it was virtually effortless. The remainder, however, were still practising some degree of conscious self-control in a variety of ways, but usually the degree of effort decreased as time went on. Obviously, all these women considered the effort involved to be worthwhile or they would not make it. Talk to some successful slimmers and immediately you will be struck by the enthusiasm with which they describe the pleasures and compensations that had sustained their efforts to get slim and stay that way. They usually feel more confident, assertive, attractive and outgoing as a result of losing weight. Their social lives may broaden, too, as they make new friends and try out new sports and activities thanks to their increased confidence. Getting slim may change your outlook on life and your attitude to other people and brings its own rewards.

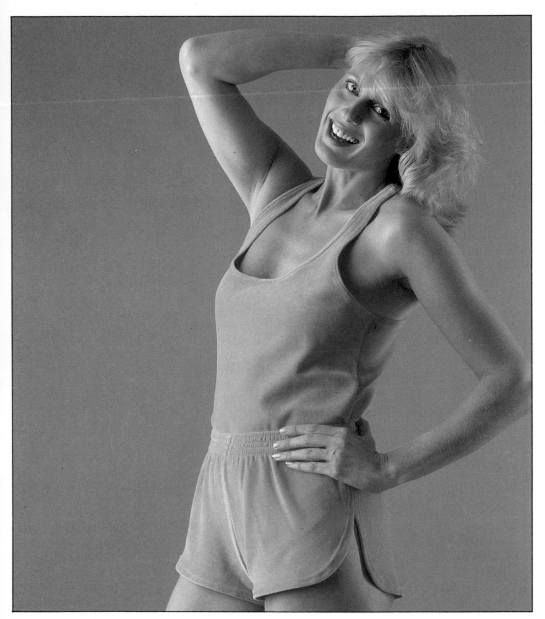

Not only do you feel healthier and fitter but you can also enjoy buying and wearing new clothes and feel proud of your new figure.

The most encouraging fact that emerges from surveys of slimmers is that normal women, who are subject to fluctuating moods and emotions and are rarely iron-willed enough to resist all food temptations, can succeed nevertheless in staying slim permanently. Although they may gain a little weight on holiday or at traditional feasting times like Christmas, they soon shed the extra weight again. Nearly all still turn to 'comfort foods' after a hurtful remark, family argument or at the end of a tiring day.

You need to be the sort of person who is prepared to practise fairly consistent self-discipline for a limited period of time to lose weight. This is not easy but, with sufficient determination, it is certainly possible. While you are losing weight, by whatever dieting method you follow, you also need to learn about calories to equip you for the stay-slim

period ahead. When you finally reach your target weight, you must be prepared to continue to make some conscious effort, at least at first, in order to maintain this indefinitely. Eating sensibly, dieting for a few days every time you gain a little weight and generally watching and controlling your calorie intake will make this possible. What you need not be is the kind of iron-willed paragon who can keep to a rigid dieting routine, day-in, day-out, for the rest of her life, and never indulging in any tempting calorie-laden foods or mopping up her tears in a delicious cream bun.

Unlike a slim person, the overweight person does not have a 'stop mechanism' when encountering tempting foods. This means that the slim woman will eat as much as she needs and then stop eating, whereas the overweight woman will not stop eating until she has cleared her plate and even then may come back for more. Whenever and whatever you eat, always stop and ask yourself at some stage during the snack or meal whether you have had enough or need to carry on eating. On some occasions, you will find that you may not be quite as hungry as you imagined yourself to be at the start of the meal and stop eating. This decision will lead to considerable conflict in your mind because, often, all you can safely and sensibly do is to throw away what is left on your plate. Do not hesitate in throwing leftover food in the rubbish bin. This is how you will gradually develop a stop mechanism which will lead you to controlling your weight. Here are some other stay-slim hints.

Don't be a calorie squanderer

If you want to keep your new slim shape you must stop being a caloric squanderer. Many people squander as much as two-thirds of their daily calories, and if they were to cut out this mindless habit-based eating, they would find the solution to their weight-gaining problems. Never eat a single calorie unless you really want and need to eat it, and staying slim will be far, far easier. When you cut out the calories you do not really want, you no longer have to resist those you yearn for. You are not squandering calories by eating a biscuit, or even a chocolate bar, when that is what you are longing to eat. Look at these classic examples of calorie squandering and develop a new awareness of the wasteful ways in which we carelessly overspend calories. They include:

● Helping yourself to another slice of toast, just so that you can neatly finish off that last teaspoonful of marmalade and therefore get rid of that sticky jar.

● Using full cream milk (extremely high in calories) in your cups of tea and coffee when skimmed milk would taste little different.

● Deciding when you try out a disastrous new recipe or a disappointing restaurant dish that you will eat it regardless of flavour because it never occurs to you to stop.

● Eating while so deeply absorbed in a book or newspaper that you are barely aware of what you are eating or even whether you are eating at all.

● Gathering up the little trimmings of pastry from the family pie and making, baking and eating the resultant little jam tart (probably at least 200 calories) to avoid wasting a little bit of raw pastry.

● Putting fat on breadcrumbed fish before you grill it. It cooks just as well and tastes just as good without it.

● Drinking an extra half-glass of wine just to finish off the bottle.

● Finishing up the last piece of pastry (often the thicker, outer edge) from a slice of pie, when you have already demolished the inner part with the tasty filling and are just carrying on eating to be neat.

● Finishing the extra-large supper you cooked because you were feeling enormously hungry. Do not allow that peak-hunger-time compulsion to commit you to eating everything that you cooked — your appetite will be more under control mid-way through the meal.

● Saying an automatic 'Yes, please!' when the waiter offers to pour more cream on a deliciously fattening dessert, without considering whether this would make it truly more enjoyable.

● Slavishly pre-frying all the vegetables for stews and casseroles without discovering whether this really does make a difference to the family's favourite dishes. Although the flavour of onions does change on being fried, you might find the flavour difference in other vegetables, such as carrots, barely detectable in a stew

● Eating the dry tasteless bun after you have had a hot-dog frankfurter.

● Grabbing a snack and eating it standing up when you are in a hurry. The food you eat this way is rarely enjoyed and often scarcely noticed.

● Eating before you go out, in case you get hungry when you arrive at your destination.

● Almost doubling the calories in your gin or whisky by using an ordinary mixer, just because you have been careless enough to run out of the low-calorie kind. Stock up for such 'emergencies'.

● Drinking glucose drinks when you are suffering from a minor illness. Drinking calories (all you are doing) will not help to cure your cold.

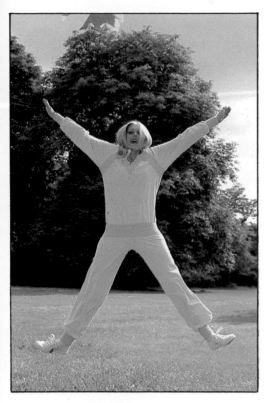

● Eating the last bun, scone or biscuit left by visitors just to save putting it away.

● Piling up a sandwich with more cheese than you need only because you grated too much accidentally.

● Poaching eggs in an egg poacher with a generous knob of butter instead of poaching them in water only.

● Eating the crusts you cut off toast and sandwiches. Do not swallow any calories in the cause of tidying up.

● Drinking the sugary milk left at the bottom of the bowl after finishing your cereal.

● Buttering the toast before you grill any cheese on top to make a toasted cheese sandwich. With a food as fatty as cheese, you would not miss extra butter calories.

● Scraping out and eating what is left in the custard pan, from sheer habit or to avoid custardy washing-up water.

● Eating all the food you have ordered in a restaurant, mainly because you will have to pay for it, anyway.

● Not skimming fat off casseroles and stews, and not draining the fat off minced meat.

● Serving yourself a double helping of cereal or muesli, because the packet is nearly empty and it would seem silly to put such a big box away with such a little inside.

● Pouring cream in your coffee when you would just as soon have milk. Never hesitate to save about 50 calories per cup simply by asking the waiter to bring milk.

● Nibbling a couple of biscuits to pass the time while you wait for the kettle to boil.

● Scraping out cooking bowls with a metal spoon, thus leaving tasty bits of mixture on the side which beg to be 'removed' by a willing finger. Use a flexible spatula instead to clean the bowls thoroughly so that there are no leftovers to tempt you.

● Accepting a drink from your friends and neighbours, just to be sociable and not because you are thirsty.

Stick to these simple rules
Keep active: when you are busy your mind dwells less on food and temptation is easier to pass by. Keep active and burn up enough calories to combat potential weight gains. Inject more activity generally into your daily life. Get into the habit of moving quicker, walking to the shops and running upstairs, getting up to fetch and carry things yourself instead of asking other people to do so while you remain seated.

Your mind matters: this concerns your attitude to dieting and to yourself. Your mind plays a vital role in getting your body in good shape so do not be too hard on yourself or aim for perfection. Make sure that you are not indulging in too many excuses for failures either. The occasional binge can be forgiven and cancelled out by more disciplined eating the following day, without wallowing in a sea of guilt. Beat boredom before it gets the better of you. If your mind is pleasantly occupied, your desire to look for comfort in the kitchen cupboard or refrigerator wanes. The new and livelier you that emerges will work wonders for your confidence.

Weigh regularly: that extra weight that can creep up on you unnoticed *can* be spotted and eliminated before it is too late by regular weighing (weekly rather than daily) and immediate action to reduce calories. Cut out the highest calorie foods first (such as fats) to speed up your weight loss.

Develop habits that can provide positive steps towards your goal of becoming permanently slim. Food habits die hard and, however adult we are, we still tend to be subconsciously influenced by those things that were drummed into us during our childhood. If you have weight problems, then you must change your habits because carrying on eating in the old way is sure to make you fat again.

CHAPTER 11

Illustrated calorie dictionary

Here's an up-to-date and comprehensive guide to the calorie content of the basic foods you are most likely to eat in your daily menus. Calorie counting remains the classic method of slimming because, for most people, it has one great advantage: you can eat anything you fancy and still lose weight as long as you keep to the right daily total. The majority of women and all men will shed weight if their calorie intake is reduced to 1,500 a day. A dieter who has successfully lost a great deal of weight but finds the last little bit difficult to shift may have to cut down to 1,000 calories a day in order to achieve her ideal weight.

Include some low-fat, protein-containing foods, such as chicken, lean meat, liver, kidney, white fish, eggs, cottage cheese and skimmed milk, in your daily menus. Fill up with lots of vegetables and fresh fruits. Also include some whole-grain cereal foods, such as wholewheat bread, or wholewheat or bran breakfast foods. Remember to count all calorie-containing drinks in your daily total. Some drinks are calorie-free: water, black tea and coffee (without sugar), and these can be consumed in unlimited quantities. Some soft drinks (labelled as 'low-calorie') have counts low enough to make little difference to your quota. Check with the label on the bottle as calories are given always on low-calorie products.

All weights are given in both metric and imperial measures. Some foods are measured also in teaspoons and tablespoons and, in these instances, calories for metric measuring spoons are given. As the Australian tablespoon is slightly larger than the 15ml version used in Great Britain, we have also given calories for a 20ml tablespoon.

ALMONDS
Shelled, per 28g (1oz)	160
Ground,	
per 15ml (1 level tablespoon)	30
per 20ml (Australian tablespoon)	40
Per almond, whole	10
Per sugared almond	15

ANCHOVIES
Per 28g (1oz)	40
Per anchovy fillet	5

ANCHOVY ESSENCE
Per 5ml (1 level teaspoon)	5

ANGELICA
Per 28g (1oz)	90
Per average stick	10

APPLES
Eating, per 28g (1oz)	10
Cooking, per 28g (1oz)	10
Medium whole eating, 142g (5oz)	50
Medium whole cooking, 227g (8oz)	80
Apple sauce, sweetened, per 15ml (1 level tablespoon)	20
per 20ml (Australian tablespoon)	25
Apple sauce, unsweetened, per 15ml (1 level tablespoon)	10
per 20ml (Australian tablespoon)	15
Apple pie, average slice with pastry top and bottom, 113g (4oz)	420

APRICOTS
Canned in natural juice, per 28g (1oz)	13
Canned in syrup, per 28g (1oz)	30
Dried, per 28g (1oz)	52
Fresh with stone, per 28g (1oz)	7
Per dried apricot half	10
Per apricot half, canned in syrup	15
Per whole fruit	7

ARROWROOT
Per 28g (1oz)	101
5ml (1 level teaspoon)	10

ARTICHOKES
Globe, boiled, per 28g (1oz)	4
Jerusalem, boiled, per 28g (1oz)	5

ASPARAGUS
Raw or boiled, per 28g (1oz)	5
Per asparagus spear	4

AUBERGINES (Eggplants)
Raw, per 28g (1oz)	4
Sliced, fried, 28g (1oz) raw weight	60
Whole aubergine, 198g (7oz)	28
Whole aubergine, sliced, fried, 198g (7oz) raw weight	405

AVOCADO
Flesh only, per 28g (1oz)	63
Per half avocado, 106g (3¾oz)	235

BACON (see also gammon)
Per 28g (1oz)
Back rasher, raw	122
Collar joint, raw, lean and fat	91
Collar joint, boiled, lean only	54
Collar joint, boiled, lean and fat	92

Streaky rashers, raw	118
1 streaky rasher, well grilled or fried, 21g (¾oz) raw weight	50
1 back rasher, well grilled or fried, 35g (1¼oz) raw weight	80
1 bacon steak, well grilled, 99g (3½oz) average raw weight	105

BAKING POWDER
Per 28g (1oz)	46
Per 5ml (1 level teaspoon)	7

BAMBOO SHOOTS
Per 28g (1oz)	10

BANANAS
Flesh only, per 28g (1oz)	22
Flesh and skin, per 28g (1oz)	13
Small whole fruit 142g (5oz)	65
Medium whole fruit, 170g (6oz)	80
Large whole fruit, 198g (7oz)	93
Whole fruit, peeled and fried in batter, 170g (6oz) raw weight	170

BARCELONA NUTS
Shelled, per 28g (1oz)	181

BARLEY
Pearl, raw, per 28g (1oz)	102
Pearl, boiled, per 28g (1oz)	34
Per 15ml (level tablespoon) raw	45
Per 20ml (Australian tablespoon)	60

BASS
Fillet, steamed, per 28g (1oz)	35

BEAN SPROUTS
Canned, per 28g (1oz)	3
Raw, per 28g (1oz)	5

BEANS
Per 28g (1oz)
Baked, canned in tomato sauce	20
Black-eye beans, raw weight	93
Broad, boiled	14
Butter, boiled	27
Butter, raw wieght	78
French, boiled	2
Haricot, boiled	26
Haricot, raw weight	77
Kidney, canned	25
Kidney, raw weight	77
Lima, raw weight	93
Mung, raw weight	92
Runner, boiled or raw	7
Snap, raw, green	10
Soya, dry weight	115

BEECH NUTS
Shelled, per 28g (1oz)	160

BEEF
Per 28g (1oz)
Brisket, boiled, lean and fat	92
Brisket, raw, lean and fat	71
Ground beef, lean, raw	45
Ground beef, lean, fried and drained of fat	55
Ground beef, lean, fried and drained of fat, per 28g (1oz) raw weight	40
Minced beef, raw	63
Minced beef, well fried and drained of fat	55
Minced beef, well fried and drained of fat per 28g (1oz) raw weight	45
Rump steak, fried, lean only	54
Rump steak, well grilled, 170g (6oz) raw	270
Rump steak, medium grilled, 170g (6oz) raw	290
Rump steak, rare grilled, 170g (6oz) raw	310
Rump steak, raw, lean and fat	56
Silverside, salted, boiled, lean and fat	69
Silverside, salted, boiled, lean only	49
Sirloin, roast, lean and fat	80
Sirloin, roast, lean only	55
Stewing steak, raw, lean only	35
Stewing steak, raw, lean and fat	50
Stewing steak, stewed, lean and fat	63
Topside, raw, lean only	35
Topside, raw, lean and fat	51
Topside, roast, lean and fat	61
Topside, roast, lean only	44

BEEFBURGERS
Beefburger, fresh or frozen, well grilled, 57g (2oz) raw weight	90
Beefburger, fresh or frozen, grilled 113g (4oz) raw weight	245

BEETROOT
Raw, per 28g (1oz)	8
Boiled, per 28g (1oz)	12
Per baby beet, boiled	5

BILBERRIES
Raw, per 28g (1oz)	16

BISCUITS
Per average biscuit
Chocolate chip cookie	60
Digestive, large	70
Digestive, medium,	55
Digestive, small	45
Fig roll	65
Garibaldi, per finger	30
Ginger nut	40
Ginger snap	35
Jaffa cake	50
Lincoln	40
Malted milk	40
Marie	30
Morning coffee	25
Nice	45
Osborne	35
Petit Beurre	30
Rich tea finger	25
Rich tea, round	45
Sponge finger	20

BLACKBERRIES
Raw, per 28g (1oz)	8
Stewed, without sugar, per 28g (1oz)	7

BLACKCURRANTS
Fresh, per 28g (1oz)	8
Stewed without sugar, per 28g (1oz)	7

BLACK PUDDING
Raw, per 28g (1oz)	78
Sliced, fried, per 28g (1oz) raw weight	85

Black pudding

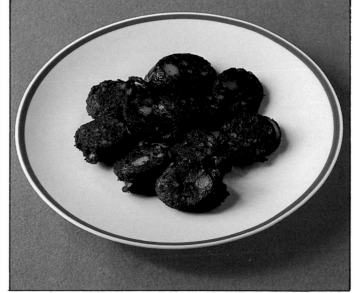

BLOATERS
Fillet, grilled, per 28g (1oz)	71
On the bone, grilled per 28g (1oz)	53

BRAINS
Per 28g (1oz)
Calves and lamb's, raw	31
Calves', boiled	43
Lamb's boiled	36

BRAN
Per 28g (1oz)	58
Per 15ml (level tablespoon)	10
per 20ml (Australian tablespoon)	15

BRANDY BUTTER
Per 28g (1oz)	170

BRAWN
Per 28g (1oz)	43

BRAZIL NUTS
Shelled, per 28g (1oz)	176
Per nut	20
Per buttered brazil	40
Per chocolate brazil	55

BREAD
Per 28g (1oz) slice
Black rye	90
Bran	65
Brown or wheatmeal	63
Currant	70
Enriched	110
Fried bread, 28g (1oz), unfried weight	160
French	65
Fruit sesame	120
Granary	70
Light rye	70
Malt	70
Milk	80
Soda	75
Vogel	65
Wheatgerm	65
White	66
Wholemeal (100%)	61

Per slice, white bread
Thin slice from a large sliced loaf	75
Thin slice from a long sliced loaf	60
Medium slice from a large sliced loaf	85
Medium slice from a large, long loaf	75
Thick slice from a large sliced loaf	100
Thick slice from a long sliced loaf	90

Rolls, buns etc., each
Baby bridge roll, 14g (½oz)	45
Bagel, 40g (1⅜oz)	150
Bap, 50g (1¾oz)	130
Bath bun, 50g (1¾oz)	120
Bread stick	15
Brioche roll,45g (1⅝oz)	215
Chelsea bun, 92g (3¼oz)	230
Croissant, 64g (2¼oz)	245

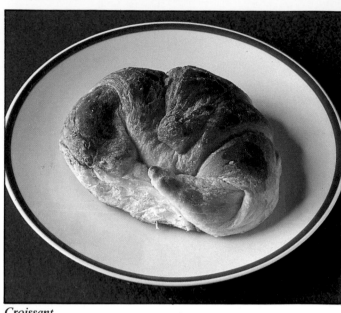

Croissant

Crumpet, 42g (1½oz)	75
Crusty roll, brown or white, 50g (1¾oz)	145
Currant bun, 50g (1¾oz)	150
Devonshire split, 71g (2½oz)	195
Dinner roll, soft, 43g (1½oz)	130
French toast, average slice	50
Hot cross bun, 57g (2oz)	180
Hovis roll, 45g (1⅝oz)	115
Muffin, 64g (2¼oz)	125
Pitta, 71g (2½oz)	205
Scone, plain, 57g (2oz)	210
Soft brown roll, 50g (1¾oz)	140
Soft white roll, 50g (1¾oz)	155
Tea cake, 57g (2oz)	155

Per 15ml (level tablespoon)
Breadcrumbs, dried	30
Breadcrumbs, fresh	8
Bread sauce	15

Per 20ml (Australian tablespoon)
Breadcrumbs, dried	40
Breadcrumbs, fresh	10
Bread sauce	20

BREAKFAST CEREALS
Per 28g (1oz)
All Bran cereal	70
Cornflakes	100
Muesli or Swiss style	105
Porridge oats	115
Puffed wheat	100
Sultana bran	90
Weetabix or whole wheat biscuits, per biscuit	55

BROCCOLI
Raw, per 28g (1oz)	7
Boiled, per 28g (1oz)	5

BRUSSELS SPROUTS
Raw, per 28g (1oz)	7
Boiled, per 28g (1oz)	5

BUTTER
All brands, per 28g (1oz)	210

C

CABBAGE
Per 28g (1oz)
Raw	6
Boiled	4
Coleslaw	40
Pickled red	3

CAKES
Home-made, per average slice or small cake
Butterfly cake, 35g (1¼oz)	202
Cherry cake, 85g (3oz) slice	335
Chocolate cake, filled with butter icing and topped with chocolate glacé icing 113g (4oz)	525
Christmas cake or wedding, with marzipan and royal icing, 99g (3½oz)	350
Eccles cake, 57g (2oz)	290
Flapjack, 43g (1½oz) piece	300
Fruit cake, plain, 85g (3oz) slice	300
Jam tart, 28g (1oz)	110
Madeira cake, 85g (3oz)	335
Mince pie, 43g (1½oz)	185
Scone, plain, 57g (2oz)	210
Sponge sandwich, jam filled, whisked fatless method, 43g (1½oz) slice	130

Victoria sandwich, jam
  filled, 57g (2oz) slice 260

Fresh cream cakes
Per average cake
Chocolate éclair
  71g (2½oz) 275
Cream doughnut,
  71g (2½oz) 260
Cream slice, with puff
  pastry and glacé icing
  99g (3½oz) 420
Meringue, 71g (2½oz) 195
Strawberry tart,
  85g (3oz) 200

CANDIED PEEL
Per 28g (1oz) 90
Per 15ml (level
  tablespoon) 45
Per 20ml (Australian
  tablespoon 60

CAPERS
Per 28g (1oz) 5

CARROTS
Raw, per 28g (1oz) 6
Boiled, per 28g (1oz) 5
Per average carrot,
  57g (2oz) 12
Sliced, fried, 28g (1oz)
  raw weight 30

CASHEW NUTS
Shelled, per 28g (1oz) 160
Per nut 15

CASSAVA
Fresh, per 28g (1oz) 45

CAULIFLOWER
Raw, per 28g (1oz) 4
Boiled, per 28g (1oz) 3

CAVIAR
Per 28g (1oz) 75

CELERIAC
Boiled, per 28g (1oz) 4

CELERY
Raw, per 28g (1oz) 2
Boiled, per 28g (1oz) 1
Per stick of celery 5

CHEESE
Per 28g (1oz)
Austrian smoked 78
Babybel 97
Bavarian smoked 80
Bel Paese 76
Blue Stilton 131
Bonbel 102
Boursin 116
Bresse bleu 80
Brie 88
Caerphilly 120
Caithness Morven 110
Caithness full fat soft 110
Camembert 88
Cheddar 120
Cheese spread 80
Cheshire 110
Cheviot 120
Cotswold 105
Cottage cheese, plain,
  or with chives, onion,
  peppers or pineapple 27
Cream cheese 125

Curd cheese 40
Danbo 98
Danish blue 103
Danish Elbo 98
Danish Esrom 98
Danish Fynbo 100
Danish Havarti, 117
Danish Maribo 100
Danish Molbo 100
Danish Mozzarella 98
Danish Mycella 99
Danish Samsoe 98
Derby 110
Dolcellata 100
Double Gloucester 105
Edam 88
Emmenthal 113
Fetta 54
Gorgonzola 112
Gouda 100
Gruyère 132
Ilchester Cheddar
  and beer 112
Jarlsberg 95
Lancashire 109
Leicester 105
Norwegian blue 100
Norwegian Gjeost 133
Orangerulle 92
Orkney Claymore 111
Parmesan 118
Philadelphia 90
Port Salut 94
Processed 88
Rambol, with walnuts 117
Red Windsor 119
Riccotta 55
Roquefort 88
Sage Derby 112
Skimmed milk soft
  cheese (quark) 25
St Paulin 98
Tôme au raisin 74
Wensleydale 115
White Stilton 96
Per 15ml (level tablespoon)
Cottage cheese 15

Grilled chicken joint

Cream cheese 60
Curd cheese 20
Parmesan cheese,
  grated 30

CHERRIES
Fresh, with stones,
  per 28g (1oz) 12
Glacé, per 28g (1oz) 60
Per glacé cherry 10

CHESTNUTS
Per 28g (1oz)
Shelled 48
With shells 40
Unsweetened chestnut
  purée 30

CHICKEN
Per 28g (1oz)
On bone, raw, no skin 25
Meat only, raw 34
Meat only, boiled 52
Meat only, roast 42
Meat and skin, roast 61
Chicken drumstick,
  raw, 99g (3½oz)
  average raw weight 90
Chicken drumstick
  fried, 99g (3½oz)
  average raw weight 105
Chicken drumstick,
  fried in egg and
  breadcrumbs 99g
  (3½oz) average raw
  weight 130
Chicken drumstick,
  grilled and skin
  removed, 99g (3½oz)
  average raw weight 65
Chicken drumstick,
  grilled, 99g (3½oz)
  raw weight 85
Chicken joint, raw
  227g (8oz) average
  weight 410
Chicken joint, grilled
  and skin removed,
  227g (8oz) average
  raw weight 165

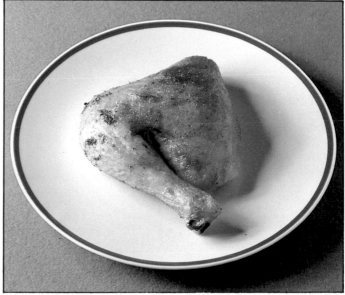

Chicken continued

Chicken joint, grilled 227g (8oz)	250
Chicken joint, fried 227g (8oz) average raw weight	285

CHICORY

Raw, per 28g (1oz)	3
Essence, per 28g (1oz)	60

CHILLIES

Dried, per 28g (1oz)	85

CHIVES

Per 28g (1oz)	10

CHINESE LEAVES

Raw, per 28g (1oz)	3

CHOCOLATE
Per 28g (1oz)

Milk or plain	150
Cooking	155
Filled chocolates	130
Vermicelli	135

Per 5ml (level teaspoon)

Chocolate spread	20
Drinking chocolate	10
Vermicelli	20

CLAMS

With shells, raw, per 28g (1oz)	15
Without shells, raw, per 28g (1oz)	25

COB NUTS

With shells, per 28g (1oz)	39
Shelled, per 28g (1oz)	108
Per nut	5

COCKLES

Without shells, boiled, per 28g (1oz)	14

COCOA POWDER

Per 28g (1oz)	89
Per 5ml (level teaspoon)	10

COCONUT
Per 28g (1oz)

Fresh	100
Desiccated	172
Coconut ice	110
Coconut milk, per 28ml (1floz)	6
Creamed coconut	218
Desiccated, per 15ml (level tablespoon)	30
Per 20ml (Australian tablespoon)	40

COD
Per 28g (1oz)

Fillet, raw	22
Fillet, baked or grilled with a little fat	27
Fillet, poached in water or steamed	24
Frozen steaks, raw	19
On the bone, raw	15
Fillet in batter, deep fried, 170g (6oz) raw weight	460

COD LIVER OIL

Per 28g (1oz)	255

COD ROE

Raw, hard roe, per 28g (1oz)	32
Fried in egg and breadcrumbs, per 28g (1oz)	55

COFFEE
Per 28g (1oz)

Coffee beans, roasted and ground	80
Instant	28
Coffee and chicory essence	60
Instant coffee, per 10ml (1 rounded teaspoon)	0

COLEY
Per 28g (1oz)

Raw	21
On the bone, steamed	24
Fillet, steamed	28

COOKING OR SALAD OIL

Per 28g (1oz)	255
Per 15ml (1 level tablespoon)	120
Per 20ml (Australian tablespoon)	160

CORNED BEEF, CANNED

Per 28g (1oz)	62

CORNFLOUR

Per 28g (1oz)	100
Per 15ml (1 level tablespoon)	33
Per 20ml (Australian tablespoon)	44

CORNISH PASTY

Per average pasty, 150g (5¼oz)	500

CORN OIL

Per 28g (1oz)	255
Per 15ml (1 level tablespoon)	120
Per 20ml (Australian tablespoon)	160

CORN ON THE COB

Fresh, boiled, kernels only, per 28g (1oz)	35
Average whole cob	85

COUGH SYRUP

Thick, per 5ml (1 teaspoon)	15
Thin, per 5ml (1 teaspoon)	5

COURGETTES (Zucchini)

Raw per 28g (1oz)	4
Per courgette, 70g (2½oz)	10
Sliced, fried, per 28g (1oz)	15

CRAB

With shell, per 28g (1oz) boiled	7
Meat only, per 28g (1oz) boiled	36
Average crab with shell	95

CRANBERRIES

Raw, per 28g (1oz)	4

CRANBERRY SAUCE

Per 28g (1oz)	65
Per 15ml (1 level tablespoon)	45
Per 20ml (Australian tablespoon)	60

CREAM
Per 28g (1oz)

Clotted	165
Double	127
Half cream	35
Imitation	85
Single	60
Soured	60
Sterilized, canned	65
Whipping	94

Corn on the cob

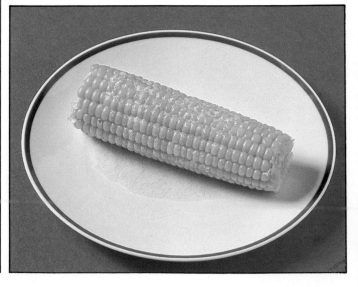

Per 15ml (1 level tablespoon)

Clotted	105
Double	60
Half cream	20
Imitation	55
Single	30
Soured	30
Sterilized, canned	35
Whipping	45

Per 20ml (Australian tablespoon)

Clotted	140
Double	80
Half cream	25
Imitation	75
Single	40
Soured	40
Sterilized, canned	45
Whipping	60

CRISPBREADS

Per average crispbread	30

CRISPS (potato)

All flavours, per 28g (1oz)	150

CUCUMBER

Raw, per 28g (1oz)	3

CURRANTS

Per 28g (1oz)	69
Per 15ml (1 level tablespoon)	21
Per 20ml (Australian tablespoon)	28

CURRY PASTE OR CONCENTRATE

Per 28g (1oz)	40

CURRY POWDER

Per 28g (1oz)	66
Per 5ml (1 level teaspoon	12

CUSTARD

Per 142ml (¼ pint) serving, made with custard powder, sugar and skimmed milk	110
Per 142ml (¼ pint) serving, made with custard powder, sugar and whole milk	155

CUSTARD APPLE

Flesh only, per 28g (1oz)	25

CUSTARD POWDER

Per 28g (1oz)	100
Per 15ml (1 level tablespoon)	33
Per 20ml (Australian tablespoon)	44

D

DAMSONS

Fresh, with stones per 28g (1oz)	10
Stewed, no sugar, per 28g (1oz)	8

DATES

Per 28g (1oz)

Dried, with stones	60

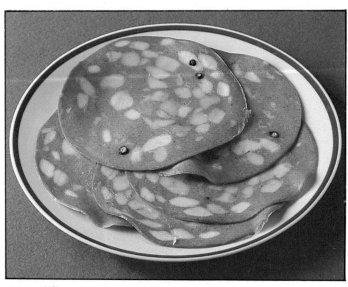

Mortadella sausage

Dried, without stones	70
Fresh, with stones	30
Per date, fresh	15

DELICATESSEN SAUSAGES

Per 28g (1oz)

Belgian liver sausage	90
Bierwurst	75
Bockwurst	180
Cervelat	140
Chorizo	140
Continental liver sausage	85
Frankfurter	78
French garlic sausage	90
Garlic sausage	70
Ham sausage	50
Kabanos	115
Krakowska	80
Liver sausage	88
Mettwurst	120
Mortadella, Italian	105
Polish country sausage	60
Polony	80
Pork boiling ring, coarse	110
Salami, Belgian	130
Salami, Danish	160
Salami, Hungarian	130
Salami, German	120
Saveloy	74
Smoked Dutch sausage	105
Smoked pork sausage	130
Smoked ham sausage	65

DRIPPING

Per 28g (1oz)	253
Per 15ml (1 level tablespoon)	125
Per 20ml (Australian tablespoon)	165

DUCK

Per 28g (1oz)

Raw, meat only	35
Raw, meat, fat and skin	122
Roast, meat only	54
Roast, meat, fat and skin	96

DUCK EGGS

99g (3½oz) egg	170

E

EEL

Meat only, raw, per 28g (1oz)	48
Meat only, stewed, per 28g (1oz)	57
Jellied eels plus some jelly, 85g (3oz)	180

EGGS, each	raw	fried
Size 1	95	115
Size 2	90	110
Size 3	80	100
Size 4	75	95
Size 5	70	90
Size 6	60	80
Yolk of size 3 egg	65	
White of size 3 egg	15	
Scrambled eggs, made with two (size 3) eggs 7g (¼oz) butter and 15ml milk	225	
Omelet, plain, made with two (size 3) eggs and 7g (¼oz) butter	215	

EGG PLANTS
see aubergines

ENDIVE

Raw, per 28g (1oz)	3

F

FAGGOTS

Per 28g (1oz)	76

FIGS

Dried, per 28g (1oz)	60
Fresh, green, per 28g (1oz)	12
Per dried fig	30

FISH CAKES
Per average fish cake, grilled or baked without added fat — 60

FISH FINGERS
Per average fish finger, grilled without added fat — 50

FLOUNDER
On the bone, raw, per 28g (1oz) — 20
On the bone, steamed, per 28g (1oz) — 15

FLOUR
Per 28g (1oz)
Wheatmeal — 93
White, plain — 99
White, self-raising — 96
White, strong — 96
Wholemeal — 90
Buckwheat — 99
Cassava — 97
Granary — 99
Maizemeal (96%) — 103
Maizemeal (60%) — 101
Rice — 100
Rye (100%) — 95
Soya, low fat — 100
Soya, full fat — 127
Yam — 90
Per 15ml (1 level tablespoon)
White — 32
Wholemeal — 29
Per 20ml (Australian tablespoon)
White — 42
Wholemeal — 38

FRENCH DRESSING
Per 15ml (1 tablespoon) — 75
Per 20ml (Australian tablespoon) — 100

FRUIT
Crystallized, per 28g (1oz) — 75

G

GAMMON
Per 28g (1oz)
Gammon joint, raw, lean and fat — 67
Gammon joint, boiled, lean and fat — 76
Gammon joint, boiled, lean only — 47
Gammon rashers, grilled, lean and fat — 67
Gammon rashers, grilled, lean only — 49

GARLIC
One clove — 0

GELATINE, powdered
Per 15ml (1 level tablespoon) — 30
Per 28g (1oz) — 96
Per 20ml (Australian tablespoon) — 40
Per 10g envelope — 35

GHEE
Per 28g (1oz) — 235

GHERKINS
Per 28g (1oz) — 5

GINGER
Ground, per 28g (1oz) — 73
Ground, 5ml (1 level teaspoon) — 8
Stem, per 28g (1oz) — 80

GOOSE
Roast, on bone, per 28g (1oz) — 55
Roast, meat only (without skin), per 28g (1oz) — 90

GOOSEBERRIES
Fresh, ripe dessert, per 28g (1oz) — 10
Fresh, cooking, per 28g (1oz) — 5

GRAPEFRUIT
Per 28g (1oz)
Canned in syrup — 17
Canned in natural juice — 11
Flesh only — 6
Flesh and skin — 3
Juice, unsweetened, per 28ml (1floz) — 9
Medium whole fruit, 340g (12oz) — 36
Sweetened canned juice, 113ml (4floz) — 45
Unsweetened juice, 113ml (4floz) — 35

GRAPES
Black, per 28g (1oz) — 14
White, per 28g (1oz) — 17
Per grape — 4

GRAVY
Per 15ml (1 tablespoon), thick — 20
Per 15ml (1 tablespoon), thin, no fat — 5
Per 20ml (Australian tablespoon), thick — 25
Per 20ml (Australian tablespoon), thin — 6

GREENGAGES
Fresh, with stones, per 28g (1oz) — 13
Stewed, with stones, no sugar, per 28g(1oz) — 11

GRENADINE SYRUP
Per 28g (1oz) — 72

GROUSE
Roast, meat only, per 28g (1oz) — 50

GROUND RICE
Per 28g (1oz) — 100
Per 15ml (1 level tablespoon) — 33

Per 20ml (Australian tablespoon) — 44

GUAVAS
Canned, per 28g (1oz) — 17

GUINEA FOWL
Roast, on bone, per 28g (1oz) — 30
Roast, meat only, per 28g (1oz) — 60

H

HADDOCK
Per 28g (1oz)
Fillet, raw — 21
Fillet in breadcrumbs, fried — 50
On the bone, raw — 15
On the bone, in breadcrumbs, fried — 45
Smoked fillet, steamed or poached in water — 29
Fillet in breadcrumbs fried, 170g (6oz) raw weight — 435
Fillet in batter, deep-fried, 170g (6oz) raw weight — 460

HAGGIS
Cooked, per 28g (1oz) — 89

HAKE
Per 28g (1oz)
Fillet, raw — 20
Fillet, steamed — 30
Fillet, fried — 60
On the bone, raw — 10

HALIBUT
Per 28g (1oz)
Fillet, steamed — 37
On the bone, raw — 26
On the bone, steamed — 26
Steak, 170g (6oz) — 155

HAM
Per 28g (1oz)
Chopped ham roll or loaf — 75
Ham, boiled, lean — 47
Ham, boiled, fatty — 90
Honey roast ham — 50
Old smokey ham — 65
Maryland ham — 55
Virginia ham — 40
Ham steak, well grilled, 99g (3½oz), average raw weight — 105

HARE
Stewed, meat only per 28g (1oz) — 55
Stewed, on bone, per 28g (1oz) — 39

HASLET
Per 28g (1oz) — 80

HAZEL NUTS
Shelled, per 28g (1oz) — 108
Per nut — 5
Chocolate hazelnut whirl, each — 40

HEART
Per 28g (1oz)

Lamb's, raw	34
Ox, raw	31
Pig's, raw	26
Whole lamb's heart, roasted, 113g (4oz) average raw weight	270

HERRING
Per 28g (1oz)

Fillet, raw	66
Fillet, grilled	56
Fillet in oatmeal, fried	66
On the bone, grilled	38
On the bone in oatmeal, fried	60
Rollmop herring	47
Rollmop herring, 70g (2½oz) average weight	120
Whole herring, grilled, 128g (4½oz) average raw weight	170

HERRING ROE

Fried, per 28g (1oz)	69
Raw, soft roe	23

HONEY

Per 28g (1oz)	82
Per 5ml (1 teaspoon)	18

HORSERADISH

Fresh root, per 28g (1oz)	17
Horseradish sauce, per 15ml (1 level tablespoon)	13
per 20ml (Australian tablespoon)	17

HUMUS

Per 28g (1oz)	50

HUNDREDS AND THOUSANDS

Per 5ml (1 level teaspoon)	15

I

ICE-CREAM
Per 28g (1oz)

Chocolate	55
Coffee	50
Cornish dairy	52
Raspberry ripple	50
Soft ice-cream	43
Strawberry	52
Vanilla	47

ICING

Butter icing, per 28g (1oz)	125
Royal, per 28g (1oz)	85

J

JAM

Per 28g (1oz)	74
Per 5ml (level teaspoon)	17

JELLY

Cubes as sold, per 28g (1oz)	73

Grilled kipper

Made up with water, per 142ml (¼ pint)	85
Per cube	29

K

KIDNEY

All types, raw, per 28g (1oz)	25
Lamb's kidney, grilled, 57g (2oz) average raw weight	50
Lamb's kidney, fried, 57g (2oz) average raw weight	65

KIPPERS

Fillet, baked or grilled, per 28g (1oz)	58
On the bone, baked, per 28g (1oz)	32
Whole kipper, grilled, 170g (6oz) raw weight	280

L

LAMB
Per 28g (1oz)

Breast, boned, raw, lean and fat	107
Breast, boned, roast, lean and fat	116
Breast, boned, roast, lean only	72
Leg, raw, lean and fat, without bone	68
Leg, roast, lean and fat, without bone	76
Leg, roast, lean only, without bone	54
Scrag and neck, raw, lean and fat, weighed with bone	54
Scrag and neck, raw, lean and fat, weighed without bone	90
Scrag and neck, stewed, lean only, weighed with bone	38
Scrag and neck, stewed, lean only, weighed without bone	72
Scrag and neck, stewed, lean and fat, weighed without bone	83
Shoulder, boned, roast, lean and fat	89
Shoulder, boned, roast, lean only	56
Chump chop, well grilled, 142g (5oz) raw weight	205
Leg steak, boneless, well grilled, 227g (8oz) raw weight	370
Loin chop, well grilled, 142g (5oz) raw weight	175

LARD

Per 28g (1oz)	253

LAVERBREAD

Per 28g (1oz)	15

LEEKS

Raw, per 28g (1oz)	9
Average whole leek, raw	25

LEMON

Flesh and skin, per 28g (1oz)	4
Whole lemon, 142g (5oz)	20
Lemon juice, per 15-20ml (1 tablespoon)	0

LEMON CURD

Per 28g (1oz)	80
Per 5ml (1 level teaspoon)	13

LEMON SOLE Per 28g (1oz)

Fillet, steamed or poached	26
On the bone, raw	23
On the bone, steamed or poached	18

215

LENTILS
Raw, per 28g (1oz) 86
Boiled, per 28g (1oz) 28

LETTUCE
Fresh, per 28g (1oz) 3

LIVER
Per 28g (1oz)
Chicken's, raw 38
Chicken's, fried 55
Lamb's, raw 51
Lamb's, fried 66
Ox, raw 46
Ox, stewed 56
Pig's, raw 44
Pig's, stewed 54
Lamb's, fried,
  113g (4oz)
  raw weight 235
Lamb's, grilled without
  fat, 113g (4oz) raw
  weight 205

LOBSTER
With shell, boiled,
  per 28g (1oz) 12
Meat only, boiled,
  per 28g (1oz) 34

LOGANBERRIES
Fresh, per 28g (1oz) 5
Canned in syrup,
  per 28g (1oz) 28

LOW-FAT SPREAD
All brands, per 28g (1oz) 105

LUNCHEON MEAT
Per 28g (1oz) 89

M

MACARONI
White or wholewheat
  raw, per 28g (1oz) 105
Boiled, per 28g (1oz) 33
Macaroni cheese, per
  average serving,
  227g (8oz) 390

Macaroni cheese, per
  206g (7¼oz) can 255

MACADAMIA NUTS
Per 28g (1oz) 188

MACKEREL
Per 28g (1oz)
Fillet, raw 63
Fillet, fried 53
On the bone, fried 39
Kippered mackerel 62
Smoked mackerel 70
Whole raw mackerel,
  227g (8oz) 318

MAIZE
Whole grain, per
  28g (1oz) 103

MANDARINS
Canned, per 28g (1oz) 16
Fresh, with skin,
  per 28g (1oz) 5
Medium whole fruit,
  70g (2½oz) 20

MANGO
Raw, per 28g (1oz) 17
Canned, per 28g (1oz) 22
Mango chutney,
  per 15ml (1 level
  tablespoon) 35
  per 20ml (Australian
  tablespoon) 45

MAPLE SYRUP
Per 28g (1oz) 70
Per 5ml (1 level
  teaspoon) 17

MARGARINE
All brands except those
  labelled low-fat,
  per 28g (1oz) 210

MARMALADE
Per 28g (1oz) 74
Per 5ml (1 level
  teaspoon) 17

MARRON GLACÉ
Per 28g (1oz) 74

MARROW
Raw, per 28g (1oz) 5
Boiled, per 28g (1oz) 2

MARZIPAN
(Almond Paste)
Per 28g (1oz) 126
Petit fours 126

MAYONNAISE
Per 28g (1oz) 205
Per 15ml (1 level
  tablespoon) 95
Per 20ml (Australian
  tablespoon) 125

MEDLARS
Flesh only, per 28g (1oz) 12

MELON
Per 28g (1oz)
Cantaloupe, with skin 4
Honeydew or Yellow,
  with skin 4
Ogen, with skin 5
Watermelon, with skin 3
Slice of Cantaloupe,
  Honeydew or
  Yellow, with skin,
  227g (8oz) 32

MILK
Per 568ml (1 pint)
Buttermilk 232
Channel Island or
  gold top 432
Evaporated milk, full
  cream, reconstituted 360
Goat's 400
Homogenized or red top 370
Instant dried skimmed
  milk with vegetable
  fat, reconstituted 280
Longlife or UHT 370
Pasteurized or silver top 370
Pasteurized or silver top
  with cream removed,
  510ml (18floz) 240
Skimmed or separated 200
Soya milk, diluted as
  directed 370
Sterilized 370
Untreated farm milk or
  green top 370
**Per 15ml (1 level
  tablespoon)**
Channel Island or
  gold top 15
Condensed full cream,
  sweetened 50
Condensed, skimmed,
  sweetened 40
Evaporated full cream 23
Homogenized,
  pasteurized, green top
  silver top and
  sterilized 10
Instant low fat milk, dry 18
Instant low fat milk,
  reconstituted 5
Skimmed or separated 5

Lobster

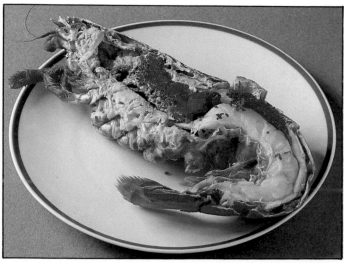

Canned milk,
**   per 28g (1oz)**

Evaporated full fat milk	45
Condensed, skimmed, sweetened	76
Condensed, full fat, sweetened	91
Condensed, unsweetened	40

MINCEMEAT

Per 28g (1oz)	67
Per 15ml (1 level tablespoon)	40

MINT

Fresh, per 28g (1oz)	3

MINT SAUCE

Per 15ml (1 level tablespoon)	5
Per 20ml (Australian tablespoon)	7

MOLASSES

Per 28g (1oz)	78
Per 15ml (1 level tablespoon)	45
Per 20ml (Australian tablespoon)	60

MUESLI

Per 28g (1oz)	105
Per 15ml (1 level tablespoon)	30
Per 20ml (Australian tablespoon)	40

MULBERRIES

Raw, per 28g (1oz)	10

MULLET

Raw, per 28g (1oz)	40

MUSHROOMS

Raw, per 28g (1oz)	4
Button, fried whole, 57g (2oz) raw weight	80
Button, sliced and fried, 57g (2oz) raw weight	100
Flat, fried whole, 57g (2oz) raw weight	120
Flat, sliced and fried, 57g (2oz) raw weight	150

MUSSELS

With shells, boiled, per 28g (1oz)	7
Without shells, boiled, per 28g (1oz)	25
Per mussel	10

MUSTARD AND CRESS

Raw, per 28g (1oz)	3
Whole carton	5

MUSTARD

Dry, per 28g (1oz)	128
Made mustard, per 5ml (1 level teaspoon)	10

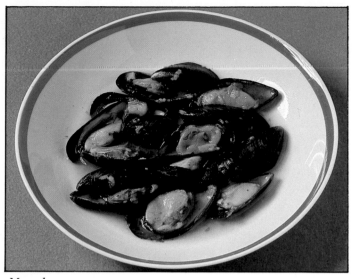

Mussels

N

NECTARINES

With or without stones, per 28g (1oz)	14

NOODLES

Cooked, per 28g (1oz)	33

NUTMEG

Powdered, per 28g (pinch)	0

O

OATMEAL

Raw, per 28g (1oz)	114
Per 15ml (1 level tablespoon) raw	38
Per 20ml (Australian tablespoon), raw	50

OCTOPUS

Raw, per 28g (1oz)	20

OKRA (ladies' fingers)

Raw, per 28g (1oz)	5

OLIVE OIL

Per 28ml (1 floz)	255
Per 15ml (1 level tablespoon)	120

OLIVES

Stoned, in brine, per 28g (1oz)	29
With stones, in brine, per 28g (1oz)	23
Per stuffed olive	5

ONIONS
Per 28g (1oz)

Raw	7
Boiled	4
Fried	98
Onion rings in batter, fried	145
Dried, per 15ml (1 level tablespoon)	10
Fried, per 15ml (1 level tablespoon)	25
Whole onion, raw, 85g (3oz)	20
Pickled onion, each	5
Cocktail onion, each	1

ORANGES

Flesh only, per 28g (1oz)	10
Flesh with skin, per 28g (1oz)	7
Whole fruit, small, 142g (5oz)	37
Whole fruit, medium, 227g (8oz)	56
Whole fruit, large 284g (10oz)	74

ORANGE JUICE
Per 28ml (1floz)

Canned, sweetened	15
Unsweetened	11

OXTAIL

Stewed, without bone, per 28g (1oz)	69
On the bone, stewed and skimmed of fat, per 28g (1oz)	26

OYSTERS

With shells, raw, per 28g (1oz)	2
Without shells, raw per 28g (1oz)	14
Per oyster	5

P

PARSLEY

Fresh, per 28g (1oz)	6
Parsley sauce, per 15ml (1 level tablespoon)	45
per 20ml (Australian tablespoon	60

PARSNIPS
Per 28g (1oz)

Raw	14
Boiled	16
Roast	30

PARTRIDGE

Roast, on bone, per 28g (1oz)	36
Roast, meat only, per 28g (1oz)	60

PASSIONFRUIT

Flesh only, per 28g (1oz)	10
With skin, per 28g (1oz)	4

217

PASTA
All shapes, raw, per 28g (1oz)	105
Boiled, per 28g (1oz)	33

PASTRY
Per 28g (1oz)
Choux, raw	61
Choux, baked	94
Flaky, raw	121
Flaky, baked	160
Shortcrust, raw	129
Shortcrust, baked	150

PAW PAW (Papaya)
Canned, per 28g (1oz)	18
Fresh, flesh only, per 28g (1oz)	11

PEACHES
Canned in natural juice	13
Canned in syrup, per 28g (1oz)	25
Fresh, with stones, per 28g (1oz)	9
Whole fruit, 142g (5oz)	45

PEANUTS
Per 28g (1oz)
Shelled, fresh	162
Dry roasted	160
Roasted and salted	168
Peanut butter	177
Per peanut	5

PEARS
Per 28g (1oz)
Cooking pears, raw, peeled	10
Dessert pears,	8
Canned in natural juice	11
Canned in syrup	22
Canned in syrup, drained, per half pear	30
Whole fruit, medium, 142g (5oz)	41

PEAS Per 28g (1oz)
Fresh, raw	19
Frozen, boiled	15
Canned, garden	13
Canned, processed	23
Dried, raw	81
Dried, boiled	29
Split, raw	88
Split, boiled	34
Chick, raw	91

Per 15ml (1 level tablespoon)
Dried, boiled	30
Fresh, boiled	10
Pease pudding	35

Per 20ml (Australian tablespoon)
Dried, boiled	40
Fresh, boiled	13
Pease pudding	45

PECANS
Per nut	15

PEPPER
Powdered, per pinch	0

PEPPERS (capsicums)
Red or green, per 28g (1oz)	4
Average pepper, 142g (5oz)	20

PERCH
White, raw, per 28g (1oz)	35
Yellow, raw, per 28g (1oz)	25

PHEASANT
Meat only, roast, per 28g (1oz)	60
On the bone, roast, per 28g (1oz)	38

PICKLES AND RELISHES
Per 28g (1oz)
Mixed pickles	5

Roast pheasant

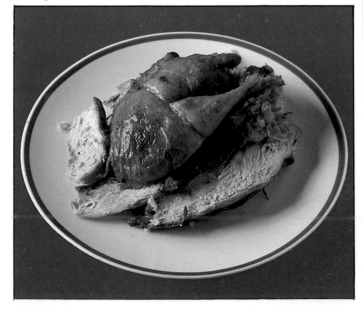

Piccalili	15
Ploughmans	35
Sweet pickle	35

PIGEON
Meat only, roast, per 28g (1oz)	65
On the bone, roast, per 28g (1oz)	29

PIKE
Raw, per 28g (1oz)	25

PILCHARDS
Canned in tomato sauce, per 28g (1oz)	36

PIMENTOS
Fresh, per 28g (1oz)	4

PINEAPPLES
Canned in natural juice, per 28g (1oz)	15
Canned in syrup, per 28g (1oz)	22
Fresh, per 28g (1oz)	13
Ring of canned, drained pineapple in syrup	35
Ring of canned, drained pineapple in natural juice	15
Ring of canned, drained pineapple in syrup, fried in batter	65

PISTACHIO NUTS
Shelled, per 28g (1oz)	180
Per nut	5

PLAICE
Per 28g (1oz)
Fillet, raw or steamed	26
Fillet, in batter, fried	79
Fillet, in breadcrumbs, fried,	65
Whole fillet in breadcrumbs, 170g (6oz) raw weight	435

PLANTAIN
Per 28g (1oz)
Green, raw	30
Green, boiled	35
Ripe, fried	76

PLUMS
Per 28g (1oz)
Cooking plums with stones, stewed without sugar	6
Fresh dessert plums, with stones	10
Cooking plums, with stones	7
Victoria dessert plum, each	15

POLLACK
On the bone, raw, per 28g (1oz)	25

POLONY
Per 28g (1oz)	80

POMEGRANATE
Flesh only, per 28g (1oz)	20

Whole pomegranate,
205g (7¼oz) | 66

POPCORN
Per 28g (1oz) | 110

PORK
Per 28g (1oz)
Belly rashers, raw,
lean and fat | 108
Belly rashers, grilled,
lean and fat | 113
Fillet, raw, lean only | 42
Leg, raw, lean and fat,
weighed without bone | 76
Leg, raw, lean only,
weighed without bone | 42
Leg, roast, lean and fat | 81
Leg, roast, lean only | 53
Crackling | 190
Scratchings | 185
Crackling, average
portion, 9g (⅓oz) | 65
Pork chop, well grilled,
184g (6½oz) raw
weight | 240
Pork chop, well fried,
184g (6½oz) raw
weight | 290
Pork pie, individual,
142g (5oz) | 535

POTATOES
Per 28g (1oz)
Raw | 25
Baked, weighed
with skin | 24
Boiled, old potatoes | 23
Boiled, new potatoes | 22
Canned, new potatoes
drained | 20
Chips (average
thickness) | 70
Chips (crinkle cut) | 80
Chips (thick cut) | 40
Chips (thin cut) | 85
Average portion
chips from fish and
chip chop, 198g (7oz) | 455
Oven chips or grill chips | 55
Crisps | 150
Roast, large chunks | 40
Roast, medium chunks | 45
Roast, small chunks | 50
Sauté | 40
Instant mashed potato
powder, per 15ml
(1 tablespoon) dry | 40
Jacket-baked potato,
198g (7oz) raw weight | 170
Jacket-baked potato
with 14g (½oz)
knob butter | 275
Mashed potato,
142g (5oz) raw
weight, mashed
with 45ml
(3tablespoons)
skimmed milk | 140
Mashed potato,
142g (5oz) raw weight
mashed with 45ml
(3 tablespoons) whole
milk and 7g(¼oz)
butter | 205
Potato salad per
28g (1oz) | 50
Roast potato, medium
chunk, 49g (1¾oz) | 75

PRAWNS
With shells, per
28g (1oz) | 12
Without shells, per
28g (1oz) | 30
Per shelled prawn | 2

PRUNES
Per 28g (1oz)
Dried | 46
Stewed, without sugar | 21
Prune juice | 25
Per prune | 10

**PUDDINGS AND
DESSERTS**
Per portion
Apple crumble
142g (5oz) | 295
Apple pie, pastry top
and bottom,
113g (4oz) | 420
Bread and butter
pudding, 142g (5oz) | 225
Christmas pudding,
85g (3oz) | 260
Custard tart, 85g (3oz) | 245
Fruit pie, pastry top
only, 113g (4oz) | 205
Jelly, 142ml (¼pint) | 85
Lemon meringue pie
113g (4oz) | 370
Milk pudding, home-
made rice, semolina
or tapioca, 170g (6oz) | 220
Rice pudding, canned
170g (6oz) | 155
Sponge pudding,
steamed, 142g (5oz) | 485
Suet pudding, steamed,
142g (5oz) | 470

Lemon Meringue Pie

Treacle tart,
113g (4oz) | 420
Trifle, 142 (5oz) | 225

PUMPKIN
Raw, per 28g (1oz) | 4

Q

QUICHE
Average slice,
113g (4oz) | 445

QUINCES
Raw, per 28g (1oz) | 7

R

RABBIT
Per 28g (1oz)
Meat only, raw | 35
Meat only, stewed | 51
On the bone, stewed | 26

RADISHES
Fresh, per 28g (1oz) | 4
Per radish | 2

RAISINS
Dried, per 28g (1oz) | 70
Per 15ml (1 level
tablespoon) | 25

RASPBERRIES
Fresh or frozen,
per 28g (1oz) | 7
Canned, drained,
per 28g (1oz) | 25

REDCURRANTS
Fresh, per 28g (1oz) | 6
Redcurrant jelly, per
5ml (1 level teaspoon) | 15

RHUBARB
Raw, per 28g (1oz) | 2
Stewed without sugar,
per 28g (1oz) | 2

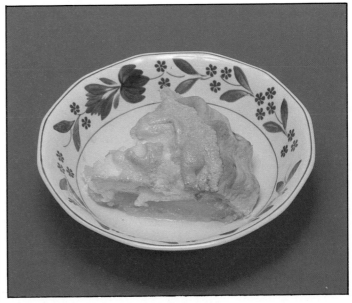

RICE Per 28g (1oz)

Brown, raw	95
White, raw	103
Boiled	35
Pudding, home-made	37
Pudding, canned	26

Per 15ml (1 level tablespoon)

Boiled	20
Fried	35
Raw	35

Per 20ml (Australian tablespoon)

Boiled	25
Fried	45
raw	45

ROCK

Seaside rock, per 28g (1oz)	95

ROCK SALMON (Dogfish)

Fried in batter, per 28g (1oz)	75

S

SAGO

Raw, per 28g (1oz)	101

SAITHE (Coley) Per 28g (1oz)

Fillet, raw	21
Fillet, steamed	28
On the bone, steamed	24

SALAD CREAM

Per 28g (1oz)	110
Per 15ml (1 level tablespoon)	50
Per 20ml (Australian tablespoon)	65
Low-calorie salad cream, per 28g (1oz)	50
Low-calorie salad cream, per 15ml (1 level tablespoon)	25
per 20ml (Australian tablespoon)	35

SALMON Per 28g (1oz)

Canned	44
Fillet, steamed	56
On the bone, raw	52
On the bone, steamed	45
Smoked	40

SALSIFY

Boiled, per 28g (1oz)	5

SALT

Per 28g (1oz)	0

SARDINES

Canned in oil, drained, per 28g (1oz)	62
Canned in tomato sauce, per 28g (1oz)	50

SAUSAGES Each

Beef chipolata, well grilled	50
Beef, large, well grilled	120
Beef, skinless, well grilled	65
Pork chipolata, well grilled	65
Pork, large, well grilled	125
Pork, skinless, well grilled	95
Pork and beef chipolata, well grilled	60
Pork and beef, large, well grilled	125

SAUSAGE ROLL

Small, 28g (1oz)	135

SCALLOPS

Steamed, per 28g (1oz)	30

SCAMPI

Fried in breadcrumbs, per 28g (1oz)	90

SEA KALE

Boiled, per 28g (1oz)	2

SEMOLINA

Raw, per 28g (1oz)	99
Per 15ml (1 level tablespoon)	35
Semolina pudding per 28g (1oz), home-made	37
Semolina pudding, canned per 28g (1oz)	26

SESAME SEEDS

Per 28g (1oz)	160

SHEPHERD'S PIE

Per average portion, 227g (8oz)	270

SHRIMPS Per 28g (1oz)

Canned, drained	27
Fresh, with shells	11
Fresh, without shells	33

SKATE

Fillet, in batter, fried, per 28g (1oz)	57

SMELTS

Without bones, fried, per 28g (1oz)	115

SNAILS

Flesh only, per 28g (1oz)	25

SOLE Per 28g (1oz)

Fillet, raw	23
Fillet, fried	61
Fillet, steamed or poached	18
On the bone, steamed or poached	18

SPAGHETTI Per 28g (1oz)

Raw	107
Wholewheat, raw	97
Boiled	33
Canned in tomato sauce	17

SPINACH

Boiled, per 28g (1oz)	9

SPRATS

Fried without heads, per 28g (1oz)	110

SPRING GREENS

Boiled, per 28g (1oz)	3

SPRING ONIONS

Raw, per 28g (1oz)	10

SQUID

Flesh only, raw per 28g (1oz)	25

STRAWBERRIES

Fresh or frozen, per 28g (1oz)	7
Canned, drained, per 28g (1oz)	23
Per fresh strawberry	2

STURGEON

On the bone, raw, per 28g (1oz)	25

SUET

Shredded, per 28g (1oz)	235
Per 15ml (1 level tablespoon)	78
Per 20ml (Australian tablespoon)	105

SUGAR

White or brown, caster Demerara, granulated, icing, per 28g (1oz)	112
Per 5ml (1 level teaspoon)	17
Large sugar lump	17
Small sugar lump	10

SULTANAS

Dried, per 28g (1oz)	71
Per 15ml (1 level tablespoon)	25
Per 20ml (Australian tablespoon)	35

SUNFLOWER SEED OIL

Per 28g (1oz)	255
Per 15ml (1 level tablespoon)	120
Per 20ml (Australian tablespoon)	160

SWEDES

Raw, per 28g (1oz)	6
Boiled, per 28g (1oz)	5
Boiled, per 15ml (1 level tablespoon)	5
per 20ml (Australian tablespoon)	7

SWEETBREADS

Lamb's, raw, per 28g (1oz)	37
Lamb's, fried, per 28g (1oz)	65

SWEETCORN

Canned in brine, per 28g (1oz)	22
Canned, per 15ml (1 level tablespoon)	10
per 20ml (Australian tablespoon)	15

Fresh, kernels only,
   boiled, per 28g (1oz) 35
Frozen, per 28g (1oz) 25
Whole cob 85

SWEETS
Per 28g (1oz)
Barley sugar 100
Boiled sweets 93
Butterscotch 115
Filled chocolates 131
Fudge 111
Liquorice allsorts 105
Marshmallows 90
Nougat 110
Nut brittle or
   crunch 120
Peppermints 110
Toffee 122
Cough sweet, boiled,
   each 10
Cough pastille, each 5

SYRUPS
Per 28g (1oz)
Golden 85
Maple 70
Rosehip 66
**Per 5ml (1 level
   teaspoon)**
Cough syrup, thick 15
Cough syrup, thin 5
**Per 15ml (1 level
   tablespoon)**
Golden 60
Maple 50
**Per 20ml (Australian
   tablespoon)**
Golden 80
Maple 65

T

TANGERINES
Flesh only, per 28g (1oz) 10
Flesh with skin,
   per 28g (1oz) 7
Whole fruit, 85g (3oz) 20

TAPIOCA
Dry per 28g (1oz) 102

TARAMASALATA
Per 28g (1oz) 135

TARTARE SAUCE
Per 15ml (1 level
   tablespoon) 35
Per 20ml (Australian
   tablespoon) 45

TEA
All brands, per cup,
   no milk 0

TOMATOES
Per 28g (1oz)
Raw, 4
Canned 3
Fried, halved 20
Fried, sliced 30
Ketchup 28
Purée 19
Whole medium tomato,
   57g (2oz) 8
Per 15ml (1 level tablespoon)
Chutney 45

Ketchup 15
Purée 10
**Per 20ml (Australian
   tablespoon)**
Chutney 60
Ketchup 20
Purée 13

TONGUE
Per 28g (1oz)
Lamb's, raw 55
Lamb's, stewed 82
Ox, boiled 83

TREACLE
Black, per 28g (1oz) 73
Per 15ml (1 level
   tablespoon) 50
Per 20ml (Australian
   tablespoon) 65

TREACLE TART
Per average slice,
   113g (4oz) 470

TRIPE
Dressed, per 28g (1oz) 17
Stewed, per 28g (1oz) 28

TROUT
Fillet, smoked, per
   28g (1oz) 38
On the bone, poached
   or steamed, per
   28g (1oz) 25
Whole trout, poached
   or grilled without
   fat, 170g (6oz) 150
Whole smoked trout,
   156g (5½oz) 150

TUNA
Per 28g (1oz)
Canned in brine, drained 30
Canned in oil 82
Canned in oil, drained 60

TURKEY
Per 28g (1oz)
Meat only, raw 30
Meat only, roast 40
Meat and skin, roast 49

TURNIPS
Raw, per 28g (1oz) 6
Boiled, per 28g (1oz) 4
Per 15ml (1 level
   tablespoon), mashed 4
Per 20ml (Australian
   tablespoon), mashed 5

V

VEAL Per 28g (1oz)
Cutlet, fried in egg and
   breadcrumbs 61
Fillet, raw 31
Fillet, roast 65
Jellied veal, canned 35
Escalope, fried in egg
   and breadcrumbs,
   85g (3oz) raw weight 310

VENISON
Roast meat only, per
   28g (1oz) 56

VINEGAR
Per 28ml (1floz) 1

W

WALNUTS
Shelled, per 28g (1oz) 149
Per walnut half 15

WATERCHESTNUTS
Per 28g (1oz) 25

WATERCRESS
Per 28g (1oz) 4

WATERMELON
Flesh only, per 28g (1oz) 6
Flesh with skin, per
   28g (1oz) 3

WHEATGERM
Per 28g (1oz) 100
Per 15ml (1 level
   tablespoon) 18
Per 20ml (Australian
   tablespoon) 24

WHELKS
With shells, boiled,
   per 28g (1oz) 4
Without shells, boiled,
   per 28g (1oz) 26

WHITEBAIT
Fried, per 28g (1oz) 149

WHITE PUDDING
As sold, per 28g (1oz) 129

WHITING
Per 28g (1oz)
Fillet, fried 54
Fillet, steamed 26
On the bone, fried 49
On the bone, steamed 18

WINKLES
With shells, boiled,
   per 28g (1oz) 4
Without shells, boiled,
   per 28g (1oz) 21

WORCESTERSHIRE
SAUCE
Per 28ml (1floz) 20
Per 15ml (1 level
   tablespoon) 13
Per 20ml (Australian
   ablespoon) 17

Y

YAMS
Raw, per 28g (1oz) 37
Boiled, per 28g (1oz) 34

YEAST
Fresh, per 28g (1oz) 15
Dried, per 28g (1oz) 48
Dried, per 5ml (1 level
   teaspoon) 8

YOGURT
Per 28g (1oz)
Low fat, natural 15
Low fat, flavoured 23
Low fat, fruit 27
Low fat, hazelnut 30

YORKSHIRE
PUDDING
Cooked, per 28g (1oz) 60

Index

Numbers in *italics* refer to illustrations

Index of recipes

Index of recipes

continued

Picture credits
All photographs are the property of Slimming Magazine
except for the following:
All-Sport Photographic: page 44
Belinda Banks: cover
Patrick Blake: page 55
Spectrum Colour Library: pages 42, 48
Susan Griggs Agency: pages 53, 70, 170-71
Vital Magazine: pages 13, 37, 38, 39, 41, 43, 49
50, 51, 59, 188-89, 190-91